How a Neurological Disorder Changed My Life for the Better

The Science Behind Nerve, Muscular, and Neuromuscular Disorders and Their Effects on Cycling

Patrick Bohan

How a Neurological Disorder Changed My Life for the Better

The Science Behind Nerve, Muscular, and Neuromuscular Disorders and Their Effects on Cycling

by

Patrick Bohan

Patrick Bohan

ISBN: 9798700307710
Inside Edge Publishing
www.insideedgepublishing.com
Printed in the United States of America

Contents

Patrick Bohan

Chapter 1: Introduction and Preface

- Disclaimer
- The Book's Purpose
- Differentiating this Book from Other Books
- Who Should Read the Book?
- Scope and Organizational Methods of the Book
- The Book's Benefits
- Unique Features of the Book

Disclaimer

Before writing this book, I would like to outline four disclaimers: First, I am not a doctor. My interpretation of events and articles is different from medical professionals. Case in point, a neurologist's knowledge may allow him or her to intuitively rule out many disorders from my diagnosis.

Second, if you have a peripheral nerve hyperexcitation (PNH) disorders, please do not be alarmed by this text and do not let it cause you any stress or fear! Part of what makes my story unique is that my case was misdiagnosed and mismanaged. The problem is, as we shall learn, I do not fit in any one bucket of defined disorders. One doctor said, "We listen to their stories, and we try to fit them into the box, but millions of people do not fit into a box." Furthermore, for these people, "Science has not caught up yet." [1] Of course, those people with extremely rare disorders provide "medical gifts" because they hold the key to medical breakthroughs to resolve other mysteries of medicine. [2]

I jokingly refer to my condition as Patrick's Syndrome, a combination of PNH and a form of neuropathy called chronic inflammatory demyelinating polyneuropathy (CIDP) or multifocal motor neuropathy (MMN). Yes, my symptoms have worsened and become more problematic over the years, but this is due to CIDP or MMN and not the PNH.

Third, I will donate any profits from this book to the Foundation for Peripheral Neuropathy https://www.foundationforpn.org/. I also need to thank all of the major contributors to this project because without their generosity, this venture would have been very difficult to complete: Ross Teggatz, Rex Teggatz, Maureen Durkin, Molly Bohan, Andy Lowther, Leon Damonze, Shawn Gillis (Absolute Bikes, https://www.absolutebikes.com/), Matt Wells and Lindsey Lighthizer (Black Burro Bikes, https://www.blackburrobikes.com/), Joe Parkin and Simon Stewart (Boneshaker Cycles, https://www.boneshakerbv.com/), Michelle Wolins (Big Ring Cycles, https://www.bigringcycles.com/), Michelle Main, Carl Newberg, Mark Wolfe, Stephen Seccombe, and Deborah and Ken Miller.

Fourth, I started this text primarily to resolve a few hypotheses. My research aimed to improve my cycling performance and find medical relief for my disorder. Also, I needed to understand if the limited athletic genetic composition and neurological disease are preventing me from winning a US cycling national time trial championship. The findings were affirmative on point one, but negative on point two. As I delved into my mysterious illness and resolving these hypotheses, I uncovered a vast wealth of useful information.

Purpose

For books like this one to fulfill a purpose, they need to solve a problem or improve a condition. Although people now live longer, they increasingly suffer from higher rates of morbidity. Further complicating matters, the medical community frequently targets and treats symptoms rather than the illness, thereby allowing people to live longer but with a reduced quality of life. Most reasons for morbidity result from our genes' exposure to new environments not previously experienced during the million-year evolutionary process of humankind.

Consider examples such as the use of manufactured drugs—both legal and illegal, alcohol consumption, poor sleep, smoking, exposure to toxins, stress, new illnesses, and highly processed and chemical-laden foods. The result is disease and, in many cases, autoimmune disorders. According to Daniel Lieberman, there is a relatively high probability of dying from a disease caused by genetic mismatches with the environment. [3] The CDC reports that there are approximately 600 rare diseases, and the prevalence rate of all 600 in the United States alone exceeds 10%. Taking all diseases into account, about 25 to 33% of the United States is sick or will be sick in the next few years. That figure is extraordinary because many disorders are avoidable through a well-balanced diet and exercise.

In this book, I describe my struggle with two rare neurological disorders, both of which I believe modern environmental conditions influenced. I also share my passion for cycling, which can reduce the chance of morbidity and help enthusiasts to maintain a higher quality of life. The purpose of the book is outlined below in a five-fold approach. Although PNH and neuropathy disorders can be debilitating and wreak havoc on the lives of those inflicted, it is still possible to have a productive, successful, and meaningful life. In fact, many neurological diseases are not necessarily an end to our lives, but instead if we can change our attitude and mind set, it can be a new beginning. A new beginning is merely a healthier lifestyle focusing on new objectives and goals. The essential facets of my story include the five As, which include acceptance, advocacy, adaptation, attitude, and action.

- **Acceptance** is to love your life and find as much joy in your current circumstances as possible.
- **Advocacy** and education for oneself when family, friends, and medical personnel are of little assistance are invaluable. When those in the medical field cannot provide the answers needed to alleviate fears, find acceptance, provide treatment options, and explain how to move forward, it is imperative to advocate for oneself through education.
- **Adaptation**—or evolving—is to change your life's course to overcome adversity. Evolving is understanding personal limitations and boundaries that result from adversity, such as a neurological

disorder. I evolved to cycling when other activities were too painful or became a safety concern. Thus, I learned that cycling was safer than rock climbing, and the pain was more tolerable and manageable than running. Evolving or adapting is difficult because it involves changing habits including working harder and making sacrifices. Sacrifices include eliminating bad habits such as smoking, alcohol, a poor diet, and stressful situations. Sacrifices also means working harder such as increasing exercise activity to keep the disorder at bay. What's more, positive changes in habits and behavior can lead to epigenetic alterations in our genetic expression making evolution and adaption long lasting. In other words, there is no magic formula to end adversity and pain. The best solution is always hard work and sacrifice.

- **Attitude** is about making the most out of a difficult situation. Attitude is pushing the envelope by focusing on positives instead of harping on negatives. Attitude is what drives core personality traits like gratitude, grit, perseverance, mental toughness, motivation, and resiliency.

- **Action** on your part must be proactive, which means being practical by focusing on the present, future, and forgetting the past. It is vital to learn from past mistakes, but also to move forward to implement what you learned. Proactivity puts us in control of our situation; whereas, harping on the past makes us powerless and leads to unwanted stress and anxiety.

In this book, I aim to:

1. Educate the public about my experiences and what I learned from my medical and cycling journey about a plethora of subjects, including anatomy, physiology, neuromuscular disease, environmental factors, pain, fear, stress, acceptance, adaptation, mental toughness, and endurance training, to name a few.

2. Provide the reader with novel information not found in other books such as techniques for acceptance, motivation, resiliency, and adaptation as well as coping mechanisms for pain, fear, stress, and depression. Also included in the text are novel training and racing tips for people with physical limitations from neurological disease, an epidemiology study of PNH disorders, and new medical theories and hypotheses as to what may precipitate PNH disorders.

3. Demonstrate that not only is vigorous exercise achievable, but so is athletic improvement and success in the presence of a debilitating neurological disorder. Furthermore, athletic achievement is possible without athletic genes.

It is my hope that this text:

- Motivates and encourages others, so they may find the strength and perseverance to excel at whatever they choose to do
- Helps people with PNH or neuropathy to evolve and to live life to its fullest

- Informs doctors to be as knowledgeable as my last neurologist who never gave up trying to find answers
- Provides persons with useful data about PNH disorders (Appendix 1)
- Encourages cyclists to adapt when life throws them a curveball

Differentiating This Book from Other Books

There are many books about people overcoming adversity to compete in athletics, including cycling. Two famous and highly publicized stories about overcoming adversity in cycling are about Greg LeMond and Lance Armstrong. LeMond overcame a gunshot wound to win the Tour de France just ten months later. Cheating aside, Armstrong overcame testicular cancer to win 7 Tour de France titles. Despite cheating, Armstrong's feat is quite remarkable, especially understanding almost everyone competing in the Tour de France was cheating at that time. My story is uniquely different from that of LeMond and Armstrong for many reasons. For instance, they are professionals, whereas I am an amateur.

Most importantly, they overcame their ailments, yet mine persists. There is, however, one commonality between Lance and me. Since we both participated in various sports before our illnesses, the illnesses assisted us to restructure our body's muscle composition to better conform to cycling.

This book is unique from other similar books because it provides an epidemiology study on PNH disorders to classify and characterize these syndromes better. There are no books about cycling achievement by overcoming debilitating neurological disorders such as both PNH and neuropathy. Books that address overcoming adversity among cyclists over the age of 50 are incredibly rare, and even fewer books address individuals who experience a misdiagnosis or feel ignored and dismissed by medical professionals. The combination of these reasons makes the book unique. Below are some examples of books that use similar search words on Amazon:

- *Overcoming Functional Neurology Symptoms: A Five Area Approach*, Allen Carson et. al. CRC Press, 2011. This book focuses on cognitive therapy; whereas, my book focuses on exercise to overcome neurological symptoms.

- *Back in the Game: Why Concussion Does not have to End Your Athletic Career*, Jeffery S Kutcher MD, Oxford University Press, 2017. This book deals with upper motor neuron dysfunction and is written by a doctor and not an athlete; whereas, my book concentrates on lower motor neuron dysfunction, and its perspective is from an athlete.

- *The Courage to go Forward: The Power of Micro-communities*, David Codani et al., Morgan James Publishing, 2018. This book describes how support groups can change lives. David went from not being able to run a half-mile to complete the Ironman triathlon. My book focuses more on individual coping mechanisms when support from friends, family, or the medical community is not enough.

There are many books about overcoming and coping with various neurological conditions, snone of these books include athletic success, specific exercise training, or novel new scientific theories that may cause their disorders.

Who Should Read the Book?

Those with a neurological disorder: About 18% of the U.S. gross national product (GDP) goes toward healthcare, equating to about 8,000 dollars annually per person. In other words, "lower mortality is being replaced by higher morbidity (illness)." [4] One of the fastest-growing healthcare crises contributing to increased GDP is neurological disorders. Any of the 25 million people in the United States suffering from neurological disorders will find the book beneficial.[5] The reason any person with a neurological condition may be interested in this text is that many symptoms of neurological disorders, syndromes, and diseases overlap. Another reference reports, as many as 20 million Americans have neuropathy.[6] There are no published estimates for people with PNH disorders, but it is safe to assume that one hundred percent of the population will experience PNH symptoms from time to time. I have conservatively estimated the number of individuals with chronic PNH symptoms at 1 to 3% or 3 to 10 million people in the United States, which may encompass a large portion of estimated 20 million people with neuropathy.

Master or senior athletes: Such individuals may find the book helpful for training and performance tips. Unfortunately, there has been a steady growth in sedentary people in society. However, at the same time, there has been a boom in senior or master athletes primarily from the baby boom generation.[7] [8] Over 14,000 athletes competed in the National Senior Games in New Mexico in 2019. [9] About 1,000 athletes competed at the 2019 USA cycling master's nationals in Colorado Springs.

Any person with rare disorders: There are about 6000 known rare disorders, and they account for about 30 million people in the United States or nearly 10% of the population.[10]

Family members or friends of individuals with neurological disorders: It can be estimated that this market is at least 50 million based on the large population of people identified with neurological conditions outlined in the first bullet point.

Anyone with chronic pain may find the information in this text useful: Those individuals with chronic pain are directly proportional to increasing age. The age factor explains why chronic pain is probably due to normal wear and tear, which may be exacerbated by daily exercise. I have talked with hundreds of athletes over the years, and just about every senior or master's athlete is coping with a medical issue. Pain is the most likely culprit. An estimated 50 to 100 million Americans with chronic pain, and about 20 million adults are dealing with what is called high impact chronic pain. [11] [12] Most individuals with high impact chronic pain have difficulty doing any daily activities.

Medical professionals: Anyone in healthcare might want to learn more about PNH so they can better inform patients about the condition. One reference found that there are nearly 16,000 neurologists in the United States and about 28%, or over 4,000, are neuromuscular specialists who specialize in PNH disorders.[13]

Coaches, fitness experts, and trainers: This group will likely benefit from the book, particularly if they have clients with neurological disorders or medical ailments. USA cycling alone lists over 1,000 certified coaches, and the Bureau of Labor Statistics estimates that there are 355 thousand fitness trainers in the United States in 2018.[14] [15]

Anyone misdiagnosed, mismanaged, or ignored by the medical profession: It may surprise many, but 12 million people are misdiagnosed each year at outpatient clinics. Of course, most of these are probably non-serious ailments. What is worse, many more patients receive no diagnosis.[16] Studies of neurological conditions suggest that approximately 5% of all cases are misdiagnosed.[17]

Anyone interested in cycling, competition, and training philosophies, especially for time trials: According to USA Cycling, there were about 6,500 Americans to participate in a time trial event in 2019. Of course, thousands more participate in criteriums, road races, and other types of events such as mountain biking or cyclocross.[18]

One person in four in the United States (80 to 85 million) may find this information interesting. Approximately 1 in 12 (25 to 30 million) will have an interest in most of the information provided in the text.

Scope and Organizational Methods of the Book

This section explains why I am a qualified author to author a book on PNH, neuropathy, and cycling and concludes by outlining each of the final twelve chapters of the book.

Scope and My Qualifications [19]

Let me briefly explain why just as many patients are experts about neurological disease as their doctors. *Differential diagnosis* is the process of eliminating other similar disorders from a patient's diagnosis. Most people with autoimmune conditions that result in neurological disorders can take up to five years or longer before they are correctly diagnosed. I postulate there are two reasons for the outrageous length of time to uncover a diagnosis. The first is due to the complex and mysterious nature of differential diagnoses for neurological conditions. The second is that some doctors have difficulty accepting or believing patients who may have sensory symptoms. The reason for this skeptical behavior is because sensory symptoms cannot be seen or verified in an exam such as pain, numbness, tingling, or fatigue. This reality is unfortunate because an extended period for a diagnosis generally means that most patients have experienced irreversible damage. Treatment for most neurological conditions encompasses treating symptoms since few disorders are curable, which is alarming information. However, it is not overly surprising considering the medical arena did not even believe autoimmune disorders were possible just 60 to 70 years ago.

The bottom line is that science and research are in their infancy and has much catching up to do when it comes to autoimmune disease and neurological disorders. The bottom line, when it comes to diagnosing patients with neurological and autoimmune conditions if doctors would listen to patients, then the diagnosis process would not only go much faster, but it would be more accurate. My current neurologist is outstanding. She asks me questions such as "What would you like to do?" or "What worries you the most?" Unlike most doctors I encountered during my diagnosis process, she is seeking my advice and thoughts instead of ignoring my ideas and concerns.

I have studied the human body since I was diagnosed with PNH over a decade ago. In that time, I collected data on over 500 people from around the globe, claiming to have been diagnosed with benign fasciculation syndrome (BFS) using a Google Docs survey. The statistical analysis and correlation results from the data collected in this survey are posted in Appendix 1. PNH disorders encompass BFS, cramp fasciculation syndrome (CFS), Isaac syndrome (IS), and Morvan's syndrome (MoS). Some PNH patients who fear their neuromuscular disorder might be something more sinister would often contact me looking for answers their doctors are unable to provide. Unfortunately, I do not have all the answers. However, I can merely highlight the results of the survey, my research, and my personal experience. At the same time, my insight is more informative than that of neurologists who tell patients that their condition is "no big deal," which is unfortunate because PNH is a big deal, and it changes the lives of those afflicted.

My experience and research have inspired me to blog about PNH disorders. My blog post, "The Misconceptions of Benign Fasciculation Syndrome," has garnered 150,000 reads, and other blog posts have reached into the thousands. Several years back, I also participated in a forum on paresthesia symptoms on a Huffington Post webcast. I am not a doctor and do not hold a Ph.D. in any educational field (I have a B.S. in electrical engineering). Nonetheless, I have had several doctors stricken with PNH reach out to me, asking for my advice. For instance, I sent the section on "Fear" to one doctor suffering from BFS, and he wrote me back saying, "The Fear component of the book is fabulous." My communication with patients, my independent research for this text, my blogs, and my survey have provided me a clearer picture of what is going on, but I am certainly no expert (I may know more than most, but no one is an expert). At the same time, I can speculate with more certainty about what is going on with me. I attempt to unravel the mystery of PNH and my disorder in this book.

As far as expertise in cycling is concerned, I have been competing in cycling the past seven years and have been on the podium in over 100 races, including national and state titles in time trial events. Yes, I have many cycling achievements, but what makes these accomplishments unique is that I attained them while battling a debilitating neurological condition that impaired both strength and power.

Book Outline and Overview
Chapter 2: Exercise, My Story, My Genome, and Aging
- Exercise Guidelines
- My Story
- Genome Testing
- What makes an Athlete Elite?
- The Effects of Aging

In Chapter 2, or the first approach of the journey to understanding PNH and mu neuropathy, I provide information about exercise guidelines for healthy and non-healthy people outlines by national and world organizations. I share my story about my progressive disorder and how I evolved to cycling. In particular, I describe why I compete in master's level cycling and the difficulties of training rigorously while coping with a neurological condition. Furthermore, the chapter explains genome testing and how my genome results may affect my neurological condition, training, and diet.

Chapter 3: The Science of Skeleton Muscle Function

- Skeleton Muscle Function
- Muscle Disorders
- Creatine Kinase
- Energy Sources
- Muscle Contraction

In Chapter 3, I address the second approach to understanding PNH and my neuropathy. I provide an in-depth look at the science behind skeleton muscle function. In Chapter 3, I explore the specific science behind muscle protein and enzyme makeup, contraction, and energy sources required for a muscle contraction.

Chapter 4: Skeleton Muscle Function and Effects of Exercise on Muscular Performance

- The Effects of Training on Muscle Performance
- Negative Effects of Exercise
- Positive Effects of Exercise

In Chapter 4, I address the third approach to understanding PNH and my neuropathy. I provide an in-depth scientific look at both the positive and negative effects of exercise on muscular performance.

Chapter 5: Cycling 101

- Why Compete
- Cycling Science
- My Training Philosophy

In Chapter 5, or the fourth approach of the journey to understanding PNH and my neuropathy, I explain the science behind time trials. I address aerodynamics, heart rate, cadence, power, fatigue, power impairment, and pain endurance. The chapter concludes with an in-depth overview of my training philosophy since I have many more physical limitations than healthy riders.

Chapter 6 and 7: The Science of Autoimmune Disease, the Immune System, and the Endocrine System

- Blood
- Immune System
- Stress
- Lymphatic System
- Endocrine System

In Chapter 6 and 7, I discuss the fifth approach to understanding PNH and neuropathy. In doing so, I provide an in-depth look at human physiology. I provide background into the immune and endocrine systems including autoimmune disease. A thorough understanding of ***human physiology*** (e.g., the science behind pain, stress, and autoimmune disorders) is necessary to explain PNH or similar neurological disorders medically.

Chapters 8, 9, and 10: My Symptoms

- Autonomic Symptoms
- Sensory Symptoms
- Motor Symptoms

In Chapters 8, 9, 10, I discuss the sixth approach to understanding PNH and my neurological condition. Specifically, I discuss all my symptoms associated with autoimmune and neuromuscular disorders. My health provides a good example that sheds light on neurological disorders since I have many unusual symptoms. For instance, I experience Dupuytren's contracture, hyperhidrosis, atrophy, hyporeflexia, cold hands and feet, temperature regulation dysfunction, irritable bowels, dry mouth, hair loss, and delayed muscle relaxation. I also experience many common symptoms found in PNH and similar neurological disorders, such as fasciculations, fatigue, weakness, stiffness, pain, vibration sensations, and paresthesia. My health is a comprehensive example since my symptoms are broad and cover all nerve sizes and functions, including autonomic, sensory, and motor. My goal in this chapter is to differentiate between PNH-related symptoms, another neurological disorder, and those tied to some other reason.

Chapter 11: Environmental Factors: What are the causes (etiology) of PNH and other Neurological Disorders?

- Alcohol
- Digestive Dysfunction
- Bacterial Infections
- Viruses
- Toxins
- Child Abuse
- High Cholesterol
- Intense Exercise

- Altitude
- Food Sensitivities and Allergies

In Chapter 11, or the seventh approach to understanding PNH disorders or my neurological condition, I detail those environmental factors that may trigger an autoimmune disorder affecting the nerve, muscle, or neuromuscular junction. An environmental trigger of an autoimmune disease may happen in two manners:

1. Individuals may have a genetic predisposition for a particular disorder that may be triggered by some environmental factors.
2. Individuals may not have a genetic predisposition; however, exposure to some environmental factors may initiate a mutation or expression change in their DNA genetic code, triggering a disorder (epigenetics).

The bottom line is this: if I am genetically predisposed to PNH and neuropathy, then I have also faced many environmental factors throughout my life that likely contributed to triggering the disorders, including bacterial infections, viruses, strenuous exercise, exposure to toxins, child abuse, living at a high altitude, and alcoholism.

Chapter 12: Initial Diagnosis Theories
- Nerve Conduction Study and EMG Testing
- Myotonia
- Neuromuscular Junction Disorders
- Initial PNH Theory

In Chapter 12, or the eighth approach to understanding PNH or my neurological condition, I review my initial diagnosis theory. Specifically, I reflect on and evaluate my initial diagnostic testing and how differential diagnosis focused on myotonia and neuromuscular disorders. I conclude the chapter with a detailed discussion about Isaac Syndrome (IS), including etiology, symptoms, facts, and characteristics. In particular, the chapter focuses on why I believed IS was my correct diagnosis and ultimately why it turned out not to be correct.

Chapter 13: Current Diagnosis Theories
- Myelopathy
- Neuropathy
- Myopathy
- My Diagnosis
- Treatment Options
- Summary

In Chapter 13, or the ninth approach to understanding my neurological disorder, I examine current diagnosis theories of my illness. My third EMG and nerve conduction study debunked the original Isaac syndrome hypothesis and brought to the forefront other ailments for evaluation, including various neuropathies, myelopathy, and myopathies. Since my symptoms did not fit any specific disorder, it is now theorized that I have multiple neurological disorders. I reveal my current diagnosis, as well as progress in various treatment options.

Appendix 1: Epidemiology Study of PNH

- Introduction
- Methods
- Results
- Conclusion / Discussion
- Acknowledgments

In Appendix 1, or the final approach to understanding my neurological conditions, I reveal the results of an epidemiology study about peripheral nerve hyperexcitation (PNH) disorders. The epidemiology study and its findings are critical for three reasons:

1. First, this study helps to define and characterize PNH disorders. This study's results include statistical analyses, and the organization of the survey questions is as follows: (1) general information (age, gender, regional residence, and other demographic information); (2) symptoms and intensity (fasciculations, cramps, weakness, numbness); (3) location and frequency of symptoms (where felt in the body and how severe); (4) remedy effectiveness (prescription drugs, supplements, massage, acupuncture, and dietary changes); (5) etiology (illness, prescription drugs, stress, family history, toxins, exercise, and neck or spine injury, vaccination); (6) conditions or events that may exacerbate symptoms (exercise, stress, or illness); and (7) other information (time of day symptoms worsen, improve, or progress)

2. To eliminate the fear factor, I do not recommend that people with peripheral nerve disorders compare themselves directly to others with PNH. [20] Individual comparisons can produce fear because each person has such unique symptoms, frequency, and intensity. Worse yet, remedies that may provide relief are also unique to each patient. However, a comparison of oneself to a statistical average of a large population is a better practice to suppress fears, which is true because averages better represent the entire population than comparisons to specific individuals. The bottom line, comparisons to an entire population will more than likely be closer to an individual's symptoms than comparing symptoms to an individual person.

3. Finally, to provide medical professionals with more information to help them understand PNH.

The Book Benefits

The overarching benefit of this book is that it illustrates both good and bad things happen for a reason. A positive outlook in the face of adversity means that we can evolve and make the most of an unfortunate situation. After all, our personalities are ultimately shaped by how we handle adversity.

Patients reading this book can benefit from learning about the following:
- Evolving by changing habits, practices, or lifestyle
- Eliminating fear through acceptance

Understanding that acceptance does not mean giving up trying to find relief and answers; it merely suggests moving forward and not dwelling on the negative aspects of the adversity we may face.

- Knowing how to advocate for oneself, even when no one else is helping them cope with their adversity.
- Being grateful or enjoying the freedoms we have and not dwelling on those freedoms that an adverse situation may inhibit, such as freedom to work or travel [21]
- Setting goals or establishing and building a life plan
- Taking advantage of the immense benefits that come from exercise.
- How to live life to the fullest

Family members and friends reading this book would benefit from learning ways to:
- Help their loved one's cope with adversity by becoming knowledgeable about their disorders
- Show patience and understanding
- Listen and believe

Medical professionals reading this book would benefit from:
- Learning the statistical facts about PNH disorders
- Helping PNH patients instead of ignoring them
- Reassuring PNH patients by answering their questions and providing them helpful information, so they do not live in fear

Unique Features of the Book

This book offers several unique features. The epidemiology study provides educational and research information not available elsewhere. My training and race methods can contextualize physical limitations. My suggestions for various coping mechanisms for fatigue, fear, depression, and pain are ones I value, not only for my neurological condition but for training and competition.

I also aim to make this book accessible, straightforward, and easy to understand. Medical books are complex and challenging to understand because of the extensive Latin terminology and other jargon. One book on the immunology insists the medical field has a glossary problem. For example, words such as "antibody" make little sense because antibodies do not work "against the body" but work "with or for the body." [i] [22] I have always found that the easiest way to learn and to teach hard to understand topics is to use clean organization and everyday language to convey information.

After thirteen years, 9 neurologists, and dozens of tests costing tens of thousands of dollars, I have no concrete diagnosis because my symptoms do not align with any particular nerve or muscular disorder. My physicians and I believe that I suffer from both PNH and neuropathy. However, even these diagnoses may not explain all my symptoms like autonomic dysfunction or denervation of the quad muscles. If I were to provide my disorder with a unique name, it would be: *chronic idiopathic prodigious and ubiquitous polyneuropathy* (CIPUP).

Finally, categorizing pain, fear, and depression as a symptom of PNH and neuropathy is unique. Imagine visiting a neurologist, and he or she says, "We need to test you for amyotrophic lateral sclerosis (ALS) and multiple sclerosis (MS)." Then, in the follow-up appointment to discuss the test results, the neurologist says everything is fine, you probably have BFS, and that is "no big deal." He or she offers you no advice or potential remedies that may alleviate the symptoms. He or she spends five minutes with you and sends you on your way. The neurologist's dismissive attitude raises more questions and leads to fear, depression, and enhanced pain, thereby compounding the effects of the disorder. In this book, I explore the science behind pain, depression, and fear, which are the worst stressors acting on the human body.

Part I

Chapter 2: Exercise, My Story, My Genome, and Aging

My most recent neurologist, who is outstanding, suggests that my exercise, in particular my intense cycling regimen, has possibly spared me from having more severe neurological symptoms. She believes my actions may have slowed the progression or even prevented it from invading my cardio and respiratory systems. At a minimum, my exercise regimen is keeping me upright and out of a wheelchair. This statement may or may not be true, but it motivates me to proceed with my cycling training and competition regardless of the pain and deteriorating symptoms for two reasons: To stay alive and prevent future debilitating symptoms.

Exercise Guidelines

There are many references for exercise guidelines for healthy adults: The World Health Organization (WHO), U.S. National Human and Health Services, the European Union, the American Heart Association, and the American College of Sports Medicine (ACSM). Most recommend at least 150min per week of brisk exercise and strength training, including curls and squats. Brisk signifies moderate-intensity or about a 3 out of 10 rating of perceived exertion (RPE). The above exercise references do not distinguish between healthy people and those with some type of chronic ailment. The fourth edition of *Chronic Disorders and Diseases* (CDD4) also does not distinguish any exercise differences between healthy people and those inflicted with many different chronic disorders.

The reason for this is it is impossible to do since there are literally thousands of disorders to distinguish among, and each person is uniquely different. Instead, the CDD4 offers exercise suggestions (limitations) for some common disorders. [23] CDD4 does not include recommendations for PNH, but it does for some disorders with similar symptoms including neuropathy.

PNH (or Isaac syndrome) symptoms are similar to other types of disorders, such as peripheral neuropathy, myopathy, and myasthenia gravis (MG), outlined in CDD4. For peripheral neuropathy, myopathy, and MG, the exercise guidelines (CDD4) for individuals capable of intense exercise suggests following ACSM guidelines. At the same time, most people with conditions such as peripheral neuropathy and MG engage in low-intensity exercise programs with the approval of a physician. The CDD4 exercise guidelines suggest modifications can be made to ACSM recommendations for safety or limitation reasons. For example, recommendations for people with peripheral neuropathy and MG include exercising in a cool environment, having symptoms treated before starting an exercise program, using physical therapy as a starting guideline, and to avoid fatigue, which usually conveys low intensity for short durations. [24] Of course, fatigue gets a bad rap because, without some fatigue, it is impossible to improve physically. [25]

One case study of an exercise plan for a patient with MG suggested easy walking for 15min, four times a week, but to build up to 30 min four times per week at a moderate intensity. The plan also included starting with fairly easy weight training, balance exercises, and flexibility exercises two or three days per week but to build resistance and intensity over time. Thus, CDD4 exercise programs for specific disorders usually recommend shorter durations with less intensity (RPE) than recommended by sources for healthy adults. Taking this into account, the ultimate goal of most plans for people with MG or peripheral neuropathy is for individual exercise plans to gradually build up to be very similar to those minimum recommended guidelines for healthy people. [26]

Interestingly, some emerging research suggests that interval training is appropriate for individuals with cardiovascular troubles. Intervals encompass short periods of intense exercise (RPE greater than 3) followed by rest or low exertion. Depending on the duration of the interval, sets of intervals may involve dozens of repeated efforts or just a few. My point is this; if interval training is appropriate for individuals with cardio concerns, it certainly can be appropriate for anyone with a neurological condition. The bottom line is that exercise, grit, and motivation are the best medicine for chronic disorders and pain. The only other recourse is a downward spiral to more health problems.[27] Simply put, strenuous and intense exercise is possible for individuals inflicted with nerve, muscle, or neuromuscular disorders.

Something that may help anyone with chronic pain or even healthy individuals remain active is to have a coach. Doctors, friends, family, physical therapists, and fitness coaches can help individuals overcome the fear of their disorder and, therefore, provide more motivation and feedback to cope with success and failure. For example, my general practitioner remains competitive, although he lost a leg in an accident. My former climbing partner, and best friend, achieves in the face of Parkinson's disease, and my stepmother remains active despite her battle with a rare neurological condition. I am fortunate to have these inspirational people in my life. They certainly will never let me feel sorry for myself or to give up fighting the good fight.

I have a certified USA cycling coach to help me improve my performance. My coach has a biomedical background and designs workouts around my limitations from the neurological condition. I provide him with my symptoms, race goals, and exercise limitations, and he develops an individualized plan that has a specific goal to improve my performance. Everyone can benefit from a coach. Finding the right coach may be difficult, but it is possible. For instance, many coaches go by the one size fits all philosophy. Alternatively stated, they have one plan that works for them, and they expect that same plan to work for all their clients. It is never that simple since we are all vastly different and have unique goals. As we will learn, each person has different genes, and the trainability of those genes varies depending on the exercise program. Hence, it is important to find a personal trainer who builds a plan around your needs and limitations. Individual plans should also be tailored to goals and specific races identified by the client.[28] A famous coach of Olympian and Ironman champions, Brett Sutton, argued, "Every athlete [is] psychologically and physiologically unique" and builds a training plan around their uniqueness. Sutton warns against trying change techniques and making athletes theoretically better because, in doing so, they may initiate a decline in performance. [29]

I am convinced that exercise can help most people with neurological conditions cope with their disorder. Thus, I encourage others with exercise intolerance from neurological disorders to force themselves to walk because I am convinced that they will feel better for doing it. Besides, the good pain from exercise will mask the bad pain from the neurological condition, which is a much more desirable outcome. If it hurts too much to walk, then try lower impact sports such as swimming or cycling.

My Story

My story, or the mystery of my neurological disorder, starts as far back as grammar school when I had *staphylococcus bacterial* (staph) infections. It is also important to note that I had mononucleosis (Epstein-Barr virus–EBV) at age 19. The impact of staph and EBV on neurological disorders will be evaluated in more detail throughout the text. During my participation in athletics, especially in high school, cramping was a chronic problem. Later, at age 40, following a climbing trip, I noticed intense paresthesia symptoms in my hands and feet and continuous twitching in my lower legs. As far back as I can remember, I always had some abnormal sensations (mostly a tingling sensation) and cramping, but this was different; the symptoms were definitely worse. My initial thought was it was the result of a neck injury or mechanical compression of a thoracic nerve from carrying heavy loads on that climbing trip (80+ pound backpack). An MRI on my neck was negative and revealed that although my disks were not in great shape, they were not bad enough to warrant surgery. In other words, the doctor did not think a neck injury or mechanical compression was causing my paresthesia symptoms, but he had no recommendations other than drinking lots of water to keep my disks hydrated. So, I learned to live with the symptoms.

Following a move to Colorado, four years later, my symptoms got much worse. After doing research on muscle twitching and other symptoms, I feared the worse: I could have amyotrophic lateral sclerosis (ALS) or multiple sclerosis (MS). My general practitioner ordered blood work, which subsequently came back normal, with the exception of elevated levels of a muscle protein called creatine kinase–CK. Minerals, vitamins, and supplements failed to alleviate the symptoms. I was referred to two neurologists–one to conduct an electromyography (EMG) and nerve conduction study and the other to do a complete neurological exam, which included a brain MRI. The tests came back negative, and I was officially diagnosed with benign fasciculation syndrome (BFS) by both neurologists. A year later, I saw a third neurologist because my symptoms continued to worsen. This neurologist spent less than five minutes with me and concurred with the other neurologists' diagnosis that it was BFS. All three neurologists agreed that BFS is "no big deal" since everyone gets muscle twitching or fasciculations from time to time.

Over the course of the next year, I found myself continually complaining about my BFS. I live by the philosophy that complaining without offering practical solutions is never acceptable. I decided to use my engineering background to statistically analyze the disorder by collecting data from an online survey. My initial goal of the survey was to help BFS patients by illustrating that we are all experiencing a similar ordeal (symptoms and intensity). My second goal was to bring more attention to the disorder and disprove the notion that BFS is "no big deal."

After seeing my fifth neurologist, he changed my diagnosis from BFS to cramp fasciculation syndrome (CFS), insisting the symptoms were more severe than just BFS. This neurologist noticed that I had another unexplained phenomenon causing my muscles to relax from a contracted state much slower than a normal muscle. My quad muscles acted more like a sponge then a liquid, and the dysfunction resembled a myotonia disorder. After a plethora of tests exploring rare muscle disorders such as myotonic dystrophy Type II, stiff person syndrome, and rippling muscle disease, the delayed muscle relaxation controversy also remained unexplained. Delayed muscle relaxation is not a symptom of CFS. However, delayed muscle relaxation is a symptom of Isaac syndrome (IS) according to dozens of papers and the National Institute for Health (NIH) homepage for rare neurological disorders. This newly acquired information led me to believe that I may actually have IS and not CFS. Isaac syndrome, like other PNH disorders, affects the voltage-gated potassium channel (VGKC) at the nerve ending. [30] Antibodies against the VGKC show up in 30–40 percent of all acquired cases of IS, and I was in the majority because I tested negative for these antibodies. [31] Since 60 to 70% of all IS cases do not present with VGKC antibodies, a negative test certainly did not eliminate IS as a plausible explanation for my disorder.

With a dozen debilitating symptoms, including muscle pain, stiffness, fatigue, paresthesia, and irritable bowel syndrome (IBS), exercise intolerance can occur. I had given up on exercise because of safety and or physical pain concerns. For example, I could no longer rock climb or be a volunteer wrestling coach due to safety concerns over the lack of feeling and mobility in my hands and feet. Any running, hiking, snowshoeing, and mountaineering activities felt like someone was stabbing me in the calves and Achilles tendon with a knife, and it took at least a week to recover from this pain. I could no longer do simple tasks because my hands were no longer reliable, and the situation was and is rapidly deteriorating. Either I had to evolve or become a full-time couch potato facing the prospect of an unproductive life.

Ten years ago, the U.S. Pro Cycling Challenge came to my house. The Cycling Challenge was comprised many of the same riders and teams that participate in races such as the Tour de France and Tour of Italia. The U.S. Pro Cycling Challenge was a week-long race on the roads of Colorado. One challenging stage included climbs over both Cottonwood and Independence passes (both are over 12,000 feet). Since I live at the base of Cottonwood pass, I biked up to the pass to watch the race. I am not alone, however, as hundreds of people flock to my hometown to bike to the pass to watch the race. When I was sitting at the pass, a group of riders asked me, "How long did it take me to ride up to pass from town?" I said, "It took about two hours," which starts to push the limits of what my body can tolerate. Thank goodness I do not have to work very hard going down, which only takes a little over a half-hour. They said, "That is pretty fast on an old and heavy mountain bike." They asked me, "Do you race?" and I told them, "No, I just ride for fun." They told me, "You should race," and asked, "Have you ever used a road bike to get to the pass?" I responded, "No, I only have a mountain bike." They said, "You will cut at least 20 minutes off your time."

After other sports and activities were eliminated from my lifestyle as a result of the neurological disorder, I picked up cycling full time since the pain and other symptoms were more manageable. It is fairly easy to understand why cycling results in less pain since most of my pain and cramping are concentrated in my calves and feet. Riding a bike stresses the calves, Achilles tendon, and feet much less than strenuous hiking or other activities such as climbing and wrestling. Even riding a bike at a high-power output stresses the lower leg muscles, joints, and tendons less than walking. Running, hopping, and jumping has three to five times as much force on the Achilles' tendons than riding a bike at 270 watts. [32]

A few years after that conversation at the top of Cottonwood Pass, I entered the Nevada Senior Games and the Huntsman Senior Games (Utah) using a road bike I rented from a local bike shop. Most states have senior games for people over 50 years of age. I had no expectations, but I did very well. I made many new friends who encouraged me to race full-time, indicating that I was fast and would only improve with the right equipment and full-time training. I took their advice and have been racing for the past seven years.

Over a span of seven years, I went from recreational cycling to winning a Colorado State Time Trial Championship (50+ Age Group), the National Senior Games Time Trial Championship (50-54 and 55-59 Age Group), and placed 13th and 11th at the United States Cycling Master Time Trial National Championships (50-54 and 55-59 Age Group). When I first started to compete, I made goals to win these three races. Most people probably thought I was delusional (both doctors and other riders). It takes time to become a good racer, but my dedication and intense training paid off.

My Genome Testing [33]

The Science of Genetics [34] [35] [36]

Since many disorders may be inherited (genetic) or the outcome of a gene mutation, it is imperative to have a basic understanding of genetics, including deoxyribonucleic acid (DNA), genes, and chromosomes. Furthermore, athletic success may be tied to how well our genes respond to training:

DNA is a double *helix structure* molecule with nitrogen bases making up the rungs of the ladder of the helix structure. The four nitrogen bases are *adenine* (A), *cytosine* (C), *guanine* (G), and *thymine* (T). *Uracil* (U) replaces thymine (T) in *ribonucleic acid* (RNA). Ribonucleic acid (RNA) is the same as DNA except it is a single strand (half a ladder). The only combination of nitrogen bases, via a hydrogen bond, is between A and C, and G and T. Thus, there are four possible combinations of nitrogen bases to make up one rung of the ladder in the helix structure: A–C, C–A, G–T(U), or T(U)–G. The nitrogen bases connect to the helix structure with phosphate and sugar molecules.

DNA holds the code or the genetic makeup of ***protein molecules***. Proteins are comprised of a string of ***amino acids***. The body produces 20 different amino acids. All life as we know it uses the same 20 amino acids. Every three rungs on the DNA helix ladder represents the code or codon for one amino acid. There are 64 possible combinations of codes or ***codons***. Mathematically, this is represented by four nitrogen base combinations for three ladder rungs, or 4^3 (4x4x4), or 64. One codon (AUG) can signal the start sequence of an RNA protein code, and the first amino acid in a protein code is always methionine. The opposite sequence partner of AUG is CGU.

An additional three codes signal the stop or ***nonsense codon***, which signifies the end to the code or the end of the protein synthesis: UAA, UAG, and UGA. The remaining 60 codons identify one of twenty amino acids the body manufactures. Some amino acids are identifiable via numerous codons or codes. For example, the amino acid glycine is identifiable from the codons GGU, GGC, GGA, and GGG. [37] ***Genes*** comprise DNA molecules or said differently, a segment of DNA containing the information for the synthesis of a protein molecule is a gene. One DNA molecule may contain the sequence for thousands of proteins consisting of millions of nitrogen bases (rungs of the ladder).

Chromosomes are strings of genes. Each cell has 46 chromosomes, or 23 pairs, of chromosomes in the nucleus. One chromosome pair comes from each parent, where one chromosome pair defines the sex of the person. Each of the 22 remaining chromosome pairs defines a wide range of genetic information about each person.

DNA must be able to replicate itself when cells divide via *mitosis*. When DNA does not replicate exactly, a mutation occurs. *Mutations* are essential for the adaption and evolution of living species to survive. However, mutations are also associated with disease. There are various mutations of DNA and chromosomes: [38] [39] [40]

A *misuse mutation* is one where a single amino acid code is altered, leading to one protein being substituted for another in the DNA code.

A *frameshift mutation* results when many amino acid codes become altered. A frameshift mutation is produced by the insertion or deletion of a protein in the DNA code.

A mutation may also occur in the end coding (nonsense mutation). A *nonsense mutation* would yield either a truncated protein or one that is too long.

Triplet mutations occur when diseased DNA sequences contain dozens of repeated codes instead of just a few in a normal DNA sequence. The length of the repeated mutation reveals the onset age and severity of the disorder. The length of the mutation tends to increase from one generation to the next and is also called an anticipation mutation.

Mitochondrial DNA mutations impair oxidative metabolism.

There are also various ways each chromosome may mutate, such as only having one pair or three pairs instead of two. These types of mutations are called *numerical mutations*.

The DNA replication process is summarized as follows: [41] (1) messenger RNA (mRNA), which has the transcribed code of the DNA to be replicated, leaves the cell nucleus into the cytoplasm; and (2) once in the cytoplasm, mRNA interacts with transfer RNA (tRNA) with the help of ribosomes to create proteins via a process called translation.

The Science of Epigenetics [42] [43]

Evolution is the study of how species change or adapt over time, and epigenetics is one of the branches of evolution. Specifically, *epigenetics* is the study of the role that the environment plays in genetics. While evolution proposed by Darwin is a slow process, epigenetics is a much faster evolutionary process proposed by Lamarck fifty years before Darwin. In particular, *Darwinism* is the evolutionary process that happens during good times, when civilizations do not face threats from environmental chaos like famine or disease. Conversely, the fast epigenetics evolutionary process is required during bad times when civilizations face environmental chaos. Darwinism addresses the changing of the human genome, while epigenetics refers to the changing of the human epigenome. More specifically, Darwinism is characterized by alterations to human genes, and epigenetics can be characterized by changes to gene expression, not the actual gene itself. In epigenetics, gene expression or plasticity can vary a great deal depending on the environmental situation.

Human gene expression continually changes and adapts to environmental stress. Adaptions to gene expression may happen in several ways. First, genes can be regulated by being either turned on or turned off. Sometimes when genes are turned off, the process is known is RNA silencing. Genes that are turned on generate specific proteins, while those turned off do not generate any specific protein because the RNA transcription has been silenced. Second, the rate of production of some gene proteins may be increased or slowed. Third, genes may be altered by having a different protein generated in its sequence. Fourth, *epigenetic change* may also be accomplished by affecting the shape of the DNA molecule by changing the histone proteins responsible for that task. Fifth, *lateral gene transfer* occurs when one organism invades another organism. After the invasion is complete epigenetic changes happen during a process called "gene jumping." In lateral gene transfer, the two organisms learn to not only survive but to coexist.

Many epigenetic changes that come from environmental stress are not favorable. Even worse, these unfavorable genetic outcomes (*epigenomes*) can pass on to future generations. For instance, when genes turn off, or protein expression change, the mechanism causing this process is methyl molecules that disrupt the RNA transcription of proteins. This process is called *methylation*. Conversely, positive changes in protein and enzyme production levels can be increased or decreased from exercise. Thus, not all epigenome outcomes are adverse. Some epigenetic changes are a necessity for the survival of species. More specifically, positive epigenetic outcomes happen during times of environmental chaos and stress, such as famine, disease, abrupt climate changes, meteor strikes, pandemics, and mass extinction. During these chaotic times, epigenome changes occur, and new life forms evolve quite rapidly. This process is much different from Darwinism, which states new life forms evolve slowly, which can still happen during less stressful times. Moreover, once epigenome traits evolve from a chaotic environmental situation, Darwinism may take hold and evolve the new traits into new genes for future generations.

Most geneticists believe that not only human features and characteristics are affected by epigenetics and evolution, but so too are behavioral traits such as fear, depression, anger, happiness, and more. Furthermore, behavioral traits are hereditary and can be passed on to future generations. Consider one example; children who experience abuse can develop behavioral traits via epigenetics, including anger, high risk-taking, criminal behavior, and depression, as well as become more prone to cancer and other diseases. Abused children may not have favorable expressions for the VMAT2 gene, commonly referred to as the *God gene*. VMAT2 transcribes the protein responsible for neurotransmitters, such as dopamine. People with favorable VMAT2 expression not only tend to believe in God but live healthier lives and are less affected by disease and bad behavioral traits such as anger and depression. The reason for the favorable effects of VMAT2 is that it comes from a more positive attitude, like believing in good over evil, which prioritizes pleasure genes over stress genes. The converse is true for the unfavorable effects of the VMAT2 gene in abused children who may prioritize stressful genes over pleasure genes.

Epigenetic changes occur during many modern-day environmental stress factors, including alcohol, smoking, marijuana, drugs, prescription drugs, exercise, toxins, and illnesses. Toxins include a plethora of heavy metals, organophosphates, and anything that may contaminate the air and water. Remember, during the evolutionary history of man, he has never experienced exposure to these toxins until the last 100 years or less. Thus, the human body is responding with epigenetic changes. Indeed, human DNA and the genome may not be affected by exposure to toxins. However, if the epigenome or gene expression is affected in a negative manner then it may result in behavioral and intellectual declines.

Because of the introduction of toxins and processed foods, the human body is evolving faster in the last hundred years than the previous million years. In other words, humans are becoming more distinct, dissimilar, and unique. May this be the reason humans are more polarized than ever? It is an exciting hypothesis that warrants further exploration, but it is beyond the scope of this text. It remains to be seen what long-term effects social media and do-it-all cell phones will have on humans. However, it is easy to speculate that there will be negative epigenetic connotations from this behavior that will be passed on to future generations. For instance, bad eyesight and tooth decay are more common in modern humans due to epigenome changes to reading small print, computers, and the introduction of sugars.

Gene alterations may be short-term or long-term, which is an epigenetic change. Genes are made up of both proteins and a "control panel". Proteins are not subject to direct epigenetic changes, but instead the control panel is the mechanism allowing for a change in protein expression levels. The control panel is where other chemicals such as methyl may bind to the gene. Methyl generally attaches to the nucleotide cytosine when cytosine is followed by guanine in the protein genetic code. As explained earlier, genes with methyl attachments are said to be methylated and the more methyl molecules genes contain the more their expression level is reduced. Furthermore, heavily methylated genes tend to stay inactive especially those that are methylated early in human development. For instance, the methylated gene process happens when stem cells become *differentiated cells* during embryo development. *Stem cells* have the capability of becoming any type of human cell (skin, muscle, cardiac, liver, lung, etc.). Stem cells become differentiated when genes to become, say a skin cell, are turned on (no methylation), but the genes to form other types of cells are turned off (methylation).

While methylated genes are usually turned off and stay inactive during our lifetimes, *histone* proteins allow for fine tuning of gene expression. In other words, gene expression may be turned up or down at varying levels. Said differently, histone epigenic changes allow for more plasticity than methyl epigenic changes. Histones allow for a process called *acetylation* where acetyl molecules are attached to the amino acid lysine. What's more, histones respond to environmental changes such as alterations in our gut bacteria. Only two percent of the human genome is made up of protein coding genes. The remaining 98% of the human genome is comprised of various long and short chains of RNA molecules that also play a big role in epigenetic changes.

However, the role of these RNA molecules on epigenetic changes are still mostly unknown. Epigenetic changes can be passed on to future generations or they can be reset in the next generation. The bottom line, histone epigenetic regulation can be random, inherited, or caused by some environmental factor and the process is reversible because epigenetic alterations is not the same as a permanent gene mutation. All humans have the same genes, but our *phenotype* is what makes us all different. In fact, most mammals and even plant life have many of the same or similar genes as humans. In other words, phenotype is defined by methyl, histone, and non-protein RNA epigenetic changes to genes that make us all unique with different height, weight, and also internal differences. [44] [45]

Genetic testing is the process of mapping out all 22,000 genes or genome of an individual. Genome testing is not for everyone, especially knowing that it can be controversial for a few reasons. First, whenever race is introduced into a topic, it automatically becomes controversial since we live in a polarized and politically correct society. However, race and genetics are mutually exclusive because ethnicity and race are not the same things. Race is biological, and ethnicity is cultural or environmental. Furthermore, since the probabilistic outcome from any genetic testing is highly dependent on environmental factors, our future outcomes are more closely related to ethnicity, and race has a much less significant role in any findings.

Second, genome testing is only a guideline since the environment plays a big role in our future outcomes. If people accept the results of genome testing as definitive, then the test may do more harm than good by adding more unwanted stress into the lives of some. Said differently, if someone has a genetic mutation indicating a high probability, they will develop dementia, it can cause much unwanted stress, but the outcome is not guaranteed because the person can change some environmental factors to mitigate that risk.

Third, can parents use genomic testing to determine the outcome of a pregnancy (to abort or not to abort)? Determining the viability of a fetus or baby via genetic testing is very controversial. Moreover, the more genetic testing involved in the process of determining pregnancy outcomes, the more controversial it becomes. For instance, should a baby be aborted if a test reveals a high probability of having Alzheimer's after age 70? One would hope not, but who knows how some parents may think. For example, some parents may not be able to tolerate the thought of their child suffering at any age. The bottom line is that every single human being has flawed genes, and the same can be said of any fetus or baby. No one is perfect (both literally and genetically), but what defects can be used in determining pregnancy outcomes is unclear.

Fourth, many genetic variations are classified as "unknown significance." In other words, there is no data to indicate whether the gene variant may be harmful or not. How people react to unknown significant gene variations can be controversial. For example, can someone overreact and obtain a double mastectomy when they have a variant of unknown significance on a gene that may signify breast cancer? In other words, genome testing may be over-diagnosing the problem and may make people feel sick when they are fairly healthy.

Fifth, the probability of a false positive or false negative is about 2%, which is significant. Finally, privacy or property rights are a concern because DNA genome sequencing is stored in data banks for the medical community to study. Many people want reassurances; their information is protected and not sold to other companies, government agencies, groups, and organizations. For example, there is always a concern that genetic information may get into the wrong hands. For instance, insurance companies may discriminate against an individual or family member with bad genes, such as having a high chance of obtaining cancer or dementia.

However, there are laws protecting against genetic discrimination. Complicating the matter more is that genetic privacy or property rights are not a question isolated to one individual, but it involves the entire family that shares much of the same DNA information. Overall, genetic testing should only be done when the benefit outweighs the harms. If used correctly, genetic testing can be an effective tool to determine diet, training, and drug effectiveness. Furthermore, genetic testing may foster environmental changes that can alter possible negative outcomes.

I decided to obtain a full genome test to determine how my training and diet plans can be altered to be most effective to take advantage of both my genetic strengths and weaknesses.   I also wanted to see if there are any clues in my genome sequencing that may provide any insight as to what may be going on with my neurological condition. I needed to determine if there are any environmental factors that I can change to prevent any possible negative outcomes. Again, genome testing can prognosticate possible future outcomes of our medical history, but it not necessarily our destiny. Specifically, our genetic future is probabilistic and not deterministic. For instance, we may have a gene expression that may indicate a higher chance of having some type of cancer or dementia, but there may be actions that can lower the probability of occurrences such as exercise, reading, and dietary changes. One doctor astutely noticed, "Everything is environmental until you convince me it is genetic." The following are my genetic results from 24Genetics that are associated with athletic and metabolic performance:

My Athletic Genome Testing [46]

My athletic performance genome tests are defined below and grouped into 5 classifications: Genotype is favorable, genotype is slightly favorable, genotype is not affected, genotype is slightly unfavorable, and genotype is unfavorable. All information and quotes describing the tests are from 24Genetics.

Favorable Genotype

The *Muscle Strength* test checks for variations in the INSIG2 gene associated with "genetic factors have been associated with a greater benefit in increasing strength after training. "

The *Muscle Recovery* or *Resiliency* test, which checks for variations in the following genes: IL6, CRP, and SOD2 which "Research has shown that certain genetic variants are associated with a slower recovery after hard exercise."

The *Sensitivity to Insulin* test checks for variations in the LIPC gene. According to 24Genetics persons with a greater sensitivity to insulin can process glucose during exercise better.

Slightly Favorable Genotype

The *Muscle Endurance* test checks for variations in the following genes: PPARGC1A, ACE, NFIA-AS2, and HIF1A. More specifically "Studies have identified genetic variants associated with a high proportion of Type I fibers and a high supply of oxygen to muscle tissue."

The *Aerobic Capacity* test checks for variations in the following genes: NFIA-AS2, RGS18, and ACSL1. In particular, this test is focused on gene variants that may affect VO2 Max.

The *Risk of Joint Injury* test checks for variations to the following genes: GNL3, FTO, SUPT3H, and IL1A. More precisely, "Sports and high-impact activities can lead to cartilage injuries and damage to the joints. Your risk of injury is calculated on genetic variations that are associated with joint problems."

The *Metabolic* test checks for variations to the following genes: AMPD1, PPARA, ADRB2, PPARD, and PPARGC1A. According to 24Genetics, for instance, "Some genes analyzed are involved in the metabolism of fatty acids whose expression can improve the oxidative capacity of skeletal muscle during exercise, i.e. different variants result in a better or less efficient mechanisms to obtain energy from fatty acids and other nutrients."

Not Affected Genotype

The *Cardio Capacity* test checks for variations in the following genes: NPY, NOS3, ADRB1, APOE, and APOE. More specifically, "Some people are carriers of genes that make them have a better cardiac capacity, allowing them to have better strength and strength during exercise."

The *Muscular Fatigue* test checks for variations in the HNF4A and NAT2 genes. In particular, "In addition to exercise, the genetic condition is another cause of muscle fatigue. There are studies that relate certain genetic variants with a better resistance to muscular fatigue."

The *Muscle Regeneration Capacity* test checks for two variations in the IL1B gene. More precisely, "Genetic variations in several genes improve the inflammatory response that allows for a slow repair of muscle damage after exercise. "

The *Global Exercise Benefit* test check for variations in the CETP and BDNF genes. According to 24Genetics "People with certain genetic variants experience rapid results to lower cholesterol, triglycerides and blood pressure." Most people who exercise gain a health benefit such as a favorable sensitivity to cholesterol (CEPT and PPARD), and blood pressure (EDN1, NOS3, GNAS, and ADD1). For instance, some individuals respond better to exercise to lower cholesterol while others will not be able to lower their cholesterol with exercise alone.

Slightly Unfavorable Genotype

The *Muscle Power* test checks for variations in the following genes: ACE, IGF2BP2, NOS3, PPARG, AGT, PPARA, VEGFA, VDR, PPARGC1A, and HIF1A. Specifically, this test checks for muscle genes that would favor power athletes such as sprinters. In particular, these genes enhance Type II muscle fiber composition and performance. Furthermore, "It is estimated that power is inherited by 80% depending on the type of specific muscle (isometric strength of the knee, hand strength, elbow flexion). To assess the power predisposition profile, genetic markers have been used that have been associated with power sports."

The *Skeleton Muscle Performance* test checks for variations in the UCP2 gene. In particular, "The UCP2 and UCP3 proteins can negatively regulate mitochondrial ATP synthesis (energy that muscles use) and thereby influence physical performance. One study has found that genetic variants in these genes are associated with improved skeletal muscle performance with training."

The *Muscle Response to Resistance Training* test checks for variations in the following genes: BMP2, IL15RA, and INSIG2. While most people benefit from endurance training, the same is not necessarily true for weightlifting. Moreover, "Several studies have reported association between certain genetic variations and muscle size and strength. Some people gain more strength and muscle size in response to the same training as others."

Unfavorable Genotype

The *Injury Risk* test checks for variations to the following genes: GDF5, COL1A1, IL6, and CRP. More specifically, "The genetic risk of injury is calculated taking into account variations in the genes related to general inflammation, since when suffering from a soft tissue injury levels of inflammation may influence recovery."

The *Risk of Ruptured Tendons and Ligament* test checks for variations to the following genes: COL1A1, MMP3, GDF5, and COL12A1. In particular, "Achilles tendon injuries are a major obstacle to any athlete's performance; they affect athletes in a wide variety of sports (up to 20% of runners) and can often take months to heal. Individuals with favorable genetic variations may have stronger ligaments and tendons than the general population, allowing them to decrease their risk of injury."

The *Risk of Overload Fracture* test checks for variations to the following genes: FUBP3, RIN3, C17ORF53, MEPE, and ZBTB40. More precisely, "The main factor affecting one's risk to overload fractures is bone density, which has a genetic component (up to 85% of the variability is explained by genetic variations)."

The *Body Mass Index (BMI)* test checks for variants in the FTO gene. According to 24Genetics "People with a certain variant in the genetic marker of the FTO gene are more likely to be overweight, an increase in body mass index and waist circumference. However, a largescale study has shown that the genetic susceptibility to obesity-induced variant in the FTO gene can change by adopting an active lifestyle. In fact, people who are more susceptible to obesity experience greater weight loss by exercising at moderate intensity." *Weight gain* may be influenced by other variants to MC4R, ADIPOQ, and ADRB2 genes. The ANKK1/DRD2 gene affects the *Desire to Eat*, which may also be influenced by the *Emotional Eating* gene (TAS2R38), *Bitter Taste* genes (TAS2R38 and TAS2R16), and *Sweet Taste* genes (TAS2R38 and FGF21). For instance, individuals that have more desire to eat, eat when they are emotional. Furthermore, individuals that have genes that favor sweet tasting foods are more likely to overeat and eat unhealthy foods; whereas, those people whose genes favor bitter tasting foods may be more likely to eat healthier foods such as broccoli and brussels sprouts. What's more, there are many genes that may also affect the ability to *Lose Weight*: TCF7L2, PPARG, PPM1K, MTNR1B, and CLOCK. [47]

My Dietary or Metabolic Genome Testing [48]

My dietary genome tests check to see how well I may or may not metabolize certain vitamins, minerals, and various food substances and they are grouped into 5 classifications: Genotype is favorable, genotype is slightly favorable, genotype is not affected, genotype is slightly unfavorable, and genotype is unfavorable. The gene names are listed in parenthesis.

Favorable Genotype

High Carbohydrate Diet (LOC10537049 and FGF21), Excessive Fat Diet (SLC46A3), Vitamin B2 (MTHFR), Vitamin C (SLC23A1), Low Fat Diet (FTO, PPM1K, IRS1, and QPCTL), and Low Carbohydrate Diet (FTO)

Slightly Favorable Genotype

Cholesterol LDL (ABCG8, APOB, CELSR2, HMGCR, HNF1A-AS1, TIMD4, LDLR, LOC10272496 8, SUGP1 and PCSK9)

Not Affected Genotype

Mediterranean Diet (PPARG) and Cholesterol HDL (ABCA1, RAB11B, CETP, FADS1, GALNT2, HNF4A, KCTD10, NUTF2, LIPC, LIPG, LPL, TTC39B, ZPR1, CETP)

Slightly Unfavorable Genotype

Vitamin D (GC, CYP2R1, and VDR), Vitamin E (APOA5), and Triglycerides (DOCK7, APOB, FADS1, LPL, BAZ1B, CILP2, TRIB1. XKR6, and ZPR1)

Unfavorable Genotype

Omega 6 and Omega 3 Levels (FADS1), Iron (TMPRSS6, TF, and ABO), Vitamin B9 (MTRR and MTHFR), Vitamin B6 (NBPF3), Vitamin B12 (FUT2), and Vitamin K (VKORC1)

My Genome Summary

My athletic and nutrition genome results are as follows:

1. Unsurprisingly, I have a slightly unfavorable genetic composition for power and strength meaning my muscle fiber composition are primarily Type I and not Type II fast twitch (this is explained in detail in the next chapter). This would explain why I was an average athlete in wrestling, football, and baseball. Although I have endurance, I lack quickness, power, and the explosion necessary to excel at these sports. However, despite some favorable endurance genes, I was, at best, only an average endurance runner in high school.

2. My genome composition is neutral for any cardiovascular gains, muscle fatigue, and muscle regeneration. That said, my muscles have a favorable genome to recover from exercise.

3. My genome for endurance training is slightly favorable for respiratory or VO2 Max and metabolic gains such as how efficiently my body uses fatty acids, glucose, and other nutrients to increase oxidative capacity during exercise. Furthermore, my muscle fiber protein composition responds well to endurance training by evolving muscle fibers to Type I slow twitch, improving overall muscle fiber strength, and enhancing

oxidative supplies to the muscles. In other words, my body responds fairly well (not outstanding) to endurance training. That said, my slightly unfavorable genome for mitochondrial efficiency to produce ATP energy may counteract some of my favorable endurance genes.

4. I have a seemingly high risk for injury especially fractures and ligament damage.

5. I am also at high risk of being overweight, but the good news is that I can control or counteract my weight predisposition through exercise.

6. My genome for diet shows the critical nature of having a balanced diet since I am at risk for metabolizing at least nine critical vitamins and minerals poorly. Despite being predisposed to possible poor genetic outcomes for these vitamins, they all remain within normal specifications. A balanced diet does not guarantee a person will have normal vitamin levels, but the chances are much greater than eating a poor diet. In fact, I have postulated that metabolizing genes that have an unfavorable expression may be trained to do an effective job simply by eating a balanced diet.

The bottom line, I have slightly trainable skeletal muscles and respiratory system. My genome may suggest I should be a better than average endurance athlete but not an athlete capable of being on the podium in most of my time trial races.

Remember, even though I have a slightly favorable genome for endurance training, my athletic and nutrition genome show that I have just as many negative predispositions to overcome such as poor vitamin metabolization, a higher risk for injury, and a higher risk to be overweight. Thus, I have postulated that overachieving genome traits such as grit, resilience, perseverance, and determination may play a bigger role in my athletic success, but I have not been tested for any of these gene predispositions. I drew this conclusion because these are the same overachieving traits that are important to overcome neurological disease. In other words, endurance training genes don't play a very important role in overcoming neurological disease. [49]

The one thing that is interesting about epigenetic changes is that individuals can observe these changes in their phenotype. An ***epigenetic change*** occurs when one of two things happen: [50]

1. Two things are genetically identical, but the phenotype varies.
2. An organism continues to be influenced by an event long after the event occurred.

The first point may explain why my endurance trained leg muscles behave differently than my non-endurance trained muscles. Not only do my leg muscles experience more neurological symptoms such as cramping and fasciculations, but they're also much less explosive because they are comprised of more Type I muscle fibers. The second point may explain why autoimmune diseases such as MMN continue long after the environmental trigger is removed.

What Makes an Endurance Athlete Elite?

Before starting this section, it is important to define the lactate threshold, functional threshold power, and heart rate thresholds: [51]

The terms *lactate threshold*, *threshold heart rate*, and *functional threshold power* are used interchangeably. Lactate threshold, heart rate threshold, and functional threshold power are the heart rate, lactate, and power a person is able to tolerate for up to one hour without fatigue. More specifically, lactate, heart rate, and power thresholds are the point at which the body moves from aerobic to anaerobic exercise. Thus, lactate, heart rate, and power threshold are determined by what percentage of energy a person can tolerate coming from carbohydrate energy sources that produce lactate. Essentially, the lactate threshold is the point at which the body is removing an equal amount of lactate being produced from any anaerobic exercise. The bottom line, at lactate, heart rate, and power threshold, in cycling, one will be uncomfortable experiencing quad pain and heavy breathing.

The evolution of the human body shows that, unlike other land animals who were made for short term speed, humans were engineered as endurance freaks. Although the first humans were unable to outrun prey in short distances, they could wear the prey out with a steady and long chase because they had more Type I muscle fibers, fat storage for energy, and sweat glands that enabled humans to run for miles without overheating or tiring. [52] Every human has more endurance capability than most land animals, but what makes the best endurance athlete?

In high school, I was, at best, an average athlete. I overachieved because I did not have any gifted athletic talent. I would categorize an elite master level time trialist, under 60 years old, as being capable of consistently finishing races with an average speed in the range of 27 to 28 mph. I consistently post times in the 26 to 27 mph range; thus, I would consider myself a step below elite. What can make an average endurance athlete in high school become a well above average master cyclist despite a neurological condition?

It is not technology or equipment because everyone has the best that money can buy. Moreover, many books and resources, such as *Talent is Overrated* (Geoff Colvin) and *Outliers* (Malcolm Gladwell), claim that 10,000 hours or ten years of experience and practice is needed to master most sports and earn elite status. These resources also suggest that individual practice has more benefits than team practice.

I won my state title and first national senior games title with less than 500 hours of time trial training, and to this day, I have fewer than 2,000 hours total of training and practice. However, 98% of my experience and practice is of the individual variety. Obviously, there are variances among athletes in how long it may take to master a sport or talent, and this phenomenon is often referred to as the "Matthew effect" of training. The Matthew effect means that those who start training with the most talent will become elite faster than those who start training with less talent. In other words, some may become elite in only 5,000 hours of practice while it may take others 15,000 hours.

Generally speaking, natural selection evolution takes place when mastering a sport or talent. Natural selection means that those who consistently show improvement will continue on their 10,000-hour journey while those who plateaued or do not improve very much are more than likely to end their journey of mastering a talent. Genetic and environmental differences are thought to be the most important factors accounting for variances in the time that it may take to master a sport or talent. [53]

Genetics can improve an endurance athlete's performance. A person may have naturally high aerobic fitness (about 1 in 20 people), a person may be a high responder to training (about 1 in 50 people), or the person may be a super athlete and have both a naturally high aerobic fitness level as well as respond well to training (about 1 in 1,000 people). I would classify myself as a fairly high responder to training. For example, as a youth runner, I conditioned myself to have a more efficient resting heartrate by changing the expression of a gene called CREB1. [54]

I distinctly remember the alarm bells that my resting 36-heart rate set off during a high-school physical that resulted in a cardiologist visit. Maybe the alarms were warranted since prior physicals never revealed a resting heart rate below 60. The cardiologist concluded it was a "runner's heart." Conversely, some studies indicate, "Genes involved in the body's immune and inflammation process predict individual differences in aerobic trainability." [55] Since my immune system is dysfunctional, this would seem to indicate that my genes are not aerobically trainable. Further complicating matters is the conflicting information in some references. Case in point, one reference (*The Sports Gene*, Epstein) insists that muscle fiber Type is not trainable, but another reference (*The Neuromuscular Aspects of Physical Activity*, Gardiner) claims muscle fiber Type is trainable. I believe my normal muscle fiber is predominately Type I, but I also believe that training has changed my muscle fiber percentage to be even a larger percentage of Type I fibers.

I do not believe that the negative effects of my neurological disorder are a major factor in limiting my cycling performance. Keep in mind that there are many disabled cyclists that can ride a time-trial at elite speeds of 28 mph. I am referring to people with disabilities but can still ride a two-wheel bike (not handcycle or tricycle classifications). These people may have power impairment from a neurological disease, muscular disease, or lower leg amputation. For some individuals, they may overcome these disadvantages through training that teaches the body to bypass diseased cells and to generate new and alternate pathways for the brain and muscles to communicate. Just as education is the equalizing factor in society, cycling is the equalizing factor in endurance athletics. What I mean by that statement is that an individual born in poverty can be successful with a good education just as individuals with physical disabilities may find success in cycling over other endurance activities such as running or swimming for reasons I will outline in this chapter.

Genetics can certainly play a role in some athletes' success. For instance, Norwegian Eero Antero Mantyranta won seven gold medals in cross country skiing in the 1960s. Mantyranta was aided by a gene mutation that provided him with greater red blood cells (even at sea-level). Nonetheless, these types of mutations are rare, and in the case of Mantyranta, it accounted for a 0.00000003% change in his DNA. [56] An athletic genetic makeup may help some achieve athletic success but having good genes may not necessarily be a prerequisite or decisive factor in cycling excellence. [57]

There are more questions than answers when it comes to scientifically understanding athletic performance. There have been relatively no genetic studies on the success of athletes. Science better understands genes and their corresponding diseases much more than genes that may help identify athletic talent. One reason for the lack of funding in sport science is because funding to identify obesity and other health disorders is priority number one. While trying to find the gene responsible for Duchenne Becker syndrome, a scientist accidentally discovered that the ACTN3 gene responsible for transcribing the actinin protein. ACTN3 appears in Type II muscle fibers and it may indicate both athletic endurance and power capabilities. Individuals with muscles containing a favorable expression of the actinin protein can develop into sprinters, and those without the favorable expression for the actinin protein may be better suited for endurance sports. However, ACTN3 only accounts for about 2% in muscle fiber variance between individuals. Thus, there may be at least 50 other genes that may play a role in muscle fiber characteristics not fully known or understood. Unfortunately, studying sport science, genetics is avoided because our politically correct society would like to avoid conversations about athletic differences because of race. Of course, the topic of race in sports genetics can be avoided by comparing epigenetic differences brought about by ethnic, cultural, or environmental factors instead of comparing biological differences from race. [58] [59] What this means is that my epigenome results in the previous section may tell part of the story about my athletic genetic capabilities, it is probably incomplete and tells only a small part of the story since science does not understand the function of a majority of the human genes.

Cycling requires less technique than other endurance sports. In particular, peddling in cycling requires less technique than other endurance sports such as technique essential for optimal running or swimming results. Said differently, a genetic predisposition for good genes may be a bigger requirement for running and swimming success. Case in point: a person who has deformities affecting their gait may find this disability not as inhibiting on a bike as in swimming and running. This is a big reason why I refer to cycling as the equalizing factor in endurance sports.

There have been dozens of books and research articles written about identifying athletic talent by dozens of so-called experts, but there is no clear formula. The reason for this is because natural athletic ability (or good genes) is only a small part of the equation that relates to the success of athletes. It is difficult to conceptualize or measure other important qualities of the success equation, including drive, focus, determination, grit, and competitiveness. Besides, most writings on identifying and nurturing talent for a sport is a process for youths, not a process for masters and people over 50. Hundreds of people have the genetic composition to succeed in some sport but do not know it because they have no interest in the sport. In other words, there are Americans who have the genetic composition to be a much better cyclist than Greg LeMond; however, they will never know it because they have no desire to cycle. There is even evidence to support that endurance athletes who begin a sport later in life may have a better chance to succeed. However, those data suggest advantages to beginning training for a new sport at age 17 instead of before 12. More specifically, the studies indicate that athletes trying to garner 10,000 hours of training by starting before age 12 may have a better chance to plateau and see no additional improvement by age 14 to 16. [60] Whereas those athletes that start a sport after the age of 17 may not plateau or have peak performance until in their mid-twenties or later. Plateauing at an early age happen to me in running since I posted my best 5K times by age 14 or 15. Unfortunately, there are no studies about starting a new sports training program after 50!

I visited UC Irvine's lazar laboratory, and they had an opportunity to shed light on my genetic composition and answer the question of why I'm such a good cyclist despite having a chronic neurological condition. One UC Irvine lab administered fatigue tests on my lower leg muscles. Since the tests were designed for unhealthy people, I did not fatigue under their conditions. Thus, the test did not reveal any information except that my neurological disorder did not allow me to fatigue as fast as other people with other types of ailments. Another lab attempted to understand my cellular function better. One test investigated the function of my mitochondria using laser technology. Mitochondria dysfunction has been related to peripheral nerve disorders, such as peripheral neuropathy. Some evidence suggests that mitochondria dysfunction can generate symptoms found in autonomic neuropathy, which can sometimes be found in peripheral nerve disorders. [61] It is also known that mitochondria dysfunction can lead to the production of excess lactic acid leading to more muscle pain and fatigue. In other words, understanding the function of my mitochondria may explain why I have elevated levels of both resting lactate and creatine kinase. [62] However, the data was never compiled, and, without understanding the details of the test, it is difficult to discern whether they would have discovered anything to.

Another false theory is that my performance may be enhanced because I live and train at 8,000 feet. Individuals living and training at altitude have an abundance of rich oxygen-carrying red blood cells (natural doping). For that reason, some would argue that I have an unfair advantage over other athletes living at lower elevations. This theory has little credence. [63] Everyone in Colorado has some level of natural doping since most people live at a minimum of 5,000-6,000 ft. elevation. Additionally, most studies indicate that it is more ideal to live at altitude and train at sea level. This situation can be accomplished in two ways: First, to live at altitude and train with the help of supplemental oxygen and second, to live at sea level but have a pressurized room for sleep. One study indicated athletes perform anywhere from 3-8% worse competing at sea level after training and living at high altitude. How can this negative effect happen with oxygen-rich blood? Since max heart rates are higher at lower elevations, people at sea level obtain better functional training because they can raise their heart rate to a higher level. Conversely, interval workouts at altitude are seriously compromised when the max heart rate is lowered. For those reasons, studies indicate that for the best performance, athletes should live high but train low.

The effects of altitude are short-lived and wear off in a week or less when a person moves to a lower altitude. In *The Sports Gene*, Epstein writes that the sweet spot for high altitude training is between 6,000 and 9,000 feet and that for optimum benefits, it is best to be born and bred at high altitude. The most successful runners are born at altitude, which enables them to develop larger lungs. The benefit of moving to and training at altitude as an adult is negligible and probably depends on the trainability traits of genes. Increased hemoglobulin may increase oxygen transport, but altitude also increases blood viscosity, which may make some less aerobically fit. [64] I was born at an elevation of 72 feet and lived basically at sea level my entire youth. I moved to a high altitude at age 44. The advantages of training high and living high only happen when racers from sea-level compete at altitude but have not been properly acclimated to the elevation. Depending on the person, proper acclimation can take as long as three weeks.

Several traits help me succeed in cycling. For instance, I have a strong mental attitude that grew from coping with a debilitating neurological disorder and child abuse. Traumatic experiences—such as child abuse—can have long-term psychological benefits. [65] I also have a relatively low metabolic age, which is about 15 years less than my actual age. I also have the flexibility and strength to hold a fairly good aerodynamic position (low CdA – this is defined in Chapter 5) on a time trial bike while generating a decent functional threshold power. Moreover, I have an ideal body type for time trial cycling. Body type should not be underestimated in athletic success.

Specialized body types are common for most athletics: Tall for basketball, short and light for long-distance running, big and tall for offensive linemen, women that have narrow pelvic bones for swimming and sprinting, and so on. My body size (height, weight, and body mass index) correlate very well with the size of professional cyclists who excel at time trialing. Interestingly, according to Chris Carmichael, who is a famous bike trainer, bigger athletes fair better in flat time trials than smaller athletes who excel at climbing. He explains, "the hole they have to punch in the air does not grow proportionally to height and size." [66] Said differently, a smaller athlete may have a lower CdA than a larger athlete, but generally, the difference in CdA does not make up for the extra power that a larger athlete generates. Smaller riders would fare better in hilly and long races in warm temperatures, while bigger riders would fare better in flat, downhill, and shorter races in colder temperatures. Most time trials combine flat, hills, and downhill terrain, which would be suited for medium build riders. Since my body type is in between small and large, it is ideal to adjust to the different extrinsic factors in a time trial race than it would be for a smaller or larger individual. [67] The reason for this result can be better explained during the section on cycling science in Chapter 5. In essence, cycling times are most reflective of how well individuals perform in those sections of the race with the most resistance or on those parts of the race that a rider may struggle with the most.

I also have the ability to suffer and endure pain by riding above a normal threshold heart rate, as well as the privilege of having a fairly high VO$_2$ max (about 55). So, how do people over 50 improve at sports? There are three reasons, according to one source. [68] The first is the motivation to achieve. Second, they have a more efficient cardiovascular and respiratory system to provide more oxygen to the muscles. Third, the central nervous system (CNS) becomes better trained to respond to muscular stress. In other words, the CNS becomes more efficient through repetition or continual practice and training. Better CNS efficiency is accomplished by creating enhanced, new, and alternate pathways for improved ascending and descending signaling between the brain and spinal cord. Thus, the most important factor for becoming an accomplished master cyclist is focused, consistent, and dedicated training. [69]

VO$_2$ max tells us how efficiently our body is utilizing oxygen and is one of the best indicators of cycling success and endurance. Like everything else in athletics, VO$_2$ max is a function of age. Younger individuals have, on average, a higher VO$_2$ max. They generally have a lower body fat composition and increased function of the cardio and respiratory systems. However, it is possible for older athletes to improve their VO$_2$ max even with age limitations working against them. Theoretically, a 55-year-old man with 20% body fat could increase his VO$_2$ max by 10% by reducing his fat composition to 15%. [70] For a point of reference, professional cyclists have a VO$_2$ max of at least 65 to 70, and a VO_2 max above 52 is considered superior for any age. [71]

The lactate threshold may be a better indication of overall cycling performance than VO_2 max. While VO_2 max measures cardiovascular fitness and maximum oxygen uptake, lactate threshold is the percentage of VO_2 max that may be sustained for one hour. In other words, if two individuals have the same VO_2 max, but one person has a 10% better lactate threshold, then they will win a 40K time trial with all other variables being equal. Besides, it is easier to raise a lactate threshold than it is to raise VO_2 max. [72]

So, what makes an endurance athlete elite? Luck! That may not be the answer everyone wants to hear, and it sounds like a cop-out, but let me explain. Individuals must pick the right sport, and that may be mostly dictated by body type and genetic makeup. Kenya and East African nations dominate middle- and long-distance racing. However, genetic studies indicate that the Kenyan runners' Type I muscle fiber ratio, VO_2 Max, and trainability of genes were no different from distance runners from Denmark. The primary difference between Danish and Kenyan runners was their body type. Kenyans were shorter but had longer legs, and more importantly, their legs were thin and had much less mass, making them more economically efficient at running. Furthermore, smaller runners are better at keeping their bodies cool because they have a higher proportion of skin surface area (sweat glands) to weight. While the Kenyan body type is a niche for long-distance running, it is not ideal for sprinting or other endurance sports such as cycling or rowing. [73]

There is no such thing as the perfect endurance athlete. At this time, science has uncovered 23 gene variations that may have some impact on endurance athletic performance. The odds of having the right variant of all 23 genes are astronomical and a mathematical impossibility. The best a person may hope for is to have 16 of the 23 gene variants or about a one in seven billion chance. This means one person in the world may have a 70% favorable endurance genetic makeup. Hence, even if more endurance genes are uncovered, the best endurance athlete can only own about 16 of them. People with good endurance genes may also have other bad gene variants that may lead to injury, cancer, disease, or illness. In other words, a lucky person who obtains ten favorable endurance genes variants must also be lucky enough to not only stay healthy and avoid injury but also avoid any other bad gene variants that could derail any chance of athletic success. [74]

Having good gene variants is one thing but finding the optimal environmental conditions to train the genes is another. Every person responds to diets, training, medicine, and other conditions differently. To get the most out of any good genes is also luck to find that sweet spot to maximize performance. Exercise and a healthy diet are usually always beneficial, but optimizing the benefit is not always an easy task even for individuals with superior endurance genes. Genetic testing is one tool that may help athletes utilize the strengths and weaknesses of their genetic traits to optimize training plans and diets. [75]

The Effects of Aging [76][77][78]

Aging plays an important role in athletic performance and for understanding neurological symptoms. Sometimes, it is difficult to determine if some symptoms are from aging or from a neurological disorder. ***Primary aging*** refers to the gradual natural changes in organism function and structure absent any chronic disease or environmental factors. ***Secondary aging*** consists of unnatural aspect of aging caused by disease and environmental factors. For instance, childhood anxiety alone can induce premature aging on both the autonomic nervous and endocrine systems. Aging is becoming a very important issue in terms of both healthcare and politics (social security) since decreased birth rates and climbing life expectancies will double the number of people living above 60 in the next 10-20 years. [79]

According to one source, "***Aging*** is characterized by a decreased capacity of the neuromuscular system to produce strength and power." Furthermore, "Deterioration in performance can be attributed to both the aging processes per se and lifestyle factors such as a decline in the amount and intensity of physical activity." Studying master's athletes allows science to understand the effects of aging better when compared to normal aging models "influenced by confounding factors such as sedentary lifestyle and chronic diseases." [80] Interestingly, despite significant loss in neuromuscular function, the decrement in master performance for track and field and cycling events is a linear relationship with only a slight decline of about 0.25–0.35 percent in world records each year up to about 75-years-old where the decline in performance is more pronounced. [81] For example, if the world record in 100 meters were 10s (it is actually a little faster), then the world record for a 60-year-old would still be around 11s!

There are also other biological factors that influence age. The important thing to remember about fighting the effects of aging is not just remaining active, but there also must be a balance between eating right, moderate exercise, intense exercise, and rest. Advancing age only accounts for about 25% of all physiological losses in the human body or about a 2.5% decrement in body function every decade (0.25% per year). The remaining 75% of physiological losses (or up to a 7.5% decrement in body function every decade) are the outcome of bad habits such as inactivity and a poor diet. [83] By age 60, the average person's cardio output has reduced by over 20% from its peak. This phenomenon may be partly explained by the degradation of the vagus nerve that controls heart autonomic function. Regular exercise is the best way to overcome reduced cardio output. For instance, having a lower resting heart rate, conditioned by exercise, reduces the wear the tear on the cardio system, which, in turn, reduces the effects of aging.

VO_2 max diminishes from deteriorating respiratory muscles that may decline by as much as 40% by age 65. Moreover, sympathetic nerve activity acting on skeleton muscles doubles by age 65. Individuals over 65 also have compromised immune systems from many physiological changes. For instance, T-cells produce and proliferate fewer cytokines reducing their signaling function. Aging people have a higher percentage of naïve B-cells unable to class-switch from IgM to IgG, reducing infection-fighting effectiveness. Dendritic cells become less effective activating T and B-cells, and there is a decline in natural killer cells as a result of reduced muscle mass and increased obesity in older adults. Natural killer cells homeostasis depends on skeleton muscle function and interleukin 15 (IL-15). Wasting muscles stems from a decrease in interleukin 15 and, thus, a decline in natural killer cells. Exercise can prevent a decline in natural killer cells by mitigating muscle mass loss.

Exercise helps the immune system maintain the length of telomeres. *Telomeres* are located at the end of the chromosomes of immune cells, and over time they shorten from aging and disease. Maintaining the length of telomeres is important to preserve a healthy immune system. Specifically, telomeres are repeating nucleotide DNA codes of TTAGGG. Generally, there are about 10-30 repeating codes that indicate how many times a cell will divide before it is naturally programmed to death by *apoptosis*. When the repeating codes are reduced, then cells cannot divide enough times to maintain cellular homeostasis. Cancer is the exception to the rule that telomeres shorten with disease because cancer telomeres lengthen, and these cells divide uncontrollably. [84] More specifically, humans have a total of 92 telomeres that are located at each end of each chromosome. Shorter telomeres are associated with increased cellular death and aging; whereas, longer telomeres are associated with higher cancer risks. Sometimes chromosomes within cells combine at the telomeres. For example, when chromosome 9 and 22 combine it can lead to leukemia. The SIRT class of genes (SIRT1 through SIRT7) are associated with histone epigenetic modifications to telomeres that may influence their size and consequently aging and cancer outcomes. [85]

An aging body produces more noradrenaline and less adrenaline explaining why there is less blood flow in the skin, digestive tract, and urinary tract and more blood flow in the brain, skeletal muscles, and heart. By age 60, the basal metabolic rate reduces by 10%, and nerve conduction reduces by 10%. A *basal metabolic rate* is the energy required to maintain body tissue, not including the energy needed for movement or to digest food [86] and nerve conduction is the velocity at which signals travel through nerves.

The *motor cortex*, responsible for muscle movement, atrophies with age. Thus, motor cortex neurotransmitters affecting muscle movements are attenuated during the aging process. These neurotransmitters are dopamine, serotonin, acetylcholine (ACh), norepinephrine, gamma-aminobutyric acid (GABA), and glutamate. Aging clearly affects many endocrine hormones (Chapter 7), but a decline in those that affect growth and development can be slowed via exercise. Additionally, by age 65, a 40% decrease in colon nerve neurons results in lost bowel function as dead tissue is replaced with connective tissue collagen and elastin.

Aging adults also have a higher chance for diseases such as cancer and heart disease emanating from obesity, muscle weakness, and a more compromised immune response. Chronic diseases become increasingly more difficult to cope with as people age. The force and power of muscle contractions generally decline more readily than muscle mass as people age, primarily due to changes in muscle fiber type and protein properties. Aging adults have significantly less muscle and bone mass and more body fat than in their prime at age 25. After age 60, the average person losses up to 2.5% of muscle mass per year. The average 80-year-old has lost 50% of his or her muscle mass, which has in many cases been replaced with fat. Muscle mass may be lost to atrophy and also through the loss of Type II muscle fibers. Sprinters and weight trainers are better equipped to maintain Type II muscle fibers in old age. Loss of muscle mass and atrophy is attributed to changes in motor units such as decreased quantity, decreased size, changes in function, changes in membrane excitability thresholds, decreased stiffness in tendons, and a decrease in the neural activation time. The neural activation phenomenon follows a degradation of the neuromuscular junction by reactive oxygen species (ROS) and a decline in axon molecular transport capabilities (the neurological system is discussed in Chapter 8). Exercise can obviously slow aging metabolic changes, resulting in loss of muscle mass.

ROS molecules such as hydrogen peroxide, hydroxyl, or superoxide are important for immune system function and are manufactured in the mitochondria. However, aging energy supplies may also be negatively affected by ROS when mitochondria, DNA, RNA, and ATP production in the muscle cells are damaged. Furthermore, oxidative stress decreases the number of oxygen-carrying red blood cells exacerbating the aging process. By age 60, the average decline in sprint speed, vertical jump, knee extensor force, and plantar flexor force decrease about 25% from their maximum.

Chapter 3: The Science of Skeleton Muscle Function and Disease

Since muscular function and dysfunction are common traits of PNH, most neurological conditions, and aging, I decided to dedicate this physiology topic to its own chapter. This chapter will explore skeleton muscle function and characteristics, including defining muscle medical terms and then explain the function of connective tissue, motor units, muscle fibers, and muscle energy sources. But first, it is imperative to have a basic understanding of cellular function.

Cells [87] [88] [89]

The cell performs seven primary functions that are described throughout this writing: [90] Movement, conductivity, metabolic absorption, secretion and excretion, respiration, reproduction, and communication.

The cell is comprised of various components or *organelles* (see Figure 3.1). *Cytoplasm* is the fluid that surrounds the organelles. The most prominent organelle is the *nucleus*, which is responsible for cell division and genetic information. *Lysosome* organelles are essential because they contain enzymes for digestion to break down fats, sugars, proteins, and carbohydrates. Lysosomes also play a role in the death of cells by digesting dead cellular debris. Lysosomes may also regulate cell proliferation or inactivity. Specifically, enzymes are proteins that make it faster and easier (less energy) to process or modify specific molecules. Most cells contain numerous *mitochondria*, which are responsible for respiratory function and generate energy from adenosine triphosphate (ATP).

The *cellular membrane* is responsible for cellular communication, proliferation, transport, and activation. These tasks are accomplished by receptors, pores or transport channels, ion pumps, cell adhesion, and catalysts such as hormones for chemical reactions. For example, a cellular membrane may accept a protein molecule on a receptor, and that may trigger a cellular activity such as activating a voltage-gated potassium channel (VGKC) or an ion pump. Chemicals that bind to the cellular membrane are the *first messenger*. First messengers that bind to a cellular receptor generally signal a *second messenger* to complete a particular cellular function. Said differently, second messenger is a cellular molecule that responds to extracellular molecules or the first messenger, which can be protein, neurotransmitter, or hormone. The second messenger in the muscle contraction process is a substance called cyclic adenosine monophosphate (cAMP). *Cyclic-AMP* signals muscles via various hormones, such as acetylcholine (ACh), epinephrine, and adrenocorticotropic hormone (ACTH). These hormones control muscle contractions, secretion of cortisol, and the breakdown of glycogen, respectively. Cyclic AMP performs many functions by influencing enzymes, transporting molecules, and even influencing gene generation. Depending on the hormone received at the cell membrane surface, cAMP production can be stimulated or inhibited. Case in point, once a chemical reaction changes cAMP to noncyclic AMP, the second messenger signal is turned off. [91] [92]

Extracellular plasma or serum is responsible for four primary activities which are described and defined throughout this writing: [93] Cell migration, cell polarity, cell proliferation, and tissue regeneration.

Cells combine to form four types of tissues: [94] Epithelial, muscle, neural, and connective. I discuss muscle, neural, and connective tissue in detail throughout this text.

Cells also combine to form organs, and the size of an organ depends on the following three factors: [95] [96] [97]

First, cell division which takes place in one of two ways: *Mitosis* or *cytokinesis*. Second, *homeostasis maintenance* is when the number of new cells equals the number of dying cells if the number of surviving cells is to remain neutral. Homeostasis is the process of maintaining equilibrium or balance. There are two ways a cell may die: Necrosis and apoptosis. *Apoptosis* is a natural process leading to cellular death. In other words, cells can only multiply an established number of times before they reach a natural death. Apoptosis may also happen to combat severe injury, accumulation of proteins, to fight infections, and obstruction of tissue ducts. A surge in apoptosis may result in immune deficiency, liver failure, diabetes, or neural degeneration; whereas, decreased apoptosis may result in autoimmune disease, persistent infections, tumors, and developmental abnormalities. *Necrosis* is different from apoptosis because it is not a natural process, and cells can die from disease, injury, and ion imbalance. For example, cellular swelling is one manifestation resulting in cellular injury and death. Healthy cells may die from necrosis when inflammation infects cells adjacent to damaged cells.

Specifically, necrotic cell death arises from an increase in cellular sodium, elevated calcium, a rise in lactic acid, decreased levels of oxygen, exposure to oxidative free radicals (ROS), and inflammation. One example of necrotic cellular death may arise from a cascade of reactions: The consequences of a lack of oxygen (*hypoxia*) include depletion of ATP production and this leads to failing sodium-potassium (Na-K) ion pumps. This failing, in turn, leads to elevated intercellular levels of sodium that ultimately leads to cellular swelling and eventual death. One reason for necrotic cellular death resulting from hypoxia is when blood vessel constriction decreases blood flow.[98] Finally, cell growth which is controlled by various cytokines, hormones, and growth factors. [99] For example, the cytokine *Interleukin-2 (IL-2)*, which stimulates the proliferation of T-lymphocytes (T-cells) or IL-3 which promotes the proliferation of white and red blood cells. Furthermore, *Nerve growth factor (NGF)*, which promotes nerve cell growth that make up the sympathetic and sensory systems of the central nervous system (CNS).

Figure 3.1: The Cell (From bing.com/images)

HUMAN CELL

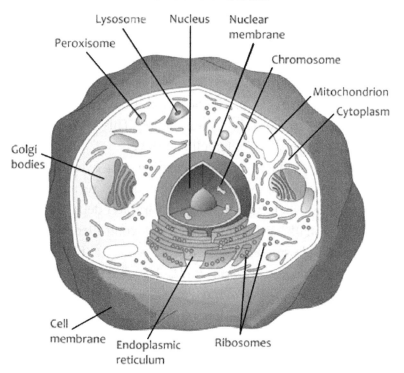

Skeleton Muscle Function

Muscle Disorder Definitions

In the upcoming chapters, there will be discussions on muscle disorders as well as references to medical muscle terminology, defined below: [100]

Myotonia is an impaired relaxation of the skeleton muscle after a contraction. In myotonia disorders, muscle rigidity may occur after a constant or involuntary contraction of muscles.

Myopathy is a muscle disease and encompasses a wide range of dystrophies, myotonias, and other types disorders

Atrophy is a massive loss of strength and increased weakness from wasting muscles.

Hypertrophy is the growth of muscle mass, usually from enlarged muscle fibers or an increase in the number of muscle fibers (hyperplasia).

Pseudohypertrophy is the apparent growth of muscle mass. However, instead of muscle expansion, pseudohypertrophy is actually from increased fat or connective tissue, giving the appearance of more muscle mass.

Hypertonia is enhanced muscle tone, which may happen after spasticity, constant muscle movements, excitability, and rigidity.

Hypotonia is a decline of muscle tone, possibly from atrophy.

Hyporeflexia refers to diminished reflexes and *hyperreflexia* to enhanced reflexes.

Hyperkinesia is an excessive but purposeful movement. Hypokinesia is characterized by the progressive slowing of muscle movements. Sometimes hypokinesia is referred to as Bradykinesia.

The *lower motor neuron system (LMNS)* generally defines those nerve cells of the motor system that originate in the spine and innervate the peripheral skeleton and visceral muscles. LMNS disorders may affect motor units, muscles, the neuromuscular junction, and nerve roots. LMNS dysfunction results in weakness, atrophy, reduced reflexes, pain, and fasciculations.

The *upper motor neuron system (UMNS)* involves those nerve cells of the motor system that innervate the brain or those points above the spinal cord such as the brain stem, pons, or medulla. UMNS dysfunction may or may not be associated with weakness, normal to increased reflexes, and atrophy or hypertrophy without the presence of fasciculations. UMNS disorders generally result in more pronounced but abnormal muscle movements, the slowing of muscle movements, no pain, and paralysis, such as those found in ataxia disorders. [101]

Several neurological disorders affecting LMNS or UMNS can affect station or gait. *Gait* refers to the ability to walk, and station describes the ability to stand from a seated position. Generally speaking, when station and or gait is affected, the source of the problem is more than likely located in the cerebellum and motor cortex of the UMNS. At the same time, a person's gait may be negatively affected by LMNS disorders arising from pain or peripheral neuropathy. Furthermore, people may have affected station and gait from an assortment of non-neurological conditions. [102]

Nerve and muscle disorders are generally classified as distal, proximal, symmetric (generalized), and asymmetric (focal). *Distal* indicates symptoms affect those muscles and nerves located the furthest from the trunk such as the hands, lower arms, lower legs, and feet. *Proximal* suggests symptoms affect those muscles and nerves located nearest the trunk, such as the hips, shoulders, upper arms, and upper legs. *Symmetrical* implies the symptoms affect those muscles and nerves located on both sides of the body in the same corresponding locations. *Asymmetrical* or focal denotes the symptoms that affect those muscles and nerves on one side of the body.

Creatine Kinase (CK) and Muscle Damage [103]

Elevated creatine kinase (CK) is a symptom of multiple neurological disorders. Hence, a basic understanding of CK function is important. There are two types of creatine kinase found in the mitochondria: Ubiquitous CK, which is present in non-muscle tissues, and sarcomeric CK, which is present in muscle tissues. Furthermore, there are three types of sarcomeric CK found in muscle tissues and the brain: Skeleton muscles (MM CK), cardiac muscles (MB CK), and in the brain (BB CK).

CK is required for muscle function, in particular, muscle contractions. Mitochondria CK produces phosphocreatine, and when it chemically reacts with adenosine diphosphate (ADP), they form adenosine triphosphate (ATP) and creatine, which is transported to the muscles for energy. After the ATP energy is used for muscle contractions, the ADP and phosphocreatine molecules are reproduced when the chemical process is reversed.

CK can be elevated when there is muscle damage from either an injury, disease or vigorous exercise. Although CK may be elevated from a muscle disorder, over time, however, CK levels may become deficient. This phenomenon is due to atrophy since there are fewer active muscle cells, motor neurons, and motor units as the muscle disorder progresses.

CK is also a building block to other important amino acids and proteins, including protein kinase. [104] Gene expression or appearance is diminished for PKC epsilon, binding proteins, and ubiquitous CK in patients with neuropathy and spinal cord injuries. This relationship has led to the understanding that PKC and CK may be linked to pain. Linking pain to sarcomeric CK may also make sense since muscles with elevated CK may be more prone to become stiff and sore.

Connective Tissue [105]

Before moving on to muscle function, a brief explanation of connective tissue is warranted. Connective tissue binds cells, tissues, muscles, and organs. Connective tissue is comprised of the following: Matrix is a noncellular component of connective tissue comprised of: *Elastin*, which is a protein molecule with high elasticity (can stretch to 200% of its length); *collagen*, which is a protein molecule with low elasticity; and *ground substance*, which is a nonfibrous component.

Connective tissue contains several types of cells: *Fibroblasts cells* are responsible for producing matrix, elastin, collagen, and ground substance; Macrophages, plasma cells, and white blood cells are responsible for fighting infection and the overall immune response; *Mast cells* are responsible for preventing the clotting of plasma cells; *Fat cells* are responsible for protective layering.

Irregular connective tissue fibers have no distinguishable pattern. There are four types of irregular connective tissue: Loose, adipose, irregular collagenous, and irregular elastic. Regular connective tissue fibers are organized in the same direction. There are two types of regular connective tissue: Regular collagenous and regular elastic.

Loose connective tissue is the most common and binds cells into tissues and tissues into muscles and organs. Loose connective tissue is commonly found in muscles and nerves, and it helps regulate the intercellular exchange of ions and molecules. Loose connective tissue has both elastin and collagen fibers making it both strong and elastic, but it contains primarily ground substance.

Adipose tissue contains a large number of fat cells and exists in the bone marrow. Adipose tissue also appears in skeleton muscles, it is essential for providing the protective padding around organs, and it is a continuous protective layer found under the skin.

Irregular collagenous connective tissue protects skeleton muscles and spinal nerves, and it provides a protective lining around some organs such as the kidney, liver, spleen, cartilage, and bones. *Irregular elastic connective tissue* is very elastic and can be found in the walls of arteries, arterioles, the trachea, and bronchial tubes. *Regular collagenous and regular elastic connective tissue* can be found in tendons and ligaments.

Muscle Function [106 107 108 109 110 111]

Muscles account for 40% of the body mass and are composed of primarily water and proteins. Since PNH and most neurological conditions are tied to muscle function, it is important to understand the very basics of muscle properties, function, and characteristics.[112]

Muscles attached to the bone are skeletal muscles. There are some differences between the operation and properties of the different types of muscles. However, this chapter will focus solely on the skeleton muscles since they are primarily affected by neurological disorders. The following are some key points about skeletal muscle characteristics, properties, organization, and function.

Muscle Fiber Proteins

This section is complicated, so it summarized in Table 3.1. There are two types of muscle fibers: Type I and Type II. There are two types of Type II muscle fibers: IIa and IIx. Type I muscle fibers have a slow contraction rate (slow twitch), allowing them to have more resistance to fatigue than Type II muscle fibers that have fast contraction rates (fast-twitch). Type IIa fibers have moderate contraction rates and fatigability, while Type IIx fibers have fast contraction rates and rapid fatigability. Specifically, muscle fiber types are identified by the ***myosin heavy chain (MyHC)*** protein predominately composes the fiber: MyHC I (Type I), MyHC IIa (Type IIa), and MyHC IIx (Type IIx).

Muscle fiber identification is much more complex than just three types. Each muscle fiber is unique for a few reasons. There are numerous variations of protein molecules that may reside in muscle fibers. For instance, there are numerous different combinations of myosin light chain (MyLC), tropomyosin (Tmy), troponin C (TnC), troponin I (TnI), troponin T (TnT), sarcoplasmic reticulum calcium ion pumps (SERCA), and myosin-binding proteins that may make up specific muscle fibers that alter their properties, including contraction rates. There are at least 31 combinations of MyHC and MyLC muscle fibers alone. Also, it's not uncommon for muscle fibers to be organized as hybrid fibers such as Type I and Type IIa and Type IIa and Type IIx. Type I and Type IIx rarely coexist.

MyLC proteins exist in multiple forms within fast muscle fibers such as MyLC 1f, MyLC 2f, and MyLC 3f as well as for slow muscle fibers such as MyLC 1s, and MyLC 2s. MyLC proteins play an important role in muscle contraction rates. More specifically, the muscle contraction rate depends on the ratio between the different MyLC proteins located in the muscle fiber. Generally speaking, MyLC 1f and 1s are associated with Type I fibers, MyLC 2f and MyLC 2s are associated with Type IIa fibers, and MyLC 3f and MyLC 2s are associated with Type IIx fibers.

Tropomyosin (Tmy) influences actin proteins, and the amount of Tmy in the muscle fiber affects both muscle tension and contraction speeds. There is both a slow muscle fiber option of Tmy, Tm alpha slow, as well as a fast muscle fiber option of Tmy, Tm alpha fast. *Troponin C (TnC)* binds with calcium during muscle contractions. There is both a fast and slow muscle fiber option of TnC: TnC fast and TnC slow. *Troponin I (TnI)* inhibit the actin–myosin-binding process in a muscle contraction. More specifically, TnI inhibits a muscle contraction when concentrations of calcium are low. There is both a fast and slow muscle fiber option of TnI: TnI fast and TnI slow. *Troponin T (TnT)* binds with Tmy and interacts with TnC and TnI. There are several options of TnT proteins for fast-twitch fibers such as TnT 1f, TnT 2f, TnT 3f, and TnT 4f as well as for slow-twitch fibers such as TnT 1s and TnT 2s. Those fibers with the highest proportion of TnT fast and Tmy fast molecules have the fastest contraction rates. TnT 1f is generally expressed with Type I fibers, TnT 2f, and TnT 3f are generally expressed with Type IIa fibers. Moreover, TnT 4f is generally expressed with Type IIx fibers. Furthermore, TnT 1s is generally expressed with Type I fibers, and TnT 2s is generally expressed with both Type II fibers. As a muscle fiber expression evolves from Type IIx to Type I, TnT fast-twitch proteins disappear in the order of 2f, 4f, 1f, and 3f. Muscle fiber expression evolution can take place from either environmental (exercise) or metabolic changes (age). SERCA 1a protein is the fast version for calcium ion pumps, and SERCA 2a protein is the slow version for calcium ion pumps. *SERCA* activity and function are closely related to the function of a protein called phospholamban.

Table 3.1: Typical Protein Variations Found in Muscle Fibers

Protein	Type I Muscle Fibers	Type IIa Muscle Fibers	Type IIx Muscle Fibers
Myosin Heavy Chain (MyHC)	MyHC I	MyHC IIa	MyHC IIx
Myosin Light Chain (MyLC)	MyLC 1f, MyLC 1s	MyLC 2f, MyLC 2s	MyLC 3f, MyLC 2s
Tropomyosin (Tmy)	Tmy alpha slow	Tmy alpha fast	Tmy alpha fast
Troponin I (TnI)	TnI slow	TnI fast	TnI fast
Troponin C (TnC)	TnC slow	TnC fast	TnC fast
Troponin T (TnT)	TnT 1f, TnT 1s	TnT 2f, TnT 3f, TnT 2s	TnT 4f, TnT 2s
SERCA	SERCA 2a	SERCA 1a	SERCA 1a

Muscle Fiber Properties

Muscle fiber properties vary along their length, even if it may only be slightly. For instance, fiber may have both

Type I and Type IIa properties. Muscle fiber properties may be influenced partly by genetics and partly by the environment. For example, the *vastus lateralis quadricep* muscle is composed, on average, of 55% Type I fibers, 30% Type IIa fibers, and 15% Type IIx fibers. However, there is a high standard deviation, with some people having as low as 15% Type I or as high as 80% Type I fibers. This difference is too much to be merely a genetic influence. As we will learn, exercise is an important environmental factor influencing the type of muscle fibers in a specific muscle.

Table 3.2: Comparison Between Type I and Type II Muscle Fibers Properties

Characteristic / Parameter	Type I Muscle Fibers	Type II Muscle Fibers
Contraction Speed	Slow	Fast, 3 Times faster than Type I
Aerobic Capacity	High	Low
Glycogen Capacity	Low	High
Power, Intensity, and Force	Low	High
Energy Needed for Contraction	Low	High
Fiber Diameter Size	Small	Large

Fiber Tension and Strength	Low	High
Atrophy	Decreased Strength and Noticeable Weakness	No Loss of Weakness or Strength
Myoglobin	Low	High
Mitochondria Count	High	Low
Fiber Color	Dark Red	Light Red
Muscle Fibers per Motor Unit	Low	High
Myosin, TnI, RyRs Receptors, Sarcoplasmic Reticulum, Traverse Tubules (T-Tubules), and Calcium Quantity Levels	Low	High
Oxidative Enzymes	100%	36 to 74% of Type I
Glycolytic Enzymes	20 – 40% of Type II	100%

Fatigue	Slow	Fast

Muscle Fiber Biological Makeup

Please refer to Figure 3.2, 3.3, and 3.4 for more clarity about this and upcoming sections. Muscle fibers encompass a membrane, myofibrils and sarcomeres, a sarcotubular system, and sarcoplasm. The ***muscle membrane*** consists of the sarcolemma and the basement membrane. The *sarcolemma* propagates electrical signals for muscle contraction and regulates the transport of molecules. The ***basement membrane's*** primary function is to maintain the muscle shape.

The *sarcoplasm* contains numerous enzymes and proteins responsible for cellular energy production, oxygen storage, and protein synthesis. For example, mitochondria, located in the sarcoplasm, regulate ATP energy conversion. The ***sarcotubular system*** is a membranous structure that communicates with the extracellular space. Specifically, the sarcotubular system is a network of transverse tubules (T-tubules) that wrap around a group of muscle fibers while also penetrating to the center of the fiber. *T-tubules* regulate electrical stimulus for contractions. The sarcotubular system is also composed of the ***sarcoplasmic reticulum***, which is responsible for calcium transport and regulation required for a muscle contraction.

A ***myofibril*** is the functional unit of muscle fibers. Myofibrils are long longitudinal fibers, cylindrical in shape, and multinucleated cells. Thousands of myofibrils are grouped together to make up a particular muscle. Each myofibril comprises repeating units called ***sarcomeres***, comprised of various proteins such as actin, myosin, titin, nebulin, tropomyosin, and troponin (I, T, and C). The myofibrils are surrounded by T-tubules and the sarcoplasmic reticulum.

A sarcomere is responsible for converting chemical energy into a contraction and is made up of several bands and various proteins. The sarcomere has a dark anisotropic band (*A-band*) and a light isotropic band (*I-band*). In the middle of the A-band is the *H-band* and in the middle of the I-band is the Z-disk. The *Z-disk* marks the end of a sarcomere and the start of a new sarcomere. In the middle of the H-band is the M-band. The A-band comprises a thick filament protein called *myosin*, and it is surrounded by the protein *actin* that makes up the I-band. Actin overlaps myosin in about half of the A-band. The A-band center (*M-band*) does not have any actin protein in a resting state. However, as the muscle contracts, the A-band myosin attracts I-band actin and thereby shortening the A-band. M proteins found in the M-band contain creatine kinase (CK).

Figure 3.2: Muscle Fiber Cross Section (From bing.com/images)

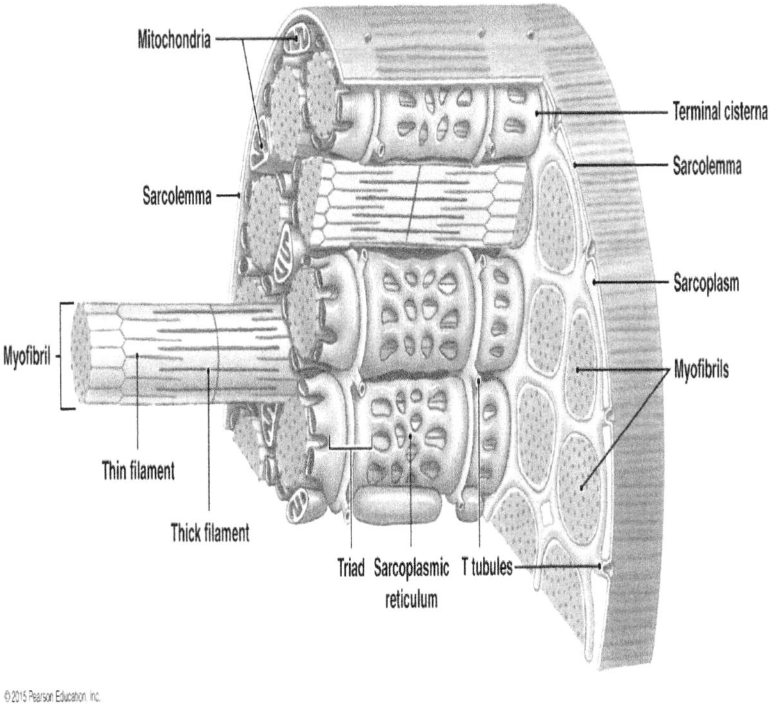

Figure 3.3: Skeletal Muscle and its Proteins (From bing.com/images)

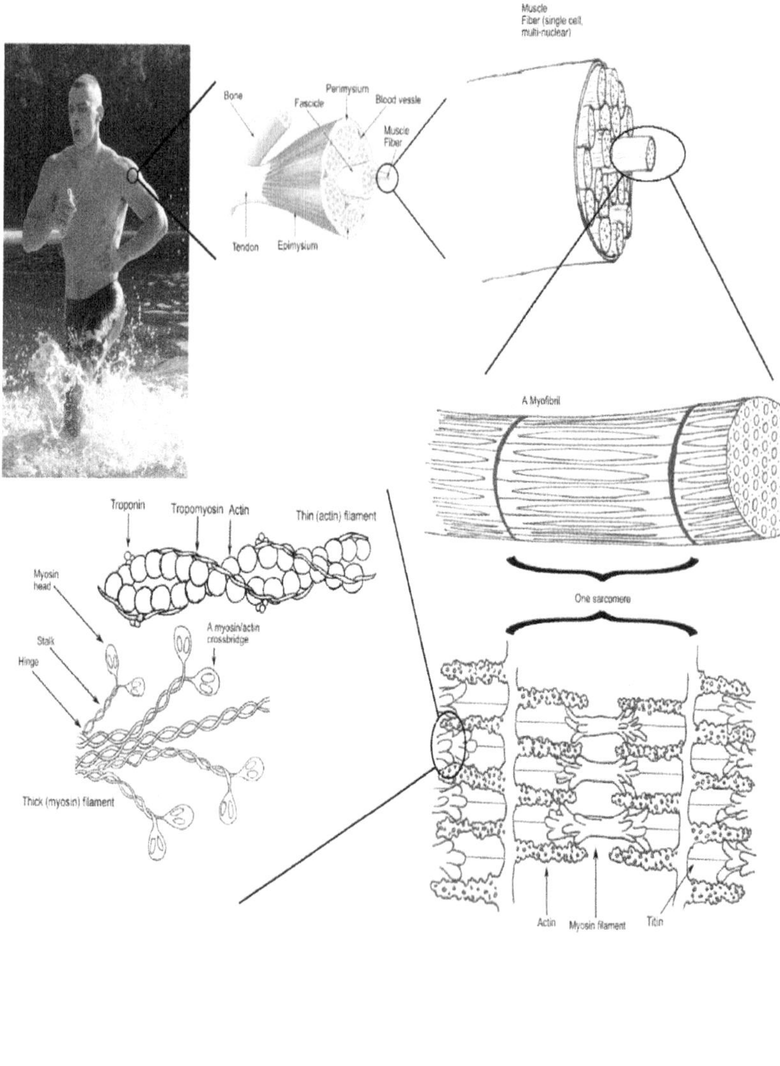

Figure 3.4: (a) Sarcomere Relaxed and (b) Contracted (From bing.com/images)

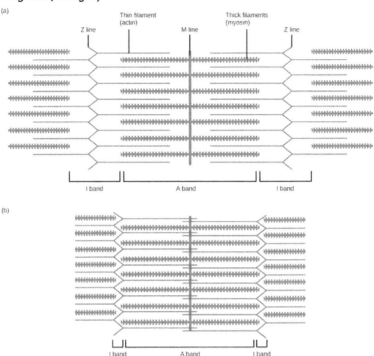

Motor Units

Figure 3.5 and Table 3.3 at the end of this section provide more detail about motor units. A ***motor unit*** encompasses the motoneuron (the nerve cell) and the muscle fibers it innervates. One motor unit or nerve cell may control several hundred muscle fibers. Each muscle has hundreds of motor units that work together to complete a muscle contraction. Motor units within muscles vary in size, and smaller motor units are recruited first in the contraction process. Smaller motor units comprise slow-twitch Type I muscle fibers, called into action before larger motor units comprised of Type II muscle fibers. Hence, rapid and fast contractions requiring a great deal of force and power will ultimately recruit both slow and fast-twitch muscle fibers. [113]

Type I motor units are characterized by slow contraction speeds, weak muscle tension strength, slow hyperpolarization recovery times, low depolarization thresholds, high input resistance, early adaption, more membrane bistability, and fatigue very slowly. Type IIa motor units are characterized by moderate contraction speeds, moderate muscle tension strength, intermediate hyperpolarization recovery times, intermediate depolarization thresholds, intermediate input resistance, intermediate adaptation, intermediate membrane bistability, and fatigue moderately. Type IIx motor units are characterized by fast contraction speeds, strong muscle tension strength, fast hyperpolarization recovery times, high depolarization thresholds, low input resistance, late adaption, low membrane bistability, and fatigue very rapidly. Hybrid motor units and muscle fibers vary between Type I, IIa, and IIx.

Higher *input resistances* and lower *depolarization thresholds* are characteristic of more excitable motoneurons ready for early recruitment. Hence, it may be hypothesized that people with a PNH disorder probably have fasciculations from Type I motor units since they are more excitable than Type II motor units because they require a lower threshold voltage for depolarization. A lower input threshold voltage for depolarization may also explain why Type I motor units are recruited first for a muscle contraction. Furthermore, since the calves have an inflated number of Type I fibers and motor units, the calves are a common location for fasciculations in PNH patients.

When a motoneuron cell repolarizes, it does not automatically go back to its initial resting cell membrane voltage. Instead, it dips below the resting membrane voltage (*hyperpolarization*) before finally recovering to its resting membrane voltage with the help of Na+ - K+ ion pumps. Type I motor units generally take more than two times longer than Type IIa and Type IIx motor units to recover from hyperpolarization.

Adaption is the process of muscle firing frequency, gradually reducing over time when the muscle is under constant and sustained excitation. Eventually, the firing frequency stabilizes in a steady-state condition. Type I motor units adapt and stabilize faster than Type II motor units.

Membrane bistability is characterized as the time between depolarization and repolarization. Motoneurons that remain depolarized longer after a single stimulus have the most membrane stability and define Type I motor units. Type II motor units have less membrane stability and are more apt to shift between depolarized and repolarized states.

Fatigue among motor units is dependent on various biophysical mechanisms and the frequency of use.

Tension strength is unsurprisingly dependent on muscle fiber quantity per motor unit and average fiber diameter. Type II fibers have thicker diameters and more fibers per motor unit than Type I fibers and are, therefore, stronger.

Nerve fibers are classified as Type I, II, III, and IV, with I being the largest and IV being the smallest. Motor units comprise groups of alpha motoneurons classified as Type Ia nerve fibers. Case in point, the calf muscle contains about 1.2 million muscle fibers, and the average motor unit (alpha motoneuron nerve fiber) controls about 2,000 muscle fibers. Said differently, one motor unit controls those fibers innervated by a single alpha motoneuron cell. The number of muscle fibers innervated by a motor unit varies in each muscle. More specifically, the deltoid, biceps, and hand muscle motor units innervate, on average, 239, 209, and 100 muscle fibers, respectively. Those motor units that control fine or precise muscle movements innervate fewer muscle fibers such as the eye muscles. It is not surprising that the motor unit size also correlates with the size of the motoneuron controlling the motor unit. A muscle twitch or fasciculation occurs when a single motor unit is excited while the remaining fibers within the muscle are not stimulated. When fasciculations become repetitive and affect more motor units, they can become more forceful and, therefore, more bothersome.

The recruitment pattern of motor units varies between isometric and dynamic types of contractions, but they all follow the mantra of recruiting slower Type I motor units before Type II motor units. *Isometric contractions* occur when muscles are contracted for long periods of time. In other words, the length of the muscles does not change during a contraction. *Dynamic or isotonic contractions* occur when muscles are constantly contracted and relaxed. In other words, the length of the muscle is constantly changing, such as in running or cycling. An isotonic contraction may be eccentric or concentric. An *eccentric contraction* is one where the muscle lengthens. A *concentric contraction* is one where the muscle shortens.

Gamma motoneurons innervate spindle muscle fibers and are classified as large Type Ib nerve fibers. The primary purpose of spindle muscle fibers is to regulate the muscle reflex system. The muscle reflex system is called the Golgi tendon organ (GTO). The GTO also regulates muscle tone and body position to maintain coordination and balance. Even in a relaxed state, the reflex system maintains muscle tone by providing resistance against gravity or by maintaining posture. Said differently, spindle muscle fibers of the reflex system help prevent injuries to muscles from, for instance, contracting too much or limiting awkward movements. The reflex system is administered by neurotransmitters such as glycine and gamma-aminobutyric acid (GAMA). The "a" and "b" designations in nerve fiber classifications describe the origin of the fibers; for instance, "a" in Type Ia nerve fibers indicates skeleton muscle fibers, and "b" in Type Ib nerve fibers indicates the Golgi tendon organ (GTO), which is responsible for sensing muscle tension. The GTO resides between the muscles and tendons.

Table 3.3: Motor Unit Properties

Parameter	Type I Motor Unit	Type II Motor Unit
Hyperpolarization Recovery	Slow, 2 times longer than Type II	Fast

Input Resistance	High	Low
Membrane Bistability	High	Low
Depolarization Threshold	Low	High
Fatigue	Slow	Fast
Recruitment of Motor Units	Early	Late
Adaption	Early	Late

Figure 3.5 The Motor Unit (bing.com/images)

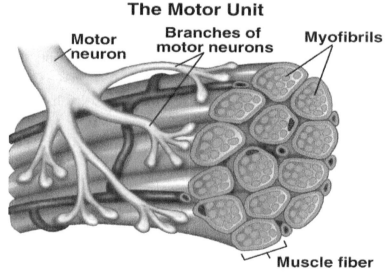

Muscle Contraction [114] [115] [116] [117] [118]

One hypothesis for muscle contraction is called the **sliding filament or cross-bridge theory**. The sliding filament theory is a four-step process that includes excitation, coupling, contraction, and relaxation (See Figures 3.2, 3.3, and 3.4). Excitation of the muscle sarcolemma membrane happens when a signal initiates **ryanodine receptor (RyRs) channels** to open, releasing calcium from the sarcoplasmic reticulum. In the coupling stage, calcium attracts myosin proteins troponin C and tropomyosin to bind with actin proteins. During the contraction stage, thin actin filaments and thick myosin filaments slide past each other, shortening the muscle or contracting it. More specifically, calcium induces an attraction between the I-band and M-band proteins, resulting in a contraction of a sarcomere. When a muscle contraction happens, it essentially eliminates the I-band, or light-colored fibers, while shortening the A-band. When the muscles relax, the sarcoplasmic reticulum reabsorbs calcium as the process is reversed.

Muscles can contract about 25 to 35% of their total length. The amount that a muscle contracts depends on the level of stimulation or the amount of power or force required for a certain contraction. Contraction also depends on how many actin and myosin proteins are available. Too many or too few proteins will decrease the contraction force. Muscles do not act alone; they act in groups. When one agonist flexor muscle contracts, the corresponding antagonist extensor muscle will relax. Muscle function is generally assessed by a CK blood tests and or an electromyogram (EMG). I will explain an EMG in more detail in Chapter 13. Over time, muscles can evolve with epigenetic changes, for instance, by decreasing or increasing muscle length through a process of adding or eliminating sarcomeres or by changing the type of muscle fibers.

Muscle Energy Sources [119] [120] [121] [122] [123]
ATP Energy

Type IIa muscle fibers have about 74% of the oxidative enzymes as Type I muscle fibers, and that number is reduced to 36% for Type IIx muscle fibers. During exercise, muscles require up to 30 times more oxygen to contract than when muscles are at rest. ATP energy is continuously needed for muscle contractions. Mitochondria are responsible for generating energy, adenosine triphosphate (ATP), using a process called oxidative phosphorylation. Oxidative phosphorylation happens when phosphocreatine and ADP react to form ATP and creatine used for aerobic exercise. The reaction is reversed after the ATP energy is consumed for a muscle contraction. Specifically, ATP energy is produced by breaking down the carbohydrates, fatty acids, and proteins. The energy used by mitochondria to produce ATP comes from the movement of charged particles moving through the cellular membranes. [124] It should come as no surprise that mitochondria are more abundant in the muscles, especially in muscles used often.

Glycolysis Energy

Under intense exercise, the body produces more oxygen from denser capillaries, activating more red blood cells, and an accelerated respiratory system. Nevertheless, under vigorous exercise, oxygen supplies can be diminished, and, therefore, glycolysis, or the breakdown of glucose, is needed to produce energy. *Glycolysis* is used for both anaerobic and aerobic exercise, but it is more dominant in anaerobic exercise.

Type IIa and Type IIx muscle fibers have anywhere from three to five times more glycolytic enzyme capacity that Type I muscle fibers. Glycolytic enzymes include creatine kinase, myokinase, lactate dehydrogenase, and adenylate kinase. Furthermore, concentrations of these enzymes are higher in Type IIx than Type IIa fibers. [125] During endurance athletics, Type I motor units are recruited for high-intensity tasks, despite having less anaerobic and power capabilities than Type II motor units. The reason for this behavior is that the recruitment of motor units follows the law that slower Type I motor units are recruited first regardless of the situation.

The body may sustain exercising at aerobic levels for long durations, but once strenuous anaerobic exercise is initiated, that state may only be maintained for short durations. During the anaerobic state, blood flow from the heart to the skeletal muscles is dependent on muscle contraction and rest. When a muscle contracts, it constricts blood flow and henceforth, oxygen from reaching the muscles. As muscles rest, they recover as blood flow and oxygen reach muscles more readily.

During glycolysis, one molecule of glucose is converted into two molecules of pyruvate, up to 36 molecules of ATP, and six molecules of carbon dioxide. Glycolysis becomes the primary energy source when more carbohydrates (anaerobic) than fats (aerobic) manufacture ATP energy. A fat molecule, used to produce oxidative energy, generates 17 times more ATP than a carbohydrate molecule produces from glycolysis. Thus, fat is a much more efficient energy source. Energy comes from both sources at all times, but the dominate energy source depends on the exercise intensity. The process of glycolysis is initiated in the cell, but outside the mitochondria.

During anaerobic exercise, skeletal muscles accumulate hydrogen ions, lactate, and phosphate ions, causing muscle fatigue. Oxygen debt is the amount of oxygen required to convert lactic acid back to glucose and pyruvate to restore those energy supplies. Slow-twitch muscles found in the calves and quads have many mitochondria for ATP production and rarely fatigue. Conversely, fast-twitch muscles found in the quads or arms have fewer mitochondria for ATP energy, making them more susceptible to fatigue. Active muscles that produce more oxygen have more blood flow, and that helps to remove metabolic waste and toxic substances such as lactic acid. Conversely, inactive muscles have less blood flow, leading to a buildup of waste and toxic substances, resulting in fatigue and pain due to stiffness, cartilage degeneration, and atrophy. [126]

Chapter 4: The Effects of Training on Muscle Performance

The science behind training on muscle performance is complex, especially when trying to understand the effects intense exercise has on individuals with neurological conditions. The positive and negative effects are summarized in Table 4.1.

Negative Effects of Exercise [127] [128] [129]

There are numerous negative effects of strenuous exercise on muscle function. Like anxiety and stress, rigorous exercise initiates the sympathetic nervous system. Thus, vigorous exercise can negatively affect the immune system similarly to how stress may impact the immune system and the brain-gut axis. However, vigorous exercise duration is short, while chronic stress duration can be long-lasting. Thus, chronic stress has a more negative impact than exercise has on the body.

Vigorous exercise increases oxidative stress, including more free radicals such as reactive oxygen species (ROS). Under normal conditions, muscles use about 20% of the body's oxygen uptake. The stress of intense exercise can increase that value to 80%. During exercise, muscles redirect blood flow away from other organs such as the gastrointestinal and the urinary systems. For example, the gastrointestinal system blood flow is decreased by up to 80% during intense exercise.

During intense exercise, the transfer of blood to the skin and muscles can initiate other problems such as compromising the gastrointestinal system by, for instance, changing the permeability of the intestinal walls. In other words, intense exercise could, in theory, stimulate a leaky gut, especially if the blood flow is not restored in a timely fashion after exercise is completed. Recovery of lost fluids from intense exercise is also problematic, possibly leaving the body in a vulnerable state longer than what is necessary. Studies indicate that both sports drinks and water do not properly support the restoration of blood flow. Both types of drinks prevent the absorption of water from the intestines to replenish extracellular fluids and bring the body back to a state of homeostasis in a timely fashion. Plain water pulls more sodium from the extracellular fluid into the intestines exacerbating the electrolyte imbalance. In other words, instead of feeling better, athletes may become bloated and have diarrhea, which further diminishes electrolytes. Thus, "exercise-associated hyponatremia (EAH), sometimes called water intoxication, refers to reductions in the body's sodium levels during or up to 24 hours after physical activity."

Positive Effects of Exercise [130]

The positive effects vigorous exercise has on muscles include improved muscle force and power through adaptations to neural, muscle, balance, force transmission, and muscle contraction kinetic physiology. One *physiological adaptation* from exercise is to elevate muscle power and force from a surge in the number of motor units recruited. It is a fact that an untrained person recruits and uses considerably fewer motor units (10–20%) to contract muscles than a trained person. For optimal neuromuscular physiological adaptations to enhance movement characteristics, including force and velocity, the training exercise should mimic the sport of interest for the best gains. Every person has a specific genetic mRNA coding sequence for MyHC proteins, but they can alter the expression of the genetic coding from both power and endurance training. In other words, an athlete may alter muscle characteristics or protein properties to have more Type I, Type IIa, or Type IIx fibers depending on their specific training goals. For example, weight training usually increases the proportion of Type IIa muscle fibers while decreasing Type I and IIx muscle fibers.

Physiological adaptations from the training include both hypertrophy and hyperplasia to increase muscle mass. *Hypertrophy* is generally brought about by increased protein synthesis and insulin growth factor (IGF), which leads to an increase in the cross-sectional area of muscles. Moreover, hypertrophy is the outcome of introducing more Type II muscle fibers while reducing the number of Type I muscle fibers. *Hyperplasia* is muscle growth that occurs from a surge in the number of muscle fibers, but this type of muscle growth is not as significant as hypertrophy. The angle at which muscle fibers are arranged with respect to the direction of the force during exercise may also evolve to be more efficient in trained athletes. In particular, a cyclist and runner have muscle adaptations that result in muscle fibers more efficiently arranged to provide maximal force and power.

Neural adaptations from the brain and spinal cord may improve coordination between muscles, so they are more efficient. In some cases, neural adaptions can teach *synchronous motor unit recruitment*, so they are faster and more powerful. Again, when one muscle contracts, another muscle must stretch. Neural adaptations control a process called coactivation. In *coactivation*, the timing between both the contracting and stretching muscle are optimized to improve joint stiffness, stability, and fatigue resistance, which ultimately improves force and power. Some evidence suggests that cell membranes may be in hyperpolarized state at rest in endurance-trained athletes, but other sources indicate that endurance trained muscles have higher threshold voltages making them contract faster. A higher threshold voltage would indicate that muscles can be more hyperexcitable at rest.

Muscle contraction kinetic adaptations from endurance exercise enhances myosin heavy chain (MyHC) muscle fiber hypertrophy, increases the speed of the myosin ATPase activity to catalyze the myosin and actin attraction process and improves the quantity and quality of the sarcoplasmic reticulum to enhance calcium uptake efficiency for faster contraction rates. *Force transmission adaptations* from exercise include improved tendon and joint stiffness, which make the transfer of muscle force to the bones more efficient. Force transmission changes may also include lateral force transmission improvements where force is transferred to adjacent sarcomeres and muscle fibers. *Lateral force transmission* is improved from elevated desmin proteins that promote transferring force from sarcomeres to the exterior of the muscle. Force transmission improvement arises from exercises that are stressful on the joints, such as running and jumping.

Improving posture and balance is also a critical physiological adaptation from exercise. There are two modes in posture control: (1) feedback mode and (2) anticipation mode. The *feedback mode* aims to restore balance through compensation reactions, and the **anticipation mode** aims to anticipate potential disturbances to posture. Both modes work together in unison to maintain balance during muscle movements. An undisturbed stance is controlled by Type Ia and II sensory nerve fibers as well as Type Ib spindle muscle sensory nerve fibers located in the GTO. For example, patients with neuropathy may have difficulty with an undisturbed stance if they have damage to Type Ia, Ib, or II sensory nerve fibers.

The good news is that balance can be improved through exercise and training to overcome disorder deficits. For instance, one-legged balance exercises on varying surfaces (flat surface, cushion surface, etc.) with the eyes open and or closed can improve balance. Improved balance happens by inhibiting or enhancing certain spinal reflexes while at the same time improving other movement control mechanisms. Furthermore, it has been proven that balance exercises may improve strength and power due, in part, by the stiffening of tendons and joints and possibly from improved neural connections for the joints. Hence, balance exercises are important for both individuals with disorders that impair coordination or for elite athletes to improve their overall performance. [131]

Physiological adaptation of the neuromuscular junction from endurance training is mixed. Fast-twitch Type II muscle fibers have larger neuromuscular junctions, resulting in more ACh receptors, more voltage-gated sodium channels, and a more negative membrane threshold potential making Type II fibers less likely to be hyperexcited. A more negative membrane potential also suggests these cells have a greater safety margin to prevent premature depolarization of cells, ultimately leading to contracture or fasciculation. Conversely, data about the size of the neuromuscular junction in endurance-trained Type I muscles are conflicting. One study suggests that both pre- and post-synaptic efficiency is improved with endurance training, leading to increased ACh neurotransmission and receptors, which also suggests a larger neuromuscular junction. [132]

The effects of endurance training on ***motoneuron activity*** from adaptations of the brain and spinal cord are vast. There is evidence to support that the transport of proteins along motoneurons is markedly increased. The increased rate of proteins toward the neuromuscular junction promotes rapid adaptations. Endurance training may also change the physical properties of motoneurons to make them more resistant to fatigue. There is evidence that the dominant hand is more efficient and more resistant to fatigue because it has lower recruitment thresholds and lower firing rates than the non-dominate hand. Motoneurons more resistant to fatigue may result when Type II neurons evolve to Type I neurons, like how muscle fibers change from Type II to Type I during endurance training. Endurance training can also promote adaptations at the spinal cord level, improving the efficiency of muscles by opening new or alternate pathways to help individuals compensate for efficiency abnormalities, including from deformities, disabilities, or disease. [133] New or alternate pathways may be achieved when, "Functional deficits caused by nerve injuries can be compensated by reinnervation of denervated targets by regenerating injured axons or by collateral branching of undamaged axons, and remodeling of nervous system circuitry related to the lost functions." Furthermore, "Peripheral nerve injuries also induce a cascade of events, at the molecular, cellular, and system levels, initiated by the injury and progressing throughout plastic changes at the spinal cord, brainstem nuclei, thalamus, and brain cortex. Mechanisms involved in these changes include neurochemical changes, functional alterations of excitatory and inhibitory synaptic connections, sprouting of new connections, and reorganization of sensory and motor central maps." [134]

Table 4.1: Positive and Negative Effects from Endurance Training

Positive Effects from Exercise	Negative Effects from Exercise
Usable Motor Units Increase	Increase in Oxidative Free Radicals
Trainable Muscle Fibers and Motoneurons	Dramatic shift in organ blood flow
Power, Force, Force Transmission, Fatigue Resistance, and Balance Increase	Stress
Muscle Mass Increase	
Coactivation and Higher Threshold Voltage Improve Muscle Contraction Speed	
Larger Neuromuscular Junction	
Protein Transport is Improved	
Neural Plasticity Improves	

Muscle Fatigue [135]

Electromyography (EMG) results for endurance exercise demonstrate that muscular force decreases over the length of a training session, but neurological stimulation surges from enhanced motor unit recruitment. However, as exercise duration persists, eventually muscle contractions slow from fatigue, and motoneuron activity is reduced as frequency, and motor unit recruitment is decreased. Moreover, during fatigue, even as new motor units are recruited, the firing frequencies in many motoneurons are still depressed and fail to be rejuvenated.

There are many possible explanations for fatigue at the neuromuscular junction: Axon conduction block, neurotransmitter depletion, and postsynaptic membrane failure. In the ***axon conduction block***, signal excitability is decreased in smaller axon branches derived from the primary axon branches. ***Neurotransmitter depletion*** results from the reduction of both ACh and ACh vesicles to transport the chemical across the synapse. Estimates suggest that a 4-fold reduction of signal intensity is required before neurotransmitter depletion affects the transmission of the signal along the muscle fibers. ***Postsynaptic membrane failure*** results from a desensitization of the membrane brought about by ACh depletion and other unknown reasons.

One potential reason for decreased motor unit frequency and recruitment, during fatigue, derives from decreased spindle muscle support as Type Ib gamma motoneuron sensory nerves become less efficient. Fatigue of the spindle muscle support system can occur for both maximal and submaximal contraction efforts. For example, I fatigue quickly despite having a large percentage of Type I muscle fibers, and this may be explained because my Type Ib nerve fibers in the Achilles tendon are not very efficient because my reflexes are absent. Thus, the transfer of power from my upper legs to the foot is diminished.

Fatigue is also believed to be related to Type III and IV alpha motoneurons. These motoneurons are responsible for a decline in motor unit frequency and recruitment, especially during maximum contraction efforts, but not necessarily during submaximal efforts practiced in endurance sports. Case in point, increased exercise excites Type IV sensory fibers, and that may stimulate the release of substances that promote fatigue such as bradykinin, lactic acid, and serotonin. Type III fibers also respond to the same chemical substances as Type IV fibers; they, too, become more sensitive during fatigue. Case in point, my fatigue may be enhanced by the neurological condition because it is associated with higher lactic acid, CK, and pain that enhance Type III and IV nerve fiber sensitivity.

Fatigue may also result from an inhibited motoneuron response from the motor cortex. The coactivation of agonist and antagonist muscles during exercise may limit the time to fatigue. At low levels of exertion (10% of maximum force), studies indicate that motor units may be rotated during the exercise process. In other words, as motor units are fatigued, they are replaced by fresh motor units as previously fatigued motor units may be recruited later in the exercise session after they had time to be rejuvenated.

The Effects of Endurance Training on the Neuromuscular System [136]

The evolution or physiological adaption of muscle protein characteristics during exercise is complex. Tables 4.2 and 4.3 illustrate both increased and decreased protein and enzyme adaptations for endurance training.

Table 4.2 Increased Protein and Enzyme Adaptations of the Muscular System During Endurance Training [137]

Early Period	Middle Period	Late Period
Activation of MAP Kinases	Type IIa and IIx Motor Units	Type I Motor Units
Heat-Shock Proteins	Oxidative Enzymes	TnT 1s/2s Ratio
Total RNA	Na+ - K+ Ion Pumps	MyLC 2s/2f Ratio
Hexokinase II	SERCA 2a	TnI slow
Capillary Density	TnT 3f/4f Ratio	TnC slow
	MyLC 1f/3f Ratio	
	Fatigue Resistance	
	Twitch Contraction Time	
	Antioxidant Enzymes	

Table 4.3 Decreased Protein and Enzyme Adaptations of the Muscular System During Endurance Training [138]

Early Period	Middle Period	Late Period
T-Tubular Volume	Parvalbumin	Type IIx and IIa Motor

		Units
Sarcoplasmic Reticulum Ca++ Uptake	Glycolytic Enzymes	TnT 1f/4f Ratio
Ca++ Ion Pumps	Calsequestrin	MyLC fast
	SERCA 1a	TnI fast
	TnT 1f/2f Ratio	TnC fast
	RyRs Content	Oxidative Enzymes
	Triadin Content	Muscle Mass
	DHPR Content	Muscle Force
	Phospholamban	

Tables 4.2 and 4.3 illustrate the evolution or adaption of the human body protein and enzyme makeup to accommodate endurance training. Obviously, not all endurance training is the same, so the evolution is unique depending on the genetic makeup of the individual and the impact of their training plan on gene expression. In Tables 4.2 and 4.3, the early period refers to the first three or four weeks of training, the middle period refers to the second three to four weeks of training, and the late period refers to the final three to four weeks of training. The following are observations from Tables 4.2 and 4.3:

First, protein and enzyme adaptations can happen in both innervated and denervated muscles. Second, adaptions to the calcium proteins are among the first to be altered, including a decline in SERCA 1a, triad, parvalbumin, and calsequestrin. Alterations in gene expression of these proteins are triggered by a decreased need for intercellular calcium required for muscle contractions. Third, oxidative enzyme adaptations increase to promote the transition of Type IIx muscle fibers and motor units to Type I muscle fibers and motor units. However, later in the process, a decline in oxidative enzymes is probably due to the fact Type I fibers and motor units are much more energy-efficient and require less ATP and mitochondria. An increase in antioxidative enzymes is also important for minimizing the effects of increased oxidative free radicals produced during training. Finally, endurance training elevates the percentage of Type I muscle fibers while decreasing the percentage of Type IIa and Type IIx muscle fibers. This is accomplished by increasing the ratio of slower muscle fiber proteins to faster muscle fiber proteins. Furthermore, the changes are only reflected in those muscle groups affected by endurance training. For instance, muscle fiber characteristics in the arm muscles are unaffected by cycling endurance training.

The Effects of Strength Training on Neuromuscular Performance [139]

The mechanisms influencing alterations in protein gene expression on the muscular and the neuromuscular system are different for strength training than endurance training. The following are some key points: ***Protein synthesis*** increases dramatically after strength training, and the effect may last several days. Insulin growth factor 1 (IGF 1) plays an important role in increased protein synthesis and muscle mass growth (hypertrophy). One plausible explanation for increased muscle fiber size derives from a growth in the number of cellular nuclei. Strength training requires more cellular nuclei for stimulated protein synthesis. Furthermore, strength trained muscle fibers are denser, resulting from a loss of collagen connective tissue and proteins unrelated to muscle contraction.

While endurance training influences gene expression adaptations to elevate the number of Type I fibers, strength training stimulates the growth of Type IIa fibers at the expense of Type IIx and Type I fibers. Endurance training focuses on metabolic changes, while strength training focuses on adaptations to the contraction of muscles. Muscle stretch and overload are the keys to initiating gene expression changes in strength training. Furthermore, some evidence suggests that eccentric exercises result in better strength-building than concentric exercises.

Muscle damage is more common in strength training and encompasses cellular membrane damage, A-band disorganization, sarcoplasmic reticulum damage, and increased cellular calcium. One reason muscle damage is more prominent in strength training is that muscle damage is more prone to occur in Type II fibers. An inflammatory response to repair muscle damage includes neutrophils, macrophages, interleukins, and tumor necrosis factor (TNF).

Sedentary Effects on Neuromuscular Performance [140]

The following are some key points about the effects of inactivity on neuromuscular performance. Unsurprisingly, inactivity has the opposite impact of what endurance training has on the neuromuscular performance triggering atrophy. *Atrophied* muscles have fewer RNA and mRNA, resulting in a decline in protein synthesis, they have a protein degradation stimulating more Type I than Type IIa muscle fibers, they have a reduction in metabolic enzymes, and atrophied muscles will eventually settle in some atrophied steady state.

Atrophy is more pronounced in those muscle groups that would generally have the most use. This would go a long way to explain my very noticeable atrophy in the hands, feet, and calves, which are high-use muscle groups. Furthermore, atrophy is more common in muscles with Type I fibers; in the extensor muscles than the flexor muscles; and it is more pronounced in muscles that remain in shortened positions and are not stretched. For example, denervated muscles have less pronounced atrophy if the muscles are stretched.

In atrophy, muscle mass, power, force, maximum motor unit firing rate, muscle hyperexcitability, fatigue resistance, and tension force decrease. Conversely, muscle twitch, and recovery from hyperpolarization is faster (more Type II fibers). About two hours of weight support per day is enough to reduce the effects of atrophy by 50%. Moreover, atrophy and a sedentary state can lead to increased visceral or belly fat. Stored belly fat does not behave like fat storage in the organs (used for energy), and it correlates to increased chances of diabetes and cancer as well as heart, kidney, and liver disease. [141]

Chapter 5: Cycling 101

Why Compete in Cycling

I always dreamed of becoming a state champion athlete. Like most kids, I dreamed of being a pro athlete, making the Olympic team and even winning a gold medal. All kids dream, but those dreams very seldom become a reality.

I was a freshman in high school in the late 70's. A student by the name of Keith Alston, from neighboring Neptune High School, won the state wrestling championship. As I read the article about Alston's conquest, I thought he was the luckiest kid on the face of the earth. I turned the page, and there was a short article about how Alston died in a car accident coming home from the event. [142] For years, I debated if Alston would have changed his destiny by giving up that state championship in exchange for the rest of life–about another 60 or 70 years. I do not think Alston would have changed his destiny because he reached the pinnacle of a sport he loved, and he obviously trained extensively to succeed. Similarly, I would not change anything that happened in my life: The abuse, the neurological disorder, and alcoholism because the adversity made me a better person. I believe there are reasons for life's challenges, and we must figure out what they are.

After winning a state masters cycling time trial championship in Colorado and Wyoming, it made me truly understand the sacrifice, love, and pain associated with athletics. It is my belief that most people do not understand the love competitors may have for a specific sport and how much suffering it takes to win a state title. Thus, I am certain that Alston would not have changed his destiny.

Being diagnosed with a neurological disorder changed how I view life. I literally thought I had ALS and would be dead in a few years. After ALS and MS were ruled out, I realized I was lucky to be diagnosed with some form of PNH and neuropathy. PNH and neuropathy are no picnic, but I have been given a second chance at life. Although exercise intolerance is one of my symptoms, I fight through it for one last chance to achieve some of my childhood dreams. The pain of training on top of a neurological disorder is intense. I tell myself I will quit once I reach my full potential, but each day and week, I keep improving. I do not understand it, and more importantly, my doctors do not understand it. Of course, I do not want to sell my coaches short; they are part of the reason for my success. Yes, people can improve at sports even in their 50s and 60s. Each year I accomplish almost all my goals. It is truly amazing and humbling since I have never had so much success at anything.

I remind myself every day that if I were never diagnosed with PNH, I would have never raced a bike and won a state championship. Thus, every day I fight through uncomfortable tightness, stiffness, and cramping on my bike is truly a blessing and wonderful day. Events in our lives transpire for a reason. By remaining positive, I was able to evolve and find success. Do not get me wrong, cycling is not easy. But nothing worth achieving is ever easy.

My message to others suffering from peripheral nerve or neurological disorders is to keep fighting and evolving.

Life is too short to miss out. I am not too sure what the future holds for me, but I will continue to take it one day at a time while remaining humble with my successes, having gratitude for being able to cycle, and learning from my failures.

My wife asks me why I put myself past so much pain and aggravation to compete in cycling. She is my biggest fan and supports my cycling adventures, but at the same time, she sees the toll that a neurological condition and training has on me. My wife is right; I do not have to compete or put myself through so much pain to race or train. After all, I have a perfect excuse not to compete. It defies logic and common sense to enhance my pain levels. One reason to torture oneself is to experience good pain from my training to mask some of the bad pain from the neurological disorder. In other words, if I am going to be in pain regardless of whether I train, then I might as well train, but there are other reasons as well. I try to explain my situation to my wife by asking her the following hypothetical questions:

- What if she knew she would eventually lose the ability to walk? Wouldn't she try to make the most out of what time she still had with the activity?
- If she was given a second chance at life, wouldn't she try to make the most of it and pursue goals and dreams that have eluded her during her lifetime?
- If she was good at cycling, wouldn't she want to know how good she can be, especially understanding it could be taken away at a moment's notice?

- You have one chance at life. Would she regret not making the most of the opportunity?
- Wouldn't it be a crime not to use her legs (although in pain) when some people literally cannot use their legs?

Sometimes, Americans fail to realize how fortunate and lucky we are to have the freedom to do almost anything we desire. Nevertheless, when we lose the freedoms we once enjoyed due to an illness or injury, it is only natural to try to make the most out of the freedoms that remain. Unfortunately, we never realize how much we miss freedom until it is too late.

The bottom line is that when I found cycling, I appreciated it more than any activity I did in the past, especially understanding that it is just a matter of time that the slow progression of my disorder may take it away from me. Therefore, I want to make the most of what time I have cycling. My appreciation and gratitude stem from understanding millions of people are suffering from ailments much more serious than what I have, and millions more will never have the opportunities I have been afforded. My neurological condition was and is a wakeup call, and I am doing my best to make the most out of a bleak situation.

I have been told my entire life that my options at success were limited. I was told that my learning experiences were limited since I had difficulties with reading and writing. I got rejected at most colleges because they said my test scores and grades were substandard. In my professional life, I was told product and test engineers were inconsequential and did not make the same impact as design and system engineers. Similarly, multiple neurologists told me my life would change for the worse, and I would not be able to do many of the activities I enjoy. I am a stubborn overachiever and do not like it when people tell me I cannot do something. It motivates me to prove them wrong. I have been proving people wrong my entire life. My wish is for everyone with peripheral nerve or other neurological disorders to also prove their neurologists or other naysayers wrong! Do not settle for what doctors or anyone may prognosticate for you! I believe most people can overcome a great deal of adversity if they put their minds to it.

Cycling Science

Cycling is a battle against oneself or intrinsic factors and the environment or extrinsic factors. Extrinsic factors include factors such as a smooth, bumpy, hilly, and flat course. Other extrinsic factors include weather conditions such as extreme heat, humidity, cold, rain, snow, allergens, pollution, altitude, and high winds. Intrinsic factors include age, aerodynamics, fitness level, technique, personality, warm-up, overtraining, sleep, diet, and strategy. [143] For example, both heat and pollution have been shown to have an adverse effect on intense training and competition for cyclists. It is still possible to try to offset some of the adverse effects of heat and pollution by using pre-cooling methods, intaking high antioxidant rich foods to fight pollutants, or training in the mornings when ozone levels and heat are less extreme. Precooling is using ice or cold water to cool the core body temperature, but that can have an adverse effect on any warm-up preparation for a race. Keep in mind that pollution may affect anyone who is doing intense training or competition more so than a sedentary person because of their need for more oxygen. Furthermore, heavy mouth breathing instead of breathing through the nose, which has more protection barriers as the air flows to the lungs, can make the impact of allergens and pollution much more detrimental. [144]

There are three competition disciplines for road cycling: road races, criteriums, and time trials. I excel at time trialing. Time trialing is unique from the other cycling disciplines because:

1. Races are short, and no drafting is allowed; it must be an individual effort. Hence, racers start individually, usually in 30-second increments, while the other disciplines are mass start races where everyone starts at the same time.

2. Time trialing is a maximum effort race, and riders are allowed to use a variety of aerodynamic equipment not found in other race disciplines, including specialized time trial bikes, disc wheels, aero bars, skin suits, shoe covers, aero helmets, and any legal item a competitor may feel may shave a few tenths of a second off their times.

3. Time trialing is known as the race of the truth because it determines the best cyclist in terms of power, speed, and fitness. [145] Moreover, those that do best in time trialing are those that can suffer. Avoiding intense suffering may also explain why a competitive cyclist is more likely to race in a road race and a criterium than a time trial. Do not get me wrong; road races and criteriums are difficult and require significant amounts of suffering. However,

strategy plays a more important role in determining the outcome of these races, which suggests that the strongest rider does not always win.

To better explain time trialing, I have attached a few photos of me competing at the end of this chapter (Figures 5.1 and 5.2). Figure 5.1 is a frontal view, and Figure 5.2 is a side view. In viewing Figure 5.2, one may surmise that the aerodynamic nature of a time trial bike and high crosswinds can be a challenge to keep the bike steady and under control. They would be correct in that assessment. Thus, wind direction and speed are other extrinsic factors to consider for races.

Aerodynamics

In time trialing, the most important place to rely on technology is for good aerodynamic equipment: Time trial bike, aero wheels, aero helmet, and a low drag skin suit and shoe covers. Due to cost, I gradually purchased items and found that each item had a significant impact on my performance. Furthermore, aerodynamic technology includes being professionally fitted on a bike every season. For time trials, positioning on the bike is the most important aspect of the aerodynamic equation. Positioning on the bike influences a parameter in the aerodynamic equation called CdA. Cd is the coefficient of drag from the air. Cd is a constant parameter but can change a little based on weather conditions such as air temperature, humidity, and altitude (air is thinner at altitude because it has less oxygen and, therefore, has less drag than air at sea level). The parameter, A, is the most important factor in the CdA formula, which is the frontal area of the cyclist, creating the wind resistance. Parameter A considers everything that can be seen in a frontal picture of the cyclist: Body, clothing, gear, and bike. Reducing A, measured in meters squared - m^2-is the goal of most time trialists. It has been estimated that lowering a CdA by as little as $0.02m^2$ can possibly improve time by up to one minute or more over 25 mi (40 km). CdA is difficult to compute or even estimate because it requires access to a wind tunnel or a specialized computer program that can count picture pixels. Many professional cyclists (time trialists) have a CdA of less than 0.22. I estimate my CdA in an air temperature of 83 degrees, a barometric pressure of 30.01 bars, and a humidity of 38% to be 0.2346. [146]

At the same time, some cyclists incorrectly believe that being in a more aerodynamic position will automatically improve race times, but that's not necessarily true. Riding in a more aero position places greater pressure on the organs of the abdominal region, thereby worsening race results. For that reason, more aerodynamic positions will be very uncomfortable, and it can make it harder to breathe and to maximize pedal stroke power. Therefore, most riders slowly work their way into a more aerodynamic position each season as their body adjusts biomechanically. Hence, lowering the aero bars (bike front end) or raising the seat by a ½ centimeter is a big change, and the body needs time to adjust to such a change. However, for people who have found a comfortable, aerodynamic time trial position, it can be the most efficient position on a bike in terms of both comfort and aerodynamics.

Aerodynamics are not as important in hill climbing as they are for low-grade climbs, flat surfaces, and downhill riding. For instance, at constant power on a flat surface, all resistance comes from the wind or the CdA parameter (plus some friction between the wheels and road). On a 2% incline, the resistance is equal between the wind and gravity. Moreover, on an 8% slope, almost all resistance comes from gravity, and very little resistance is coming from the wind or the CdA parameter. To provide the reader with an idea of what goes into engineering an aerodynamic bike and finding the best time trial position, something as simple as having dimpled rims on the wheels (as opposed to smooth) and riding with the shoulders shrugged can dramatically increase the aerodynamic performance of a rider by as much as 1-2 min over 25 mi (40 km). [147]

Heart rate

Most competitive cyclists rely on technology and data to improve their cycling performance. There is an electronic gadget for everything: Speed, cadence (revolutions per minute - RPMs), heart rate, and power. Furthermore, indoor simulators can help make boring trainer rides more exciting. Of all these gadgets, most people rely on power meter data to improve their performance. However, I only rely on a heart rate monitor for my training since I find too much data causes analysis paralysis. To be sure, monitoring cycling data has gotten completely out of hand, and the book, *Cycling Science,* suggests over three dozen potential parameters to be monitored daily.

Maximum heart rate is also a function of age. Older individuals tend to have lower maximum heart rates than younger people (see the below formula). For a competing athlete, the threshold heart rate is about 85 to 90% of their maximum heart rate. Again, the threshold is the maximum heart rate athletes can maintain for one hour. My body is unique in the sense that I can ride above a typical threshold (85–90%) and race at 92 to 96% of my maximum heart rate. For instance, my maximum heart rate (HR Max) is about 175. This is based on actual data and is not estimated by the commonly used formula:

- **HR Max = 220–Age**, which would estimate that my max heart rate is under 165. [148]

For a 175-maximum heart rate, a typical endurance athlete's threshold heart rate would be between 148 to 157. Instead, I can ride at a threshold heart rate of 161 to 168. Thus, I race more like I have a maximum heart rate of 185. A higher max or threshold heart rate equates to more speed and power output.

Cadence

Most knowledgeable cyclists suggest a high cadence of at least 90 revolutions per minute (rpm) is essential for endurance racing. The reason for this strategy is that the body saves energy by pushing an easier gear at a higher cadence than a harder gear at a lower cadence. [149] My cadence is very slow, 75 to 80 RPMs, but I have a good reason for my strategy. Since my neurological condition prevents my quad muscles from contracting and relaxing normally, having a high resistance on my legs always allows my legs to avoid the repeating action of contracting and relaxing. Hence, a low cadence always keeps my legs engaged in a contracted state while riding. Of course, this is one way to waste considerable energy and become fatigued much faster, but evolution is key to find the best course of action to cope with our limitations.

Some data indicate that higher cadence places more stress on the calve muscles than does a slower cadence. More specifically, the *soleus muscles* of the calves are stressed slightly more with a slow cadence, but the *gastrocnemius muscles* of the calves are stressed considerably less. Thus, the overall effect of a slow cadence is less stress on the calves. This is important because my calves are the site of significant pain and discomfort. Moreover, studies indicate that the pedaling technique in cycling is far less important on performance than swimming, or running technique is in those sports. One reference indicates that more than 80% of all energy generated from the joints in the lower body can be delivered to the pedals for power, but that number is much lower in walking and running activities. Moreover, physical fitness parameters such as VO_2 max, strength, lactate threshold, and aerodynamics (CdA) are better indicators of cycling performance than pedal efficiency. These findings for pedal mechanics are more significant in time trial races since the races are short, and therefore, fatigue from poor pedal mechanics is not as much a factor as in longer road races. [150]

Based on the information in the preceding paragraph, beware of the bike fitter who tries to change your body mechanics to improve pedal efficiency or aerodynamics. For example, a fitter may try to change people who are asymmetrical in their pedaling mechanics. However, there may be a very good reason a rider is more comfortable being somewhat asymmetrical in their pedal mechanics (i.e., injury, a slight difference in leg length, strength, and comfort). I had a bike fitter put a small offset in my shoe cleat to help "balance me out." I saw another bike fitter, and he was furious and threw the offset in the trash. In trying to change my mechanics, the offset was causing unnecessary pain and probably less efficiency instead of better efficiency. [151]

Power

Studies indicate that people relying on heart rate monitors or on power meters for their training plans have negligible differences in overall gains. One proposed reason to use a power meter instead of a heart rate monitor is to avoid the cardiac drift factor. What cardiac drift denotes is that heart rates will naturally increase for each subsequent training interval. The cardiac drift phenomenon is a human defense mechanism to keep the body cool or when the body becomes dehydrated. Therefore, training plans that call for shorter intervals, shorter workouts, and exercising when it is cooler can lessen the effects of cardiac drift. This makes heart rate monitors just as effective as power meters. [152]

Heart rate is said to be unreliable because many intrinsic and extrinsic factors can "distort" readings such as heat, causing cardiac drift discussed above. At the same time, heat and the same intrinsic and extrinsic factors will also affect how much power a person can generate. Chris Carmichael insists that the "validity" of heart rate measurements is less reliable than power output, but I would dispute his findings since the two are methods are highly correlated. [153] For instance, athletes have corresponding training zones for both heart rate and power. My heart rate training zones are as follows: (1) anything under 65% of my maximum heart rate is zone 1; (2) 65 to

80% of my maximum heart rate is zone 2; (3) 80–90% is zone 3, and (4) anything above 90% is zone 4.

Similarly, zones 1 to 4 have corresponding powers. Thus, using a power meter for pacing isn't necessary for anyone riding within their specified heart rate zones. If my workout called for a zone 2 level endurance ride, and as long as my heart rate remains in zone 2, I am likely to be within zone 2 power levels. In other words, a power meter is redundant information that only leads to data analysis paralysis.

Generally, heavier people generate more power than lighter people do because they have bigger muscles. Heavier people need more power than smaller people to go at the same speed, and this is most obvious when climbing a hill. Hence, power per kilogram of body mass is more important than the threshold power that a cyclist may maintain. For example, I have a threshold power to weight ratio of around 4.0 (watts per kilogram). As a point of reference, according to one source, a biker with a 4.0 power to weight ratio would rate as a borderline category two rider. Below pro cyclists, there are five categories for amateur men from elite (1) to novice or beginner (5). [154]

Most knowledgeable cyclists insist a power meter is essential for determining optimum pacing strategies during races and training sessions. However, pacing strategies for time trial races are simple, and a power meter or heart rate monitor is not essential. The most important time trial race strategy is to increase effort riding into the wind or uphill and then decrease power or heart rate on downhills or riding with the wind. When I say to decrease effort, this statement may be misleading because competitors are still going as fast as they can while at the same time trying to recover from a bigger effort after riding the uphill or headwind section of the race. There is never time to rest in a time trial, but only time to scale back a few watts for a short period of time.

Let's consider a basic example to show why bigger efforts are needed on sections of the course with the most resistance. Consider a rider completing a short 10K time trial in 15 min. The course was 5K uphill and then 5K downhill. At the top of the hill, there is a 180-degree turn. Thus, the start and finish of the race are in the same spot. For simplicity, let us assume it takes the rider 10 min (about 18.5 miles per hour - mph) to do the 5K uphill section and another 5 min to do the downhill 5K section (about 37 mph). One may conclude that the average competitor speed was 27.75 mph for the race or the mathematical average of the uphill and downhill speeds ([18.5 + 37] ÷ 2). However, the competitor for this race would average 24.8mph.

Why is there a 3mph discrepancy in these average speeds? Since the racer is taking more time to go uphill, the average speed will be closer to the uphill speed than the downhill speed, and a mathematical average is not a valid calculation. For example, if for the same race the competitor averaged 20 mph to go up the hill and 35.5 mph down the hill, the result would also be a 27.75 mph mathematical average. However, the actual average speed would be nearly 1 mph faster (25.7 mph), and the competitor would complete the race in closer to 14:30 (30 s faster). Therefore, it is imperative to race the slower sections of the course with the most resistance using a bigger effort to minimize the amount of time riding at a slower speed. The above example also shows why a medium body type is better for time trialing since smaller riders have a bigger disadvantage on flats and big riders have a bigger disadvantage on hills. Yes, smaller riders will make up time going uphill, and larger riders will make up time going on the flats, but having smaller compensations favors medium-sized people. My point is that a person can still have an effective pacing strategy by riding to feel and not worrying about the electronics but instead concentrating on the task at hand.

Another use for a power meter is to check for bilateral symmetry if a rider has a power meter on each pedal. Bilateral symmetry investigates if a rider generates the same power in each leg on their respective pedal stroke. However, as we already learned, research suggests that bilateral symmetry or asymmetry has very little effect on time trial performances. The bottom line is the research suggests that symmetrical power may be more important for sprinting than for endurance racing. [155]

The following points define the physiology behind pedal power generation in cycling: The plantarflexion calf muscles (soleus and gastrocnemius) are very important, although they only account for about 5-10% of the pedal power. Not only do the calf muscles help produce pedal power, but they are also essential to keep the ankle joint stiff, so the power generated from the hip and knee extensor muscles is efficiently transferred to the pedal. The primary function of ankle muscles is to transmit the forces from the proximal quad muscles via the Achilles tendon. Uniarticular muscles are controlled by one joint, and they are power producers, while the biarticular muscles are controlled by two joints, and they are the power distributors for any cycling activity. Normally, upper body muscles have very little impact on the power output of a cyclist. Nevertheless, an experienced cyclist riding in an aerodynamic position can better manage their upper body muscles to activate lower body muscles emanating in more cycling power. About 10% of the power generated in the pedals comes from the muscles of the hip flexor or hamstrings. [156] Hence, pulling activity in the upstroke of the pedal motion may improve effectiveness and overall power. Most of the pedal stroke power, about 80% comes from the four quadricep muscles. Hence, most cycling power comes from the knee joint which is transferred to the lower legs and feet. [157] [158]

Cycling studies found that fatigue generally begins with the calf muscles. Furthermore, it should come as no surprise that flexor muscles fatigue faster than extensor muscles. Studies also indicate that the muscles in the upper legs can offset some fatigue in the lower legs. [159] [160]

Fatigue, Recovery, and Overtraining

Fatigue refers to any exercise-induced reduction in maximum force or output power. Fatigue is common for any strenuous muscular activity, as well as from neurological and muscular disorders. Fatigue is complex and can happen anywhere along the descending motor pathways from the brain (central fatigue) to the peripheral nerves (peripheral fatigue). There are many causes of fatigue, including pain, stress, and depression. Fatigue has been associated with Type Ib nerve fibers located in the spindle muscles because fatigue reduces the effectiveness of tendons transferring power from the muscles to the bones. [161]

One form of fatigue is called delayed onset muscle soreness (DOMA). DOMA is said to be influenced by Type III, and IV nerve fibers are small, unmyelinated, or lightly myelinated fibers responsible for pain. Motor cortex involvement in fatigue may also be related to Type III and IV nerve fibers, but the etiology is unknown. [162] After a competition or intense training, there may be normal muscle damage or fatigue, which may be verified by certain blood tests. For instance, within two hours after an intense training event, blood serum indicates a surge interleukin-6 (IL-6) and leukocytes responding to muscle inflammation. Two days after the training event, blood serum may indicate elevated creatine kinase (CK), substance P, and C-reactive protein (CRP) during the healing process. [163] [164]

Since fatigue is age-related, older riders need more rest days to recover than younger cyclists. Most progress in muscle development is made during rest and recovery and not during the actual workout. However, recovery from intense or long cycling rides is a bit easier than from intense or long runs since the load on the muscles is not as extreme. Part of the reason for this is called "ground contact time," creating what is referred to as "reduced impact tolerance" that does not exist in cycling. One study showed that knee extensor strength diminished by 28% after five hours for runners, but only 18% in cyclists after five hours. [165] Monitoring morning heart rates and the heart rate during training is the best tool for understanding when rest and recovery are needed. Case in point, an elevated morning heart rate may indicate the need for a rest day. For conditioned cyclists, the recommended rest times are as follows: [166] (1) 24 hrs after low-intensity training; (2) 24 to 48 hrs after 75 min at lactate threshold training; and (3) 48+ hrs after 30-45 min above lactate threshold training.

My fatigue is difficult to gauge for a few reasons. First, I sleep worse on days off, and my morning heart rate the day after a day off is much higher than if I trained arduously the day before. For that reason, I implement lower stress workouts into my training plan. For example, on my days off from cycling, I use active rest strategies (exercise at a very low heart rate) such as walking a moderate pace for two to three miles and do other flexibility, strength, and balance exercises. Active rest strategies help me sleep better on days off. Second, my neurological symptoms ensure my muscles never feel fully rejuvenated regardless if I rest or exercise. I have learned how to live, train, and race with constant fatigue. If I input rest days into my training plan for every day I felt fatigued, I would never train.

Overreaching or overtraining, sometimes referred to as overtraining syndrome (OTS), may be the result when there is a substantial decline in race results. OTS affects many athletes, especially those with obsessive-compulsive personalities. Studies indicate that recovery from overtraining is difficult. Race results would continue to decline even after a prolonged recovery period. Overreaching is part of overtraining. For instance, overreaching is indulging in one extra interval than what is outlined in the training plan. Therefore, to avoid overreaching and overtraining, having a coach as a neutral observer to control an exercise plan is warranted. [167]

One factor involved in OTS is not only extra stress placed on the muscles during exercise but also any type of psychological stress. Most Americans cope with some sort of psychological stress daily. I cope with quite a bit of stress from a neurological condition and its unknowns. Furthermore, because of my neurological disorder, diagnosing me with OTS would be impossible since OTS is diagnosed by the process of elimination or an exclusion diagnosis. In other words, if there is no other underlying disease, then OTS could be a reason for vastly decreased performances (usually greater than 10%). However, since I have an underlying disease, OTS is an impossible diagnosis and is difficult to diagnose for any athlete. The following are some characteristics and symptoms of OTS: [168] [169]

OTS is linked to depression, chronic fatigue, lack of motivation, poor sleep, and helplessness. Furthermore, OTS has been linked to the hypothalamus, thyroid, and pituitary gland. Chronic overtraining suppresses adrenocorticotropic hormone (ACTH), prolactin, and growth hormone (GH) which is discussed in Chapter 7. Studies indicate that high variability in morning or training heart rates could also be an indicator of OTS, while increased creatine kinase (CK) and lactate are not good indicators of OTS.

Recovery is most important immediately following an intense workout. Immediately following a workout, the body needs fluids and food to start the recovery process. Remember, the body is more susceptible to illness after a challenging workout because the immune system has been depressed. [170] The bottom line, endurance training without much rest or recovery time is counterproductive and may lead to muscle atrophy and power loss. This phenomenon may explain why some individuals with chronic PNH may or may not experience muscle atrophy. For instance, if people have PNH fasciculations that never cease in a muscle, it could lead to atrophy. If, conversely, fasciculations are periodic in a muscle, then muscle hypertrophy may occur.

Power Impairment [171]

As individuals age, they naturally lose muscle strength and have power impairment. However, people may also have power impairment from other unnatural reasons, such as a neurological condition. Decreased strength is characterized as weakness or paresis. Weakness may result in the loss of speed, rapidity, or agility movements, as well as a decreased range of motion. Weakness may also result in fatigue or the loss of endurance.

Doctors measure strength by comparing results with normal muscle strength in the unaffected muscles of patients. Generally, neurologists use a non-linear scale from 0-5 to grade strength with a zero indicating no muscle strength and a five indicating normal strength. However, a person with a rating of 4 has already seen a drastic or severe change in muscle strength. This rating scale is called the medical research council (MRC) scale of muscle strength. One extreme example of power impairment would come from a lower leg amputation. Riding on a prosthetic, the cyclist must learn new cycling mechanics to overcome the loss of sensory tissue, the loss of neural communication between limbs, as well as muscular loss. The cyclist must also learn to become an asymmetric cyclist to transfer energy from one limb to the other. For instance, since the gastrocnemius calf muscle mechanics are changed from a two-joint flexor to one joint flexor muscle, the mechanics of a pedal stroke also changes. In a lower leg amputee, not only is the amount of power required from the gastrocnemius increased over normal leg muscles, but the peak power is shifted by 90 degrees in the pedal stroke. Similarly, the rectus femoris quadricep muscle generates more power in a lower leg amputee than in a normal muscle, and the peak power occurs about 90 degrees earlier in the pedal stroke. In other words, not only are stronger muscles required to generate more power in an amputee, but the mechanics behind a pedal stroke is completely changed due to the asymmetric nature of the injury. [172] The same types of compensation occur for any leg injury, including muscle disorders, but perhaps to a lesser extent depending on the severity of the injury to the muscle. All that said, prosthetic legs are certainly a disadvantage, but in many regards, modern technology has designed them to be more efficient than ever evolving human limbs that have been trying to perfect arms, hands, legs, and feet architecture for 5 million years. [173]

I never considered myself disabled, but it is becoming clear that I am progressively losing function of the hands, feet, and many muscles in the legs. Since I suffer from power impairment, my neurologist filled out paperwork for me to obtain a para-cycling classification. After the paperwork was analyzed and okayed by USA cycling, I was then scheduled for a classification meeting and doctor examination. This meeting was canceled because of Covid-19. I do not feel that my power impairment would be equivalent to a lower-leg amputee, but the two disabilities are difficult to compare. On the one hand, I do not have to make drastic asymmetrical compensations in muscle use and pedal stroke technique. At the same time, although my muscle dysfunction is symmetrical, the loss of power is not necessarily completely balanced, possibly requiring some asymmetrical compensation.

Even worse, since my disorder is evolving, my level of compensation is always in flux. Moreover, my power impairment is not confined to one lower leg, but a combination of the upper and lower portion of both legs. Complicating matters is that my loss of strength in the upper body cannot be ignored either because it does play a minor role in generating cycling power for time trialing. My power impairment is also much different than a lower leg amputee because of the fatigue factor from denervated motor units and absent Achilles reflexes. Hence, much of my power impairment is likely to develop from rapidly fatiguing motor units during the race. Said differently, a lower leg amputee has equivalent power impairment at the start and finish of a race, but my power impairment is worse at the end of the race. One important reason to obtain a para-cycling classification would be to surround myself with inspirational people. I am sure all these athletes have amazing stories that anyone would find motivational.

Pain Endurance [174]

Every study on pain indicates that highly competitive runners and cyclists endure pain better than non-competitive athletes. In many regards, my neurological situation conditions me to tolerate cycling pain. Many times, the pain from my disorder masks the pain I should be experiencing during high-intensity interval training (and sometimes the converse is true). One explanation for that phenomenon is that neurological pain is psychologically perceived worse than exercise pain because exercise pain is short-lived while the neurological pain is permanent.

Pain is relative, and therefore, it is impossible to compare one person's pain experiences to another person. However, it is possible to learn how to cope with pain through experience and wisdom. These experiences may be either intentional or beyond our control. For instance, I experienced several life events that conditioned me not only to endure pain but also to become an expert on living in pain.

I was abused as a child and suffered many broken bones that were never treated. I also suffer from a painful neurological disorder whose symptoms result in exercise intolerance (beyond my control). Additionally, wrestling taught me how to suffer during workouts (intentional). I was a mountaineer, and many expeditions to climb peaks took several days to weeks. Long expeditions are much more challenging and painful than a 30-minute time trial (even with a neurological condition) for several reasons (intentional). First, difficult weather conditions, including extreme cold as well as the effects of high altitude. Second, coping with unsanitary conditions and lack of hygiene. Third, thirst and hunger are common. Mountaineers eat what they can carry, and to limit loads, they pack the bare minimum. Furthermore, many times the only source of water was from snowmelt. Fuel for stoves is heavy, and mountaineers tend to tolerate more thirst than to break their backs carrying excess fuel. Finally, more stressful decision making and planning lead to more anxiety and less sleep.

Hard work generally outperforms natural talent until natural talented individuals resort to hard work. People may be gifted with a low metabolic age and a very high VO_2 max, but that does not indicate they would be good at time trialing. The bottom line, individuals unable to endure pain and suffering while training and competing, will be unable to succeed in the sport of time trialing. The following excerpt about pain and riding at a threshold heart rate explains cycling pain:

Pacing means riding right at the limit or threshold. This pace is difficult to maintain because the cyclist is breathing hard, the heart rate is high, the muscles are burning, and the state of being uncomfortable. To ride right at the limit, the cyclist must really want to do it and must push, suffer, and focus 100 percent on riding at the limit. One well-known cycling coach, Neal Henderson, called this exercise-induced discomfort.

Physiology and Metabolic Testing

At the University of Colorado Medical School, athletes can have their metabolism and physiology studied. [176] In short, it is a stress test on a bike. During the stress test, every five minutes, the resistance increases, and a blood sample is taken. Participants also wear a mask for additional respiration data to measure VO_2 max. The stress test continues until failure or the point at which the subject is no longer able to continue. The data provide athletes and coaches with basic information such as their functional threshold power, carbohydrate storage, and VO_2 max. However, the primary purpose of the test is to determine how efficiently the athlete uses their energy sources. The body has three primary energy sources: Protein, fat, and carbohydrates. In particular, the stress test determines the crossover point at which the body starts to burn more carbohydrates than fats or the point at which aerobic exercise is transitioned to anaerobic exercise. Said differently, the crossover point is the state when a person receives more than 50% of their energy from carbohydrates and receives less than 50% of their energy from fat.

The bad news is that I learned that my crossover point started very early in the stress test or at about 50% of my max heart rate. This means my body is not using its energy sources optimally for endurance racing. The good news is that my training plan was altered to optimize my fat and carbohydrate energy systems that changed my crossover point from 50% to better than 75%. This change was accomplished by incorporating more zone 2 endurance rides in my training plan.

My Training Philosophy

My current training philosophy or plan is not much different from the "experienced competitor" 6-hour weekly plan proposed by Chris Carmichael. Carmichael's plan which includes endurance riding, steady-state riding (up to 92% of lactate threshold), power intervals, and over/under intervals. However, Carmichael's plan is not specifically tailored for a time trial specialist. For that reason, my coach incorporates K-4 intervals into my plan. My training plan is specifically designed around my neuromuscular limitations, age, time trial specialty, and my specific race goals. [177] Before moving forward, it is important to note a couple of important facts. First, there is no such thing as the perfect diet or fitness program since we all have different gene variations that respond to foods and exercise much differently. [178] Second, my seven hours of cycling per week does not sound like much, but cycling training is more of a function of quality and not quantity. [179]

What is training? Training is generally considered a *progressive overload*. What this means is that the body is progressively stressed with more duration, intensity, and frequency for biological adaption. This is also known as the progression principle. Overload training takes a cyclist out of their comfort zone with intense exercise that stresses the sympathetic branch of the autonomic nervous system (discussed in Chapter 10). The overload philosophy is like the statement, "What does not kill you will make you stronger." For example, intense training in adverse weather conditions may be uncomfortable, but it will make any cyclist a better racer. [180]

Conversely, *chronic overload* occurs when the muscles, bones, joints, and cartilage are subject to massive amounts of work. Chronic overload can result in injury, pain, and fatigue. There are lots of factors that may lead to muscle damage and injury, including fitness level, overtraining, skeletal abnormalities, improper technique, poor warm-up, and a bad attitude. [181]

Since it is presumed impossible to maintain peak fitness all year round, training plans, overload, rest, duration, intensity, and frequency change throughout the year. Generally, the offseason encompasses low intensity riding as well as non-specific cycling cross-training. As the competition season nears, the specific cycling training intensity, duration, and frequency pick up. Since most of my races are time trials, the goal of my workouts is to increase my VO_2 max, anaerobic threshold, and lactate threshold levels. Another goal for my workout plan is to biomedically condition my muscle composition via epigenetic changes to be primarily composed of Type I muscle fibers. This transition is accomplished by influencing protein gene adaptations that convert Type II muscle fibers to Type I muscle fibers. [182]

Cycling Specific Training

Endurance Workouts

My endurance workouts are shorter than most endurance athletes to avoid muscle cramping, tightness, stiffness, excessive fatigue, and weakness. My workouts consist of one to three 1.5-hour endurance rides per week, maintaining a heart rate between 65 and 77% of my max heart rate. Traditional training methods for endurance call for three or more hours of riding. Hence, short endurance rides sound like an oxymoron. Riding with a heart rate between 80 and 90% of my lactate threshold for over an hour simulates a longer ride time. Kilojoules of energy consumed during a ride may be a better guideline than the time or distance ridden. Using more energy in shorter rides corresponds to more kilojoules simulating a longer training ride. [183] The overall goal of endurance rides is to increase VO_2 max and educate the body to burn fat instead of carbohydrates for energy production. Burning fat promotes the manufacture of less lactate and a higher lactate threshold. Fat is such an efficient energy source that even a lean person can ride for dozens of hours using fat reserves but only two hours using carbohydrate reserves.

Interval Workouts [184] [185]

Intervals condition the body to cope with pain and suffering. The primary biomedical purpose of intervals is to increase VO_2 max, evolve body function to burn fat instead of carbohydrates, elevate lactate threshold, teach the body to flush lactate out of the muscles faster, and instruct the body to tolerate higher levels of lactate while racing. Short to moderate length intervals, 30 s to 8 min in length, elevate VO_2 max, while longer over-under intervals prime the body to tolerate higher lactate thresholds. An over-under interval encompasses riding at an intense level for at least five minutes, for example, at 90% of a maximum heart rate, and then without any rest, riding at least another three minutes at an even higher heart rate (95% of maximum). For races 30 min or less, like most master level time trials, preparation methods should be dominated by sprint intervals of one minute or less.

The important facet about interval training is that power and heart rate must be higher than heart rate, power, or lactate threshold levels, or improvement will not happen. Over time, interval length may increase while at the same time, rest periods between sets may shorten. Shorter rest periods train the body for faster recovery, while longer intervals promote longer optimal efforts. VO_2 max and peak performance is improved by increasing the density or number of mitochondria responsible for producing energy. Ultimately, training for a 40K time trial encompasses two 20 to 30-minute intervals riding at threshold heart rate and lactate levels.

A training plan that includes one week of four interval workouts followed by three weeks of one interval training day and more endurance rides is optimum to improve performance. This four-week plan should be repeated three times before the start of the season. [186] Of course, it is important to note that, most exercise resources do not recommend strenuous exercise for cycling or weight training for just anyone. Part of the reason training resources recommend moderate over strenuous exercise is that moderate exercise boosts the immune system, while some evidence suggests that strenuous exercise may deplete the immune system's ability to fight free radical toxins. [187] Of course, there are other studies that indicate the more vigorous a person may exercise, the less chance they have of developing cancer.

Even overweight individuals who exercise are less likely to die from disease than sedentary thin people. For example, offensive linemen, weightlifters, and shot putters are very large but in better shape than sedentary thin people. Exercise can overcome obesity. [188] Therefore, I refer to exercise as a great equalizer for the health of a person. Just as education is a great equalizer for opportunity. For instance, a good education can overcome poverty and racial differences just as exercise can overcome other unhealthy habits such as a poor diet and lack of sleep.

K-4 Intervals

Riding uphill in a big gear with a slower cadence or what is sometimes referred to as resistance training not only builds strength and power but increases VO$_2$ max and adapts the body to burn fat instead of carbohydrates. Slow cadence exercises metabolically change (epigenetically) fast-twitch muscles into slow-twitch muscles, and slow-twitch muscles are more apt at burning fat than carbohydrates, while the opposite is true for fast-twitch muscles, which are more apt at burning carbohydrates than fats. [189]

Hypoglycemic Workouts [190] [191]

Hypoglycemic workouts or riding with just water and on an empty stomach. Most individuals can store enough carbohydrates in the muscles and liver for a 1.5-hour workout. Hypoglycemic workouts are NOT recommended by any cycling coaches. Indeed, they are frowned upon to avoid fatigue and bonking during workouts. However, cycling workouts are designed by people with normal muscle function. Even those books that discuss exercise for people with muscle dysfunction are all about avoiding fatigue. Unfortunately, I am going to have pain, fatigue, and generally uncomfortable muscle sensations than my competition regardless of the situation. Hence, I must come up with unique ways to evolve and cope with fatigue, pain, and general uncomfortable feeling that others will not experience. Hypoglycemic training accomplishes this task by building fatigue and pain tolerance. While everyone wants to run away from fatigue, I welcome it with open arms because it is a part of life. The bottom line, hypoglycemic workouts enhance both fatigue and pain resistance.

Hypoglycemic workouts educate the body to perform better when it is fully fueled. They also instruct the body to burn fat instead of carbohydrates and promote maintaining or losing weight. The higher the percentage of body fat a cyclist maintains, the more inefficient their race and training performance become. Part of the reason for this is because fat takes the place of water storage, denying the body oxygen required for energy production. Moreover, the function of insulin is to store fat and glucose, while the function of glucagon is to bring fat and glucose out of storage. [192] Therefore, anyone wanting to lose weight should not be eating small meals during the day or eating before exercise. Food prompts insulin to be pushed into the bloodstream, while hunger prompts glucagon to be pushed into the bloodstream to signal the consumption of stored glucose and fat for energy. The push and pull relationship between insulin and glucagon is how the body maintains a state of homeostasis. [193]

Hypoglycemic workouts teach the body to cope with body mass reduction during exercise. Research proves that trained athletes can tolerate more than a 3% decline in body mass without any loss in performance. However, the same cannot be said of untrained athletes. In other words, athletes can acclimate their bodies to cope with adverse conditions. Another example of training acclimation is when athletes condition their cells to reabsorb larger amounts of sodium, so it is not all lost in sweat.

Race Warm Up Strategies

The literature on the subject of cycling **warm-up strategies**, including stretching as well as warmup intensity and duration, are widely varied. [194] This is not surprising since warm-up methodology seems to be individualized. Most people do the same warmup for every race, but my warmup routines vary dramatically based on the length of the race and the temperature. My coach plans the same warm-up for me regardless of the race, but he has no idea what the weather is going to be like. For instance, longer races and hotter temperatures require shorter warmups, while shorter races and cooler temperatures require longer warmups.

I warm up on the road in warmer temperatures but warm up on a trainer in colder temperatures to better regulate my body temperature. For shorter races or if it is cold, I get my heart rate up to a 95% threshold during a warmup, while I may only get my heart rate up to 70% of threshold during a warmup for longer races or races in warmer temperatures. Why are my warmup strategies so different? Since I fatigue faster than other riders, I need to closely monitor my warmup strategy especially understanding that my symptoms are worse at colder temperatures, but not surprisingly, extreme heat exponentially increases how quickly I fatigue.

Race Pacing Strategies [195]

Without considering intrinsic or extrinsic factors, it has been proven that maintaining a constant pace is the optimal strategy. Pacing studies to combat extrinsic factors have uncovered increasing power during periods of high external resistance, and decreasing power during periods of low external resistance is the best pacing strategy. Many extrinsic factors, such as heat, may force competitors to decrease their pace. Monitoring technology during races is not an effective pacing strategy. It is easier to pace based on feel since there are too many intrinsic and extrinsic factors that competitors cannot control.

Non-Specific Cycling Training

Weight training is an example of a ***non-specific training*** activity because it focuses on objectives outside of cycling-specific training. Non-specific training is higher in the offseason, and it is tapered off as the cycling competition schedule arrives. During the cycling season, it is always best for training activities to be specific, and therefore, more workout time is dedicated to cycling. [196]

One common question about cycling training is if it should encompass weight training. A significant difference exists between endurance exercise on a bike and weight or strength training. The biggest difference is that endurance athletes have smaller muscles because they have biomechanically changed their Type II muscle fibers into Type I muscle fibers, characterized by slower contraction velocities that are more resistant to fatigue. Whereas the opposite is true for strength training. Therefore, the longstanding assumption is that weight training would be counterproductive to cycling. Dozens of recent studies indicate that two sessions a week of strength exercises can improve power output and lactate threshold. [197]

The reason cycling improvement results from strength training is related to an increased proportion of Type IIa muscle fibers at the expense of Type IIx muscle fibers. In other words, strength training also produces more muscle fibers available to resist fatigue. Interestingly, most cycling references do not recommend upper body strength training outside a few core exercises. I disagree with this philosophy because upper body strength is underestimated for time trialing. One fear of strength training for cyclists is that they will add body mass or gain weight. However, most studies indicate that muscle mass may go up, but body mass remains the same indicating muscle is replacing fat. [198]

Stretching, Strength, Balance, and Flexibility Exercises [199] [200]

There is no need to sign up for a gym membership; strength and flexibility may be maintained by doing exercises in the home. The goal of non-specific time trialing **weight training** is first, to hold the most aerodynamic position on a time trial bike and second, to improve pedal power. Accomplishing these goals requires a plan that incorporates both upper and lower body strength, balance, and flexibility exercises.

All strength and stretching exercises promote balance benefits. **Balance** is critical for cycling, but it is even more critical for anyone with a nerve or muscular disorder. Balance exercises also help develop alternate or new neural pathways to compensate for lost neural pathways in individuals with neurological disease.

My workouts focus on completing three or four sets of high repetition (about 15 per set) for each exercise. High repetition workouts avoid adding muscle mass while maintaining strength, endurance, and balance. **Strength exercises** include squats, lunges, deadlifts, curls, bench press, planks, leg lifts, sit-ups, and push-ups. Yoga poses or exercises support, stretching, balance, and flexibility.

Research on the effectiveness of **stretching** and its benefits for cycling performance has been mixed, but to achieve optimal results, leg strength exercises should be completed one leg at a time (when allowed) to mimic a bike pedal stroke. Furthermore, exercises using both legs should also mimic riding a bike; for example, one should complete squats with the legs separated by a distance equivalent to the separation of the pedals on your bike. The bottom line, task-specific strength training (for example, specific to cycling) always results in bigger gains. [201] Moreover, performing leg exercises slowly prevents a change in gene expression from Type I muscle fibers to Type IIa muscle fibers.

Miscellaneous Training Tips

The most important aspect of training is a good *diet*, especially for someone with a neurological condition. I say that because diet recommendations for training consider healthy individuals, not those inflicted with a neurological condition. Diets for competitive endurance racing have changed over the years. Moreover, diets are individualized, depending on personal preferences, allergies, and food sensitivities. The best-recommended diet for optimum time trialing performance is as follows. [202]

Many resources recommend diets high in carbohydrates (60%) with only 20% protein and 20% fats. Carbohydrate diets usually include foods rich with gluten. I disagree with the carbohydrate-rich philosophy for several reasons. First, I have food sensitivities to gluten, and second, since I have a muscular disorder, any reduction in proteins could exacerbate pain, fatigue, and atrophy. Thus, my diet comprises at most 40% carbohydrates with at least 35 to 40% protein. Tons of carbohydrates may be required for cyclists who ride hundreds of miles each week, not for time-trial specialists. Likewise, many training and racing diets include caffeine. I stay away from caffeine because it exacerbates symptoms leading to more fatigue and a higher probability of cramping. [203]

Meats, fish, vegetables, and fruits are recommended to obtain a balance of natural fats, carbohydrates, and proteins. Although fats and carbohydrates are the most important energy sources, protein consumption should not be avoided because protein can be used as an energy reserve when carbohydrates are depleted. Furthermore, protein is essential for muscle building and recovery. A lack of protein may lead to the body cannibalizing itself for nutrients, especially for people who train intensely. Of course, any cannibalization of tissue would be self-defeating for any training plan.

People should avoid carbohydrates coming from sugars, processed foods, and most starches because it can have dire performance consequences. I consume additional protein, fat, and carbohydrates from cheese, yogurt, rice, peanut butter, quinoa, potatoes, and oatmeal when healthier options are not enough. A person who exercises intensely faces no threat of heart disease from a diet high in fat or high in carbohydrates, but if the diet is not balanced, it may affect performance. Finally, I stay away from sports drinks, juices, and all flavored drinks. I am unique in that I only drink water and acquire all my nutrients from food.

Ride by yourself. Time trialing is an individual event, unlike road races and criteriums where team efforts and group riding are part of the strategy. Individual training conditions riders to push through bad days without team help or drafting off of other riders. In other words, individual workouts teach a person to cope with more pain and adversity. So, I advise spending plenty of time riding on those boring trainers for a few reasons. Trainers allow people to follow workout plans precisely because the environment is not influenced by many extrinsic factors such as weather. Also, trainers simulate longer workouts because there is no coasting since a trainer can simulate uphill riding, but not downhill riding when athletes coast.

Workout when you feel at your best. [204] For me, this means morning workouts over afternoon or evening workouts. I have more pain later in the day than at the beginning of the day, regardless if I have worked out or not.

It is okay to be selfish about your needs if you are coping with pain and other neurological symptoms. For example, after repeatably voicing my dietary concerns and temperature regulation needs to family members, they never seem to take them seriously. I went with the flow for decades before I decided to use hotels at family gatherings to provide my body the tender loving care it requires. It is not selfish or narcissistic if it is truly a necessity for your health.

Rest, and sleep. I require more rest and sleep than most. I rest throughout the day after workouts. Remember, my muscles never relax, even when I am resting. Thus, when I stress my muscles from training and racing, the need for rest and sleep is exacerbated. To maximize sleep and rest, I require a cold dark room with white noise and a humidifier. [205] I rarely rest well the day before competitions because my symptoms are worse (probably due to increased adrenalin). I generally make up for that lost sleep after the competition is over. There are two types of rest: Active and passive. **Active rest** is doing light exercise such as easy zone 1 riding, light stretching, and walking (there is no intensity). Active rest promotes the healing of sore or damaged muscles. **Passive rest** is avoiding all types of exercise. [206]

Avoid boredom when resting. Boredom happens when one loses focus. Those individuals suffering from boredom are both mentally and physically less healthy. There is some truth to the statement of being "bored to death." Hence, stimulating the brain when resting is important and can be accomplished by trying to learn something new. For example, during rest is an excellent time to meditate and focus on activities we enjoy, such as reading. Studies also indicate that meditation is a good tool to combat both stress and chronic pain. [207]

Having both *schedules and training flexibility* is important: "Many paths lead to the same goals." [208] I go into the cycling season wanting to race as much as possible, but generally, I must reduce competitions and training goals because of my neurological limitations. I am usually overly optimistic about what I can achieve. It is better to be too ambitious than too cautious. [209] In other words, setting goals are essential even if we fail to meet them in their entirety. This is not a failure; it is smart.

The Effects of Neurological Fatigue on my Race Results

Before moving on, the following example proves conclusively that I fatigue faster than other riders in longer races. On average, I lose anywhere from 3-10s for every 5 km a race is longer than 20 km. The bottom line is that whether I am faster or slower than the competition, I ALWAYS lose time in longer races. For example, comparing my results against two top rival riders over two years yields:

- My coach defeated me, on average, in 3 20K races by 1:06.

- My coach defeated me, on average, in 2 30K races by 2:00.
- My coach defeated me, on average, in 2 40K races by 2:50.
- A rival defeated me, on average, in four 20K races by 0:07.5.
- The same rival defeated me, on average, in 2 30K races by 0:22.5.
- The same rival defeated me, on average, in 2 40K races by 0:37.0.
- Other rivals, whom I defeated in these races, do better over the long haul than I do but not as good as the two listed above.
- In other words, my coach gains about an additional 10s every 5K covered over 20K, and my rival gains about an additional 5s every 5K covered over 20K.

This *fatigue factor* yields an equivalent loss of anywhere from three to eight watts of threshold power—a significant amount of fatigue only explained by my neurological condition and both denervation of motor units in various leg muscles and absent Achilles reflexes. Once motor units are lost to denervation, other motor units may be recruited to complete the task. However, fewer motor units mean that muscles will fatigue easier and generate less power over time. This analysis does not consider how much power was lost at the start of the race due to denervation, but only what fatigue and loss of power that happens after 20K. In other words, there is no point of reference or mechanism for me to measure how much power I am losing at the start of any race or even after the first 5K or 10K. Ultimately, the above analysis translates to about an overall loss of about 2% in total power. As a rule of thumb, 1% of power loss corresponds to about a loss of about one second for every mile covered.

Chronic denervation may also help explain why significant improvements in my cardio fitness over the past several years resulted in minimal gains in my race results. This past year I elevated my VO_2 max by 4%, there was a significant increase in Type I muscle fiber density, and there was a dramatic surge in the efficiency of my energy system by significantly elevating the heart rate at which I begin to burn more carbohydrates than fat. That said, I saw, at best, a 1% increase in performance.

One plausible explanation for decreased muscle power, brought about by the denervation of motor units, might be cardiac drift. *Cardiac drift* occurs when the heart rate naturally increases, although exertion and power remain constant. Causes of cardiac drift include heat, dehydration, physiological stress, and muscle fatigue. During a race, the heart has to work harder to cool the body, send more oxygen to fatiguing muscles, and compensate for lower blood pressures caused by dehydration or fatigue. [210] Although all competitors should be experiencing cardiac drift, my drift may be exacerbated by muscle fatigue.

The bottom line, my theory about the effects of my neural plasticity is that the new brain-muscle and brain-tendon communication pathways are not as efficient as the standard methods of communication between the brain and muscles and brain and tendons. In the short term, the new pathways are just as effective as the standard communication methods, but the new pathways fatigue much faster. For example, the neural plasticity mechanisms to compensate for no peroneal nerve excitation and absent Achilles tendon reflexes are short lived and begin to decline very fast due to, for instance, increased excitation from Type III and IV nerve fibers that initiate pain and pain mediating substances. This explains my loss of time in longer time trials and my inability to walk for more than 45 minutes or stand for longer than an hour without a lot of discomfort. Furthermore, neural plasticity of genes is easier to modify their expression earlier in human development and not so much as adults. Hence, much of my neural plasticity for overcoming diseased nerves may have been developed from endurance training as a youth. [211]

Conclusion

My assumption that a poor athletic genetic composition and neurological disease are significantly hindering my cycling performance was wrong. Part of the reason for this finding is five-fold. First, training can alter muscle and nerve fiber composition overcoming physical limitations from poor genetic makeup. Second, training can lessen the effects of neurological disease by creating new and alternate pathways for the brain and muscles (and tendons) to communicate. Third, cycling is a great equalizer in sports. What I mean by this is that cycling is a sport that enables older individuals and those with disabilities to remain fast and competitive. The reason for this phenomenon is that cycling does not require the technique for success as other sports such as running and swimming. Fourth, my endurance genome is above average. Finally, those genes that influence personality traits such as drive, determination, resiliency, grit, and mental toughness can also compensate for many physical limitations in cycling.

Most of the above-mentioned changes may have occurred because of epigenetics such as changing muscle fiber protein composition, opening new pathways and expanding neural plasticity so the brain and muscles can communicate when the primary pathways are diseased, or enhancing neural plasticity to promote personality changes to have more mental toughness and drive. It is quite possible I acquired the genes to be mentally tough or to have a high percentage of Type I muscle fibers, but epigenetics can further improve on those characteristics or traits. Sure, neurological disease is a disadvantage, but it is not as big as I anticipated. The biggest physical limitation and disadvantage appears to be the fatigue factor from the denervation of motor units, dysfunctional Type Ib nerve fibers affecting the tendons (particularly the Achilles tendon), and enhanced Type III and IV nerve fiber sensitivity from pain.

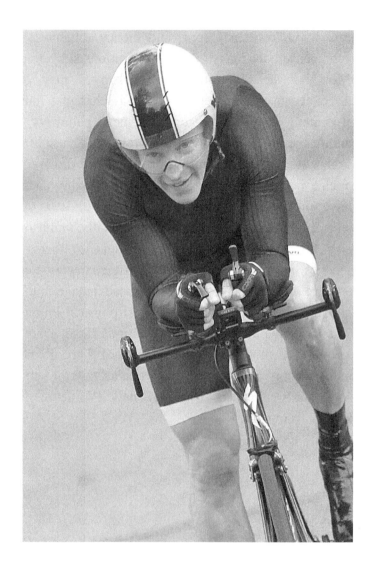

Figure 5.1: Time Trial Race in 2017 at Cherry Creek State Park, Colorado
(Photo Courtesy of Ryan Muncy:
http://www.ryanmuncyphotography.com/)

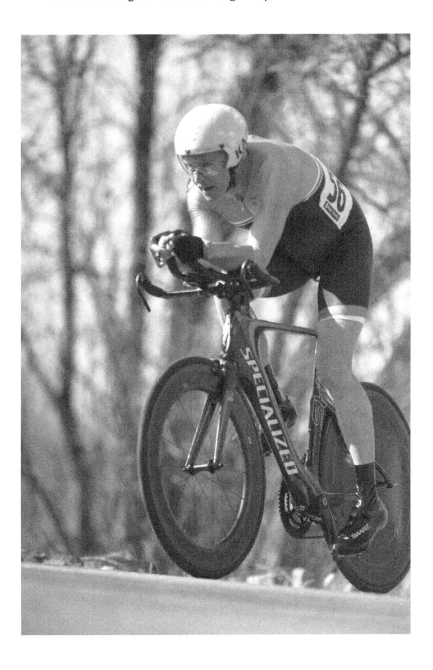

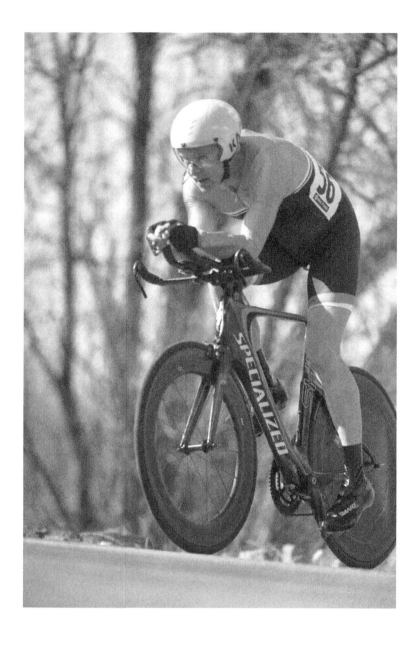

Figure 5.2: Time Trial Race in 2019 at Cherry Creek State Park in Colorado
(Photo Courtesy of Ryan Muncy: http://www.ryanmuncyphotography.com/)

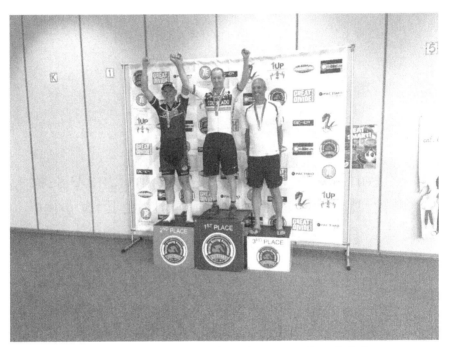

Figure 5.3: Winning the 2017 Colorado State Time Trial Championship (Masters Over 50, Category 4)
(Photo Courtesy of Kevin Craig)

Part II: The Science of Autoimmune Disease, the Immune System, and the Endocrine System

Chapter 6: Autoimmune Disease and the Immune System

The impact of the immune and endocrines system on aging and cycling performance has already been discussed. It is also important to learn the science behind these complex systems because they also play a huge role in my autoimmune neurological disorder (MMN or CIDP). See Figures 6.1 and 6.2 for more clarity about the information covered in this chapter on the immune system.

Blood

Blood is critical to human life because it carries oxygen from the lungs to other tissues and carbon dioxide from tissues to the lungs, it delivers nutrients from the gut to tissues, it transports waste products to their disposal sites, it carries hormones from their glands to target tissues, and it protects the body from invading organisms. [212]

The composition and manufacture of blood is as follows: (1) blood comprises water (92%) and solutes such as sodium, potassium, chloride, calcium, and hydrogen ions (8%); (2) blood is 55% plasma, 5% white blood cells, and 40% red blood cells; (3) the cellular composition of blood contains *erythrocytes* (red blood cells), *leukocytes* (white blood cells), and *platelets* (thrombocytes); (4) blood also contains several types of proteins, such as *immunoglobulins*, that protect the body from disease; (5) immunoglobulins make up about one-eighth of the proteins found in the blood; (6) other proteins found in the blood are essential for clotting, iron transport, or the transport of vitamins; and (7) the manufacture of red blood cells, the five different types of white blood cells, and platelets begin in the bone marrow. [213]

Red Blood Cells [214] [215] [216]

Red blood cells are responsible for tissue oxidation. Iron (Fe) is a crucial component of hemoglobin and myoglobin found in red blood cells. *Hemoglobin* transports oxygen via red blood cells to oxygen-deprived muscles, for instance, during strenuous exercise. One hemoglobulin molecule can transport four oxygen molecules to those muscles requiring additional oxygen. The hormone *erythropoietin (EPO)* is released during stages of hypoxia or when there is insufficient oxygen for muscle function. EPO supports the transport of additional oxygen molecules through the proliferation of red blood cells. Furthermore, ion concentrations within red blood cells are maintained primarily by Na-K pumps. Red blood cells have no nucleus or mitochondria. Thus, energy for the Na-K pumps cannot come from the mitochondria producing ATP energy, but instead from a process called glycolysis.

One disorder brought about by an overabundance of red blood cells is called *polycythemia*. This disorder is common among people who live at high altitudes. People living at altitude have more red blood cells to enhance oxygen circulation because there is less oxygen in the air they breathe. Blood viscosity is thicker when it has excessive red blood cells, and therefore, the blood is prone to clotting. One solution for polycythemia is for patients to have blood removed periodically. The most common red blood cell disorders are *anemias*, which result from a deficient red blood cell count or a decline in the quality of the hemoglobin.

Anemias may be the result of different reasons such as low iron reabsorption in the intestines or a shortened life span of red blood cells. Anemias are primarily hereditary, such as sickle cell anemia. However, they can also take place for immunological reasons, alcohol abuse, some medications such as anti-seizure drugs (carbamazepine), or toxins. The primary function of platelet cells is for blood coagulation or clotting. *Thrombocytopenia* is the outcome of a deficient platelet count leading to hemophilia. *Thrombocythemia* is the consequence of excessive platelet production, which escalates the risk of intravascular clotting.

White Blood Cells [217 218 219 220 221]

White blood cells are referred to as *leukocytes* and are responsible for fighting infections and to remove injured or dead cells. The different types of white blood cells are monocytes, neutrophils, eosinophils, basophils, and three types of lymphocytes (B, T, and natural killer cells). Leukocytes are also classified as *granulocytes* (neutrophils, basophils, or eosinophils) or *agranulocytes* (monocytes or lymphocytes). When *basophils* mature, they exit from bloodstream circulation and take up residence in tissue. Once in tissues, basophils become known as *mast cells*. When monocytes mature, they too exit from bloodstream circulation and reside in tissues. Once in tissues, *monocytes* become known as *macrophages*. Macrophages in the liver are known as *Kupffer cells* and in the skin or the lining of the intestinal system, known as *dendritic cells*. Malfunction of the leukocytes usually results in *leukemia*. For instance, *Epstein–Barr* virus (mononucleosis) can cause leukemia associated with B-cells.

Macrophages are responsible for removing old and damaged cells. Take one example, once suppressor T-cells and interleukin-10 turn off the immune system, this effectively programs all the immune cells, activated to fight a pathogen, to death by apoptosis. It is the job of macrophages to ingest all the dead cellular debris. *Neutrophils* are the most abundant leukocyte and account for 60–70 percent of the white blood cell count. Neutrophils primarily defend against bacterial infection. *Eosinophils* account for about 3% of the white blood cell count and have the same function as neutrophils but can also respond to allergens. *Basophils* account for about 1% of the white blood cell count and perform the same function as neutrophils but also secrete histamine during allergic reactions.

Granulocytes and agranulocytes are both known as phagocytic cells. Phagocytic cells are cells that engulf pathogens and debris in a process called *phagocytosis*. Phagocytic cells also attract lysosome enzymes that contain hydrogen peroxide to destroy pathogens and debris. The *mononuclear phagocyte system* (MPS) comprises macrophages that reside in the organs of the lymphoid system, such as the spleen, thymus, and lymph nodes. The MPS system is the first line of defense against bacteria and is responsible for removing old cells, dead cells, and pathogen-antibody complexes.

Lymphocytes reside, proliferate, and mature in both the thymus (T-cells) and bone marrow (B-cells). All other red and white cells reside, proliferate, and mature in the bone marrow. Only about 20% of all T-cells mature and proliferate. The other 80% are programmed to death (apoptosis) for failing to pass the *tolerance protocol* during their maturation process. There are two classes of T-cells: Effector cells (cytotoxic T-cells) and regulator cells (helper T-cells). *Effector cells*, such as *killer T cells*, attack pathogens directly. Regulator *helper T-cells* turn on the immune system; whereas, suppressor helper T-cells turn off the immune response. *Natural killer cells* are unique because they can identify pathogens in the absence of immunoglobulins and complement proteins that identify pathogens for other immune system cells. Hence, natural killer cells have an accelerated response to a pathogen and can, therefore, identify and destroy pathogens quickly.

Figure 6.1: Immune Cells of the Innate and Adaptive Response (From bing.com/images)

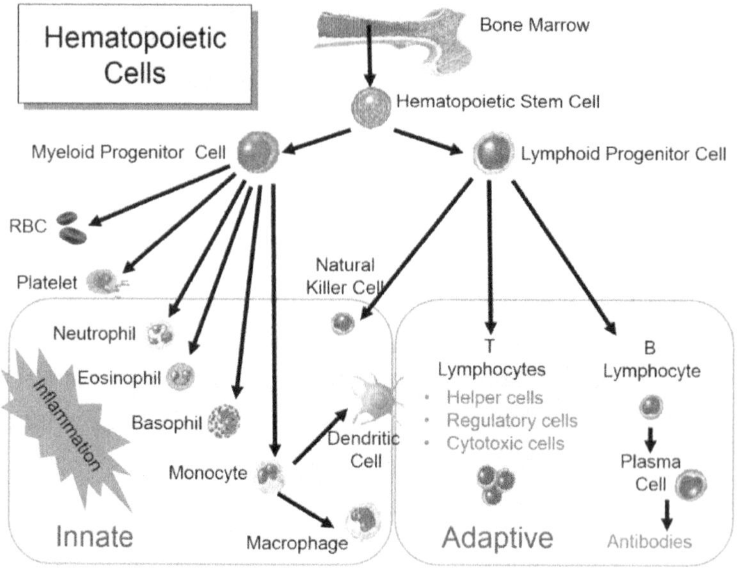

Immunoglobulins

As mentioned earlier, antibodies are classified as immunoglobulins, and there are five types: IgA, IgE, IgG, IgM, and IgD. Immunoglobulins vary widely, and there are 100 billion gene combinations. B-cells are not quite as diverse and have about 1 million genetic combinations. Each of the immunoglobulins may be defined as follows: 222

IgA

IgA primarily protects body secretions from infections and can, therefore, be found in saliva, tears, and mucous. IgA accounts for about 15% of the immunoglobulins, and they can also fight inflammation in the respiratory and gastrointestinal tract.

IgE

IgE activates white blood cells, such as mast or eosinophil cells, to fight infections and inflammation from allergies. IgE plays a pivotal role in allergic reactions to food, drugs, pollen, dust, mold. Thus, it is not surprising one mediator of an IgE is response is histamine. IgE accounts for less than 1% of the immunoglobulins, but IgE counts can surge in the face of an allergic pathogen.

IgD

The function of IgD is not yet fully understood, but it is believed that one possible role of *IgD* is to boost the maturation of B-cells. IgD is the least common and accounts for less than 1% of the immunoglobulins.

IgM and IgG

IgM and IgG are combined because they work together in the adaptive immune response as well as activate white blood cells such as macrophages and neutrophils to eliminate invading bacteria and viruses. As explained earlier (during the adaptive immune response), when faced with a new pathogen, IgM is the primary response. IgG is the secondary response with a magnitude equal to that of IgM. However, if the pathogen were to reappear, both IgM and IgG respond simultaneously, with the IgG response being at least two times greater than the IgM response.

IgM accounts for about 5% of immunoglobulins, and IgG accounts for about 80% of the immunoglobulins. They are the only immunoglobulins that activate and interact with complement. IgM is the most efficient immunoglobulin because it has ten pathogen binding sites. IgM acts as a pathogen receptor on the surface of B-cells, which is unsurprising since B-cells specifically produce IgM since it is the primary response to a pathogen. IgM can convert to IgG, IgA, IgD, or IgE through a process called *class-switching*. For instance, if the helper T-cell recognizes the pathogen on IgM; then, it releases various cytokines, including IL-21 and IL-4, to convert IgM to the appropriate immunoglobulin. Class-switching activates with the help of follicular helper T-cells (Tfh).

A simple immunoglobulin structure is Y shaped (IgG– three binding sites). Thus, IgG can bind with the pathogen, complement, and host cell. IgG can be found in the blood as well as lymph, cerebral, and cerebrospinal fluid.

Autoimmune Disorders

The immune system is extraordinarily complex, meaning it's not difficult for something to go awry. When the immune system attacks healthy tissue or benign pathogens, this is known as an autoimmune response. Autoimmune diseases originate because: [223]

1. People have a genetic predisposition to certain diseases, and this may be from MHC gene malfunctions that fail to identify them as host cells.
2. People are exposed to certain environmental conditions that can trigger a genetic predisposition to a particular disease.
3. People may not have a genetic predisposition to a specific disease. However, an environmental trigger

(toxin, alcohol, smoking, food, or prescription drug) may result in a genetic mutation or gene expression change that may result in autoimmune disease.

4. Autoimmune diseases are more likely to occur with advancing age when the immune system is compromised.

5. Many autoimmune disorders may be related to the decline in *regulatory T-cells*, which prevent the suppression of immune responses. In other words, the immune response continues long after the pathogen is gone.

Hypersensitivity reactions are inappropriate immune responses to benign pathogens. There are five types of hypersensitive reactions: [224] [225] [226] [227]

1. *Type I* is an IgE mediated immune attack. Type I reactions arise from allergens such as pollen, dust, dander, foods, or drugs that result in the excessive production of IgE and the release of mediators from basophils and mast cells. Type I reactions generally occur within minutes from the time the body is in contact with the allergen. Overproduction of inflammatory mediators can lead to serious ailments such as hay fever, eczema, and asthma. Individuals who have normal reactions to allergens will not initiate the unnecessary release of mediators from mast cells and basophils to induce a hypersensitive reaction. The overproduction of mediators from a Type I response encompasses histamine,

bradykinin, serotonin, platelet-activating factor, and cytokines such as IL-4, IL-13, and IL-5.

Histamine can stimulate nerve endings, causing itching as well as other symptoms such as abdominal cramping brought about by the contraction of smooth muscles of the gut, a rise in cardiac contractions, and a drop-in blood pressure. An increase in the production of another hormone, *bradykinin*, produces pain in the peripheral nerves. Close to 95% of all *serotonin* production is in the gut. Elevated serotonin production leads to diarrhea, fluctuations in blood pressure, migraines, and bronchial spasms. Some drugs that inhibit IgE and mediators like cytokines (in particular, interleukins) can alleviate symptoms of Type I hypersensitive allergic reactions.

2. *Type II* is an IgG-mediated immune response against pathogens circulating in bodily fluids. Type II reactions generally involve IgG and the complement system, causing the unnecessary lysis of healthy cells leading to many disorders depending upon the pathogen and the function of the cells, tissues, and organs being attacked. Disorders associated with Type II reactions include anemia, rheumatic fever, clotting dysfunction, and neutropenia (low neutrophil count). Type II reactions generally occur in hours to days from the contact with the pathogen.

3. *Type III* is an IgG-mediated immune attack against pathogens embedded in tissues and organs. Type III reactions are similar to Type II reactions. Many pathogens have multiple binding sites and, therefore, can attract many IgG molecules to bind with them. Most times, the immune system can remove these large cell clusters, but other times they may deposit in healthy tissue and organs that may lead to an unnecessary immune response. Inflammation of healthy tissue is induced when a phagocytosis process is initiated by complement and neutrophils to fight these embedded cell clusters. Disorders associated with Type III reactions include lupus, rheumatoid arthritis, myalgia, Raynaud's phenomenon, and IgA nephropathy. Type III reactions generally occur in weeks from the time of contact with a pathogen. Type III hypersensitivity reactions differ from Type II in that the antibody in Type II reactions bind to a soluble pathogen in the blood or fluids that do not deposit in body tissues.

4. *Type IV* is a T-cell-mediated immune attack. Type IV reactions can involve both cytotoxic and helper T-cells without the help of an antibody. Many skin reactions to poison oak or ivy are manufactured by an unnecessary cytotoxic or killer T-cell reaction. In these cases, reactions occur upon contact with the pathogen. Rheumatoid arthritis, diabetes, and

multiple sclerosis are examples of other, more severe kinds of Type IV hypersensitive autoimmune disorders. Type IV reactions generally occur in days from the contact with the pathogen.

5. *Type V* is when antibodies block hormone transmitters or receptor sites. Myasthenia gravis and Graves' disease are examples of autoimmune Type V hypersensitive disorders. For example, in myasthenia gravis (MG), antibodies block acetylcholine receptors, thereby restricting cellular access to acetylcholine (ACh). This concept will be discussed in more detail later in Chapter 13.

The immune system prevents hypersensitive reactions through a process called *tolerance*. For example, T-cells and B-cells learn the difference between pathogens that are a threat to host cells from those pathogens that are not a serious threat to human health. T-cells and B-cells learn tolerance during their development in the thymus and bone marrow, respectively. Those cells that fail tolerance tests (80%) are programmed to death via apoptosis before they mature and are released into circulation. Many factors will determine whether a pathogen will initiate tolerance or hypersensitive reactions, and they include: [228] (1) The maturity of the immune system. For example, younger and older person's immune systems may be immature when compared to other demographics; (2) The structure of the pathogen. Small molecules are more likely to be tolerated than a large one; (3) The pathogens' ability to react with other pathogens; (4) The presence of inflammatory signals; and (5) The duration of the pathogen exposure.

Immune Deficiency

The immune system may malfunction from both an overactive or an inadequate response. An overactive response is called hypersensitive Type I, II, III, IV, and V reactions (described earlier), which may happen, for instance, in response to an allergen. An inadequate immune system response is called immunodeficiency. [228]

Immune deficiencies can result from the inability to produce T-cells, B-cells, or immunoglobulins. Immune deficiencies, prolonged or temporary, may be produced by stress, autoimmune disease, physical trauma, antiseizure medications, and alcohol abuse. Antibody deficiencies are called *hypogammaglobulinemia*. Secondary complications from hypogammaglobulinemia are arthritis, gastrointestinal symptoms such as diarrhea, autoimmune disease, and cancer. IgG has four subclasses, and deficiency of one of the subclasses accounts for 17% of all cases of immune deficiency. The genetic mutation for IgG subclass deficiency and selective IgA deficiency is unknown. Low concentrations of IgG class 2 mitigate the ability of the immune system to fight bacterial infections. Since the complement system activates IgG, deficiencies in complement have been confused with deficiencies in IgG. Genetic mutations found in disorders such Wescott-Aldrich syndrome or ataxia-telangiectasia have diminished IgM along with absent IgA. Finally, a defect in a DNA-editing enzyme, activation-induced cytidine deaminase

(AICD), results in IgM overproduction and diminished concentrations of IgG and IgA. [229]

Take, for example, the several immune deficiency disorders that may result in *staphylococcus aureus* reoccurring infections: [230] [231]

IgA deficiency is the most common antibody deficiency for staph. However, over time, the immune system evolves and has fewer infections because IgM and IgG compensate for the low concentrations of IgA. Patients with IgA deficiency should not be treated with Immunoglobulin treatment (IVIg) because they may form antibodies that will attack IgA.

Hyper-IgM syndrome patients have high concentrations of IgM, low concentrations of IgG, and normal B-cell concentrations. Hyper-IgM syndrome is believed to result from a genetic mutation to encode protein CD40 or helper follicular T-cells. The consequences of the genetic mutation prevent IgM from being class-switched to IgG.

Hyper-IgM syndrome is similar to *common variable immunodeficiency (CVID)*, which is also characterized by low concentrations of IgG with normal B-cell concentrations. Thus, CVID is also associated with the dysfunction of helper follicular T-cells or encoding the protein CD40.

C3a and C5a *complement system deficiencies* can lead to serious Type III hypersensitive reactions causing many immune disorders, including staph.

Several phagocytic diseases weaken the body's ability to kill and ingest pathogens, such as *staphylococcus aureus*. For instance, *chronic granulomatous disorder (CGD)* is a dysfunction of the phagocytes and leads to a deficiency of hydrogen peroxide, which is needed to kill pathogens.

NOD receptor deficiency is a dysfunction of the pattern recognition receptor system. If we recall, NOD receptors identify pathogens from the host cells. When the immune system is unable to identify foreign cells, such as staph, then the body is susceptible to infections.

A *deficiency in the gene encoding* for IL-6, IL-21, and IL-23 may lead to encoding errors of Th-17 helper T-cells, in turn, inhibit B-cell antibody class-switching. The consequence of Th-17 gene encoding errors results in the elevated production of IgE and impaired function of neutrophils.

A low level of neutrophils characterizes an acquired immune deficiency disorder called *neutropenia*.

A Typical Immune Response [232] [233]

A summary of a typical nonspecific and specific immune response follows. A nonspecific immune response fights a wide variety of pathogens, viruses, and bacteria; whereas a specific immune response fights a particular pathogen learned from its adaptive memory.

A Nonspecific Response

A typical nonspecific immune response contains many pathways that depend on the type of pathogen. Several nonspecific immune responses include the following:

1. Lysosome enzymes initiate the lysis of pathogens by attacking their cellular membranes.

2. Interferons activate macrophages, neutrophils, natural killer cells, killer T-cells, B-cells, and helper T-cells.
3. Natural killer cells target and kill viruses and tumor-infected cells, as well as activate macrophages to fight bacteria pathogens.
4. Macrophages and neutrophils perform phagocytosis. They can also signal reactive oxygen species (ROS), such as hydrogen peroxide, to kill pathogens.
5. The complement system is activated, and C5 through C9 initiates the process of lysis by attacking the cellular membrane of foreign cells.
6. Killer T-cells directly attack foreign cells with the help of lysosomes and complement.
7. Complement, C3b binds with foreign cells, so they are identifiable for phagocytosis, which is generally carried out by macrophages.
8. Immunoglobulins bind with foreign cells, so they are identifiable to phagocytosis, which is generally accomplished by macrophages.
9. The complement system may also activate mast cells, basophils, or eosinophils to fight allergens.
10. Inflammation is a typical nonspecific immune response for a wound. Once a wound is cleared of any debris and foreign pathogens, the wound healing process is initiated by macrophages. Molecules called CTLA-4 and PD-1 signal the immune system to shut off (programmed to death by apoptosis), which allows for the activation of the wound healing system. Wound healing primarily

encompasses fibroblast cells stimulated by growth factors to regrow connective tissue (scaring). If the immune system fails to shut off, the consequences can be an autoimmune disease. Conversely, if the immune system shuts off in the face of a mutation, cancer cells may proliferate. For that reason, many new drugs for cancer treatment focus on reactivating the immune system, whereas, treatments for autoimmune disorders focus on suppressing the immune system. Excessive wound healing escalates the chance of a gene mutation that may lead to cancer. For instance, cigarette smoking resulting in repetitive immune system activation and wound healing of lung tissue may eventually lead to cancer.

A Specific Response

A typical specific immune system response to a particular pathogen is as follows:

1. Dendritic cells identify pathogens when they lack major histocompatibility complex (MHC) proteins on the cellular surface.

2. Lack of MHC Type I proteins signal killer T-cells. When there is a second and third signal confirmation, killer T-cells proliferate to fight the pathogen.

3. Lack of MHC Type II proteins signal helper T-cells. When there is a second signal confirmation, the T-cells proliferate and help activate macrophages.

4. Lack of MHC Type II proteins can also signal helper T-cells to activate B-cells. When the second

signal is confirmed, the proliferated helper T-cells activate B-cells that generate immunoglobulins. Depending on the nature of the foreign cell, IgM may be class-switched into the appropriate immunoglobulin. Immunoglobulins bind with pathogens, so they are identifiable for phagocytosis. Phagocytosis is generally carried out by macrophage cells.

5. Vaccines or monoclonal antibodies are exact copies of an antibody that can be injected into humans to fight a particular virus by stimulating a specific immune response.

Figure 6.2: The Immune System and Response to a Pathogen (From Bing.com/images)

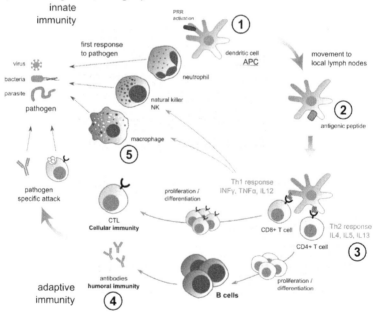

Autoimmune Disorders

This section addresses the causes or etiology of autoimmune disorders. If the immune system is too weak it may allow once friendly bacteria to go rogue. If the immune system is too strong it can attack, destroy, and destabilize gut bacteria. Either scenario is bad and may initiate the beginning of an autoimmune disease. Autoimmune disorders generally manifest when three things go awry or dysfunction: First, the balance between killer T-cells and B-cells is dysfunctional. Second, the balance between helper T-cells and regulator T-cells is disrupted. Third, the immune system is unable to differentiate pathogens from healthy host cells. There are five causes of autoimmune disease: [234] [235] [236]

1. A *genetic predisposition* happens, for instance, when certain types of MHC Type II proteins are not correctly identified on host cells. Furthermore, external factors like diet, heavy metals, toxins, infections, and stress can trigger numerous autoimmune disorders, especially in individuals with a genetic predisposition. When the immune system attacks foreign pathogens such as gluten, mercury, organophosphates, bacteria, and viruses, the body will, at times, also attack healthy tissue. Many products that humans use every day have been associated with autoimmune disorders such as antacids, ibuprofen, alcohol, gluten, processed foods, and antibiotics. In most cases, the products disrupt the flora of the intestinal system setting off a vicious cycle of events (this will be explained later). It is possible to avoid an autoimmune disorder, such

as eating a healthy diet and limiting exposure to certain toxins.

2. *Gender linkage* is common for many autoimmune disorders. For example, women are ten times more likely to acquire lupus. People with a deficient immune system are more likely to get an autoimmune disease. However, many people with healthy immune systems may also get an autoimmune disorder. Case in point, women have stronger immune systems than men, which may partly explain why they are more susceptible to autoimmune disease. About 75% of all autoimmune cases involve women. A stronger immune system sometimes means the immune system can become overactive and fail to shut off. [237]

3. The immune system makes a mistake and attacks healthy tissue. When a pathogen alters the identification mechanism of healthy cells, the corresponding immune response against those healthy cells is called the *bystander effect*. Antibodies against certain infections may "cross-react" with healthy tissue.

4. A *faulty immune system* response would explain Type I through Type V hypersensitivity reactions. Furthermore, tissue already damaged via an autoimmune disease may be more susceptible to further infections.

5. *Immunological intolerance* happens when T-cells can no longer tolerate healthy tissue. The science behind what causes intolerance is not yet completely understood.

There has been a growing epidemic of autoimmune diseases around the globe over the past several decades. From 1997 to 2010, the number of autoimmune cases has more than doubled to 50 million people in the United States. Food allergies rose between 1997 and 2011 by 50% and skin allergies by nearly 70%. The incidence of asthma, diabetes, and immune-related disorders has increased three to five-fold over the last 50 years in developed nations. Furthermore, autoimmune disease costs the United States healthcare system about 100 billion dollars annually. There are not any cures for most autoimmune disorders, and the best that doctors and patients can hope for is to be able to treat the symptoms effectively. [238] [239] [240] [241]

There are many etiology theories for increased cases of autoimmune diseases: [242] [243] [244] First, many doctors place the blame of the autoimmune epidemic on *environmental factors* such as toxins, vaccines, viruses, and heavy metals. Some evidence supports this claim since there has been a higher incidence of cases in areas that have contaminated soils and air. Furthermore, many toxins found in developed nations do not appear in underdeveloped nations with low incidences of autoimmune disease.

Another theory for autoimmune disorders suggests that children lack exposure to both good and bad bacteria. Lack of good bacteria populations is the result of two theories called the *hygiene and "old friends" hypothesis* for autoimmune disease. In the era of hand sanitizers and antibacterial cleaners, young immune systems do not fully develop. The technology era and given that children further exacerbate this anti-bacteria epidemic because they no longer go out and play, limits their exposure to good bacteria found in nature. Lack of good bacteria leads to low IgA production in the gut, and it is associated with constipation, diarrhea, gas, bloating, abdominal cramping, and reflux. The cleanliness theory has gained credence since underdeveloped countries have exceptionally low rates of autoimmune disease.

The same evidence emerged within Amish communities in the United States. The Amish lifestyle closely represents those found in underdeveloped countries (limited exposure to technology, vaccines, cleaning products, and processed foods). The result is that the Amish have fewer incidents of allergies and autoimmune disease because they tend to have more neutrophils and fewer eosinophils. The bottom line is that the Amish have both a bolstered innate and adaptive immune system. There is also evidence that allergies and autoimmune disorders may correlate to wealthier families who have more money to buy cleansers and have maids clean their homes. In the late 1980s, there was an 80% surge, not only in home and personal hygiene products, but technology also introduced newer and stronger antibacterial products, further diminishing human exposure to bacteria. The present-day Covid-19 era of germaphobia may also lead to more future cases of autoimmune disease.

Other etiology theories suggest that autoimmune disease may arise from the inability of macrophages to **remove dead immune cells**, or there may be a mutation with the FAS gene, which leads to the development of abnormal T-cells.

Elevated stress and prescription drug use are one explanation for the rise in autoimmune disorders. For example, chronic antibiotic use has led to a suppressed immune system resulting in more allergies and autoimmune disorders. In 2015, the FDA estimated that 80% of all antibiotics were used on food-producing animals in the United States. In other words, humans may be unknowingly ingesting more antibiotics than they realize.

The one thing that is known for sure, there is a strong relationship between autoimmune disorders and peripheral nerve disorders such as PNH and neuropathy. [245] [246]

Lymphatic System

Muscle activity is essential for a healthy body. Case in point, when muscles are active, they help the flow of lymph fluids to rid the body of unwanted toxins. [247] Fluid, minerals, vitamins, and other molecules and cells flow between the bloodstream and body tissue via capillaries. The mineral-rich fluid flowing through the lymphatic system is known as lymph fluid. Lymph fluid or plasma is similar to blood plasma, except it does not contain any proteins. The *lymphatic system* is the link between the blood circulation system and the immune system. The lymphatic system has three functions: [248] [249] (1) draining excess fluids that, if not released from tissues, it can induce swelling; (2) playing a role in the absorption of fats from the small intestines; and (3) supporting the immune system by transferring bacteria, viruses, and other harmful foreign objects to the lymph nodes where T and B-cells and other white cells reside

The *lymph nodes* appear in the neck, under the collarbone, in the armpit, groin area, or strategic locations near regions where pathogens may enter the body, such as in the nose, eyes, mouth, or genital region. They are primarily composed of B-cells, memory B-cells, and T-cells. *B-cells* secrete antibodies to identify foreign bacteria or viruses. *T-cells* destroy the bacteria and viruses attached to host cells and antibodies. Finally, *memory B-cells* identify bacteria, infections, or viruses that may reappear later with a faster response. For example, immunization shots prompt memory B-cells to be ready to fight similar viruses introduced at a later date. [250] [251]

Chapter 7: Autoimmune Disease and the Endocrine System

Endocrine System [252 253 254 255 256 257 258 259 260]

The *endocrine system* regulates hormones. Since many hormones have previously been discussed, some of this section will reinforce what has already been discussed. The endocrine system works hand in hand with the immune and nervous systems to respond to stressors with a protective response. Hormones may activate a cellular activity, or they may inhibit a cellular activity. The hypothalamus, located in the forebrain, releases many hormones that set off a cascade of reactions. In particular, when the hypothalamus releases liberin hormones, such as corticotrophin-releasing hormone (CRH), CRH then initiates a response from the pituitary gland that generates tropin hormones, such as adrenocorticotropic hormone (ATCH). Furthermore, ATCH then initiates a response from the adrenal cortex when it produces hormones such as cortisol. The bottom line, the *hypothalamic-pituitary-adrenal (HPA) axis*, plays an important role in the autonomic nervous, endocrine, and limbic systems. The HPA system has been employed by living species for over 500 million years and has, therefore, been able to stand the scrutiny of the evolutionary process.

The following sections outline some important glands, the hormones they secrete, and the dysfunction that may occur when the hormones they produce are out of balance. The hormones produced by the glands discussed here are generally a response to a cascade of signals usually initiated with the hypothalamus.

Pituitary Gland

The *pituitary gland* is stimulated by the hypothalamus and has several important functions. The *basophil cells* of the pituitary gland produce *adrenocorticotropic hormone (ATCH)*, which initiates the adrenal glands to regulate cortisol levels which, as we will learn, is one of the most critical hormones in human function. The basophil cells of the pituitary gland also produce *thyroid-stimulating hormone (THS)*, which initiates the thyroid to regulate thyroxine (T4) and triiodothyronine (T3). *Growth hormone* is a common hormone produced by the pituitary gland. Growth hormones initiate muscles to escalate protein metabolism. One such hormone is *somatotropin*, which is also responsible for the proliferation of various immune cells such as macrophages and killer T-cells. Excess somatotropin can be brought about by stress, lack of NREM sleep, and hypoglycemia. Furthermore, the overproduction of somatropin can lead to larger organs, tissues, and bones, as well as excessive sweating and an overactive immune system. Somatotropin deficiency is related to aging and obesity, leading to decreased muscle mass and the weakening of the immune system.

Adrenal Glands

The adrenal glands are located above the kidneys and are regulated by the thyroid, hypothalamus, and pituitary gland. Glucocorticoid hormones (GH) and mineralocorticoid hormones (MH) are two classes of adrenocortical hormones released from the adrenal glands. The adrenal glands secrete both steroid and adrenaline hormones.

Glucocorticoid hormones (GH) are involved in protein, fat, and carbohydrate energy functions. GH are released under stress, and they can negatively affect the immune system and lead to hypertension, ulcers, growth development dysfunction, muscle atrophy, glaucoma, depression, psychosis, and osteoporosis. *Cortisol* belongs in the GH classification of hormones, which is responsible for metabolism, circulation, and immune system function. In particular, cortisol plays an important role in regulating glucose and monitoring the autonomic response to stress. Cortisol can also build up or tear down the storage of fatty acids, amino acids, and glucose. *Cushing syndrome (cortisol overproduction)* and *Addison disease (cortisol deficiency)* are common disorders involving cortisol. Cushing and Addison results from either overproduction or underproduction of ACTH. Cushing's disease may be responsible for diabetes, muscular weakness, elevated cardio output and blood pressure, muscle weakness, decreased growth, neuromuscular and cardiac excitability, and ulcers. Addison's disease leads to many concerns, including hypoglycemia, sweating, decrease blood pressure, decreased neuromuscular excitability, and gastrointestinal infections. *Mineralocorticoid hormones* are involved in ion and mineral regulation and water balance (ion and PH regulation are discussed in more detail in Chapter 9). Aldosterone is an example of an MH class of hormones. *Aldosterone* regulates sodium retention as well as potassium and hydrogen excretion. In particular, aldosterone is responsible for regulating pH homeostasis. Addison's disease is also associated with the underproduction of aldosterone, resulting in a sodium ion deficiency and a potassium ion overabundance. Cortisol and aldosterone can be overproduced in response to pain, stress, histamine (allergies), various enzyme defects, hyperkalemia (overabundance of potassium), dopamine, and hypoglycemia (low sugar). Conversely, cortisol and aldosterone may be inhibited by hyperglycemia, enzyme defects, and hypokalemia.

The adrenal glands also circulate adrenaline and norepinephrine, which is stimulated by glucocorticoid hormones, the sympathetic nervous system, and adrenocorticotropic hormone (ACTH). *Adrenaline* can elevate insulin, glucagon, potassium uptake by muscles, and heart rate. Adrenalin may also slow motility in the intestines. *Noradrenalin* is responsible for reducing insulin production and converting tyrosine to adrenaline. In most cases, hormones (the first messenger) act on a second messenger such as *cyclic adenosine monophosphate (cAMP)* or calcium to carry out a cellular mission. Cyclic AMP influences cellular enzymes, transports molecules, and influences gene expression. Influences on gene expression are how stress and exercise advance epigenetic changes in proteins. Once cAMP is converted into noncyclic AMP, the second messenger signal is turned off to inhibit any further reactions. Since steroids produced by the adrenal glands can act directly on DNA, they advance protein synthesis, and that can induce muscle growth.

Thyroid Gland

The *thyroid gland* often responds to pituitary gland hormones and secretes *thyronine, triiodothyronine (T3), thyroxine (T4)*, and *calcitonin* hormones. These hormones regulate autonomic functions such as thermal regulation, cardiac rate, respiratory rate, muscle tone, and calcium serum levels. In particular, T3 and T4 are important for metabolism regulation, and calcitonin is important to inhibit calcium reabsorption.

The parathyroid gland secretes *parathyroid hormone (PTH)*, which regulates calcium and phosphate to maintain cellular PH. Alterations in the parathyroid hormone (PTH) leads to either *hypoparathyroidism* (PTH deficiency) or *hyperparathyroidism* (PTH overproduction). PTH function is the opposite of calcitonin and initiates the reabsorption of calcium. Thyroid hormones alter the metabolic function of proteins, carbohydrates, and fats. Alterations in the *thyroid hormone (TH)* can lead to hypothyroidism (TH deficiency) and hyperthyroidism (TH overproduction).

Hyperthyroidism is usually brought about by an iodine deficiency or inflammatory damage to the thyroid gland triggered by autoimmune disorders such as *Hashimoto thyroiditis* and Graves' disease. *Graves' disease* occurs when immunoglobulin IgG blocks the receptors for thyroid-stimulating hormone (THS). Hyperthyroidism results in several problems, including increased cardiac output and blood pressure, sweating, weight loss, diarrhea, hyperreflexia, insomnia, muscle weakness, lowered cholesterol, hyperglycemia, and neuromuscular excitability. Conversely, *hypothyroidism* leads to hair loss, hyporeflexia, depression, lack of drive, decreased cardio output, hypoglycemia, decrease neuromuscular excitability, weight gain, dry skin, salt and water retention, and constipation. Both hyper and hypothyroidism cannot happen at the same time, but they can occur at different times over the course of a lifetime.

Diabetes

Diabetes is probably the best and most common example of autoimmune dysfunction. Diabetes is also an example of the most common hormone malfunction - *insulin deficiency (hyperinsulinism)*. *Diabetes* is a disorder of insulin regulation, and diabetic neuropathy symptoms can closely mimic those of peripheral nerve disorders. *Polyneuropathy* symptoms from diabetes result in impaired nerve conduction of the motor, autonomic, and sensory nerves. Sensory dysfunction includes pain, numbness, tingling, paresthesia, and loss of sensation.

Motor dysfunction includes atrophy, decreased reflexes, and muscle weakness. Autonomic problems include constipation, diarrhea, erectile dysfunction, sweating, and body temperature regulation. There may also be more serious cardiac implications leading to exercise intolerance, heart-rate variability, hypotension, and even death. Insulin deficiency not only leads to diabetes, but it can also induce fatty liver, acidosis, and dehydration. Prolonged diabetes leads to skin infections, blindness, stroke, and renal failure. Diabetes can also promote collagen accumulation in blood vessels.

Diabetes may be triggered by a viral infection, autoimmune disease, a genetic predisposition, insulin insensitivity, cellular receptor dysfunction, or pancreatic disease that causes the destruction of beta cells. Diabetes occurs more readily to the aging population, mostly because of a surge in the rate of apoptosis and a decreased rate in the proliferation of beta cells. *Hypoglycemia or hyperinsulinism* can be brought about by liver failure, enzyme defects, tumors, glucose consumption from intense exercise, mutations, or alcoholism. The symptoms of hypoglycemia are sweating, tremors, loss of conscience, and seizures. Overproduction of prolactin from stress can initiate several problems such as hyperglycemia, diabetes, and impotence.

Chronic Stress [262 262 263 264 265]

A physiological explanation for chronic stress is warranted since it is related to autoimmune disease, the immune system, and the endocrine system. It is worth noting that coping with some stress is good. Even traumatic life experiences can have a positive effect on people (as well as negative). Stress can improve health and strengthen the immune system. Strengthening the immune system from stressful experiences results from resiliency that educates the body to fight future stress and pain. Just as stress is vital to developing bones and muscles via exercise, or the brain through education, psychological stress is also necessary. The body develops from both physical and mental stress, and without it, the body cannot grow and improve. The United States is a sick country, primarily because we avoid all types of stress.

There are two principles as to why people avoid stress: The comfort principle and the present principle. The *present principle* explains how most Americans and people value the present day over future outcomes. The present principle is the foundation of the *comfort principle*, where Americans will choose comfort over discomfort or stress. For instance, it is easier to access and consume convenient, comfort foods over foods often perceived as less tasty and healthful; it is more comfortable to sit in a reclining chair watching TV than it is to exercise; and it is easier to communicate via social media than it is to do it in person. Every new generation becomes increasingly conditioned to avoid stress in favor of comfort. Unfortunately, human genetics have not had enough time to evolve toward comfort and sedentary lifestyles. While medical science is doing enough to treat symptoms of diseases to keep us alive, our quality of life declines. The bottom line is that, if people want a better chance to live a high-quality life, they should do something outside their comfort zone every day and think about the future instead of filling their lives with shortsighted pleasures. People have a present-day choice of having a better life or becoming a victim or statistic. Because of the comfort principle, most people choose to be a victim of disease. Exercise is the most effective mechanism to exit one's comfort zone and initiate positive stress on the body.

Stress wreaks havoc on the body, but the good news is that controlling stress is within our reach. Experts claim the most important attributes to control stress and increasing pain tolerance is called *resiliency* or mental toughness. *Mental toughness* is associated with self-discipline, expanded will power, conscientiousness, and less worrying. People with mental toughness are better able to focus on tasks, making them less likely to be stricken by boredom. *Boredom* is a common reason for people to have obsessive thoughts that may promote stress. Some evidence suggests that resiliency and mental toughness are both influenced by genetics and the environment. Case in point, a gene called FKBP5 is likely associated with PTSD. Another gene associated with neuropeptide Y (NPY) may also be involved in resiliency. Simultaneously, environmental factors such as meditation, coping with stressful situations, and intermittent fasting can build resiliency. [266]

Stress occurs when one's experiences exceed their coping abilities or mechanisms. Chronic stress research indicates it can enlarge adrenal glands, atrophy the thymus and other lymphoid immune tissues, and result in ulcers in the gastrointestinal tract. Stress also has distinct stages, and one oversimplified model includes *alarm, adaptation, and exhaustion*. Stress is related to the hypothalamic-pituitary-adrenal endocrine system as well as the sympathetic nervous system, including the autonomic nervous system.

Acute stress has an ending point, but *chronic stress* has no definitive endpoint, and it can, therefore, persist for long periods. Said differently, acute stress is a condition under control, while chronic stress is not under control. Not only can chronic stress initiate disease, but it can also exacerbate existing disorders. Chronic stress stimulates the aging process and precipitates an imbalance of white blood cells, including too many or too few killer T-cells (cytotoxic, Th1), too many or too few helper T-cells (regulatory, Treg, or T17), or too many or too few B-cells (or helper T-cells, Th2).

Additionally, chronic stress impairs the gastrointestinal system leading to irritable bowel syndrome (IBS – discussed in Chapter 10) or inflammatory bowel disease (IBD). Specifically, it decreases the number of good bacteria in the digestive system (1) by decreasing IgA, and (2) by increasing adrenaline, which leads to an overgrowth of harmful bacteria. Chronic stress can also make the lining of the digestive tract more permeable, resulting in leaky gut syndrome. A *leaky gut* occurs when harmful bacteria and other molecules can "leak" into the bloodstream, causing allergies, sensitivities, and even autoimmune diseases. A leaky gut can occur when a molecule called zonulin is damaged. *Zonulin* is the glue that holds *gut-associated lymphoid tissue (GALT)* cells together. Zonulin may be damaged via antibiotic use, chronic stress, physical trauma, infections, chronic dysbiosis, anti-inflammatory drugs, toxins, and alcohol. A leaky gut may result in autoimmune diseases in a variety of ways: (1) the production of too many killer T-cells that attack healthy tissue; (2) the production of too many antibodies that attack healthy tissue; or (3) the inability of T regulatory cells to turn off the immune response.

Nervous and Endocrine System Response to Chronic Stress [267 268 269]

Please see Figure 7.1 after this section to better clarify stress and the endocrine system. The body reacts to stress via the nervous or endocrine systems. The nervous system's response to stress is called the *sympathetic nervous system* (discussed in the next chapter) which accelerates the heart rate, increases blood pressure, releases the hormone adrenaline, dilates lung airways, inhibits digestion and absorption of nutrients, inhibits salvation, and inhibits bladder contraction (motility).

In the absence of stress, the *parasympathetic nervous system* provides the opposite response of the sympathetic nervous system. *Glands* secrete endocrine system hormones and neurotransmitters during stress. Examples of these substances include cortisol, adrenaline, noradrenaline, and dopamine from the adrenal gland, corticotrophin-releasing hormone (CRH) from the hypothalamus, and adrenocorticotropic hormone (ACTH) from the pituitary gland. Escalated stress is a proinflammatory response signaling CRH to release cortisol. [270] High blood glucose (sugar) produces elevated insulin levels and decreased amounts of cortisol, and increased cortisol negatively affects the digestion of sugars, proteins, and fats. The outcome of elevated cortisol is an increase in body fat, diminished muscle mass, diminished bone density, elevated anxiety, a rise in depression and mood swings, and an impaired immune system and memory. A surge in cortisol may impair the immune system by diminishing the production of killer T-cells and by producing too many immunoglobulins, which can signal an unnecessary immune response. The overproduction of cortisol can also inhibit the immune system by reducing the mass of lymphoid tissue. [271]

Initial responses to stress result in large amounts of cortisol, but over time, as the adrenal glands become fatigued, cortisol production is inhibited. Moreover, insufficient cortisol can also have dire consequences on the immune system, including elevated killer T-cells concentrations, which commonly trigger autoimmune disease. [272]

Figure 7.1: The HPA Axis and the Stress Response (From bing.com/images)

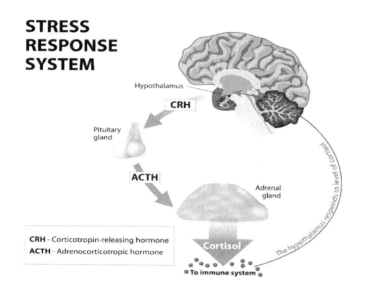

Part III: My Symptoms

Chapter 8: My Sensory Symptoms, The Science of the Nervous System

The nervous system and its response to hormones and stress was touched upon in the previous chapter. Each nerve has a specific function. For instance, one nerve can monitor temperature regulation for a specific finger. *Nerves are the human body's wiring system and provide signals from the skin, muscles, and organs to the brain and vice versa. The brain controls everything we do. In essence, we do not see with our eyes or taste with our tongue; it is the brain that controls these activities. [273]

The *nervous system* contains five parts: the brain, spinal cord, peripheral nerves, autonomic nervous system, and the enteric nervous system. The nervous system also contains two components (see Figure 8.1). First, the *central nervous system (CNS)* encompasses the brain and spinal cord. The CNS is also referred to as the *upper motor neuron system (UMNS)*. Second, the *peripheral nervous system (PNS)* encompasses the peripheral nerves, the autonomic nervous system, and the enteric nervous system (gut). The PNS administers all motor, sensory, and autonomic activity in the limbs and trunk. The PNS, also known as the *lower motor neuron system (LMNS)*; it relays information between the central nervous system (CNS), muscles, and organs via the peripheral nerves. [274]

The PNS encompasses 43 nerves, including 12 pairs of cranial nerves originating from the brain's base and 31 pairs of nerves originating from the spinal cord. The organization of these nerves is as follows: (1) the cervical nerves (C1 through C8 vertebrae); (2) the thoracic nerves (T1 through T12 vertebrae); (3) the lumber nerves (L1 through L5 vertebrae); (4) the sacral nerves (S1 through S5 vertebrae); (5) the coccygeal nerve; and (6) the 12 cranial nerves (CN I, CN II, CN III, …. CN XII) [275]

Nerves are divided into three primary categories. First, sensory nerves command all bodily feelings such as smell, taste, sight, hearing, and touch. Second, motor nerves command all bodily movements such as muscle contractions. Finally, autonomic nerves (discussed in Chapter 10) command bodily functions such as blood pressure, bowel movements, sexual function, heart rate, and breathing. The autonomic nervous system responds to stress and prepares the body to defend itself (*sympathetic nervous system*). Conversely, in the absence of stress, the autonomic nervous system can conserve energy and resources (*parasympathetic nervous system*). [276]

Figure 8.1: The CNS and PNS (From Bing.com/images)

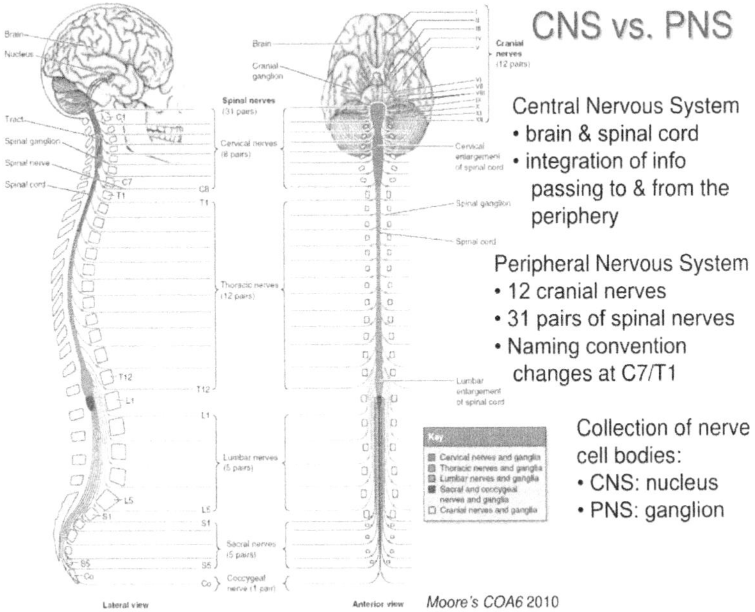

CNS vs. PNS

Central Nervous System
• brain & spinal cord
• integration of info
   passing to & from the
   periphery

Peripheral Nervous System
• 12 cranial nerves
• 31 pairs of spinal nerves
• Naming convention
   changes at C7/T1

Collection of nerve cell bodies:
• CNS: nucleus
• PNS: ganglion

Moore's COA6 2010

The following are some characteristics of nerve cells that make up the CNS and PNS (see Figure 8.2): [277] [278] [279]

First, a *nerve cell* is comprised of neurons and axons. The *neuron* is the nerve cell body, and the *axon* is the long arm of the nerve cell that conducts signals away from the cell body. One of the real mysteries of neurology is how neurons and axons communicate. The nerve cell body (or neuron) encompasses the nucleus and dendrites.

Second, a *dendrite* conducts signals toward the cell body. A *nerve cell signal* leaves the cell body via the axons and terminates at the axon terminal. Once the signal leaves the axon terminal of one neuron, the signal is transferred to the next neuron's dendrite and is relayed to its axon terminal. This process continues thousands of times as a signal relayed from the brain to the muscles and organs. Once the signal reaches the axon terminal located at the neuromuscular junction, the message is converted into a chemical signal (neurotransmitter) and then sent to the muscle cells.

Third, *glial (neuroglia) cells* appear in the connective tissue of the peripheral nervous system (PNS) and support nerve cell function. In particular, glial cells supply nutrients to the nerve cells. The *Schwann cell* (oligodendrocytes) is the only glial cell in the PNS. Some axons are protected by a layer of insulation or myelin sheath produced by Schwann cells. *Myelin sheaths* have two functions. First, myelin sheaths provide a mechanism to transport nutrients to the nerves, and second, signals propagate faster in nerves that have myelinated axons. Furthermore, axons with thin myelin sheaths transmit signals slower than axons with thick myelin sheaths. Myelin sheath protecting autonomic axons are the thinnest, myelin sheath protecting motor axons are the thickest, and myelin sheath protecting sensory axons has various sizes. The **Nodes of Ranvier** separate sections of the myelin sheath. Nodes of Ranvier are sections of axons with no myelin. Nodes of Ranvier are essential for signal propagation.

Fourth, **axonal neuropathy**, or unmyelinated nerve damage, affects the longest nerve or longest communication line first. For example, since the length of nerves in the feet and lower legs have the longest path from the spine, axonal neuropathy symptoms will emerge at these locations. This is similar to peripheral nerve (PNH) disorders; symptoms generally begin in calves and feet.[280] [281] **Demyelinated neuropathy**, such as MMN, is damage to myelinated nerves. Unlike axonal neuropathy, the onset of neuropathy symptoms from demyelination may happen in any body region. Understanding the myelin thickness of axons is important to identify demyelinated neuropathy symptoms and their order of occurrence. In particular, axons with thin myelin sheaths may show signs of neuropathy and nerve damage faster than axons with thicker myelin sheaths. The **terminus** of the nerve or the nerve endings, at the neuromuscular junction, are unmyelinated.

Finally, the nervous system encompasses both myelinated and nonmyelinated nerve fibers. Gray matter comprises unmyelinated neuron cell bodies found within the CNS, while white matter comprises the myelinated neuron cell bodies found in the CNS. Peripheral nerves may be sensory, motor, autonomic, or mixed. When nerves are mixed, a sensory neuron that conducts impulses toward the brain is called an *afferent neuron*. When nerves are mixed, a motor neuron that conducts impulses away from the brain is called *efferent neurons*.

Figure 8.2: The Nerve Cell (From bing.com/images)

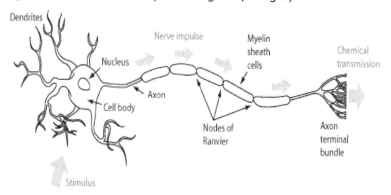

If a vertebra on the spinal cord is cut in half (transverse), it is organized as follows (see Figure 8.3). On one side of the vertebra is the *posterior horn*, which includes gray matter and afferent nerve fibers that transmit signals from the muscle to the brain. These nerve fibers originate in the peripheral nervous system's muscles and pass through the dorsal root and the dorsal root ganglion on the way to the spine. Finally, the nerve fibers in the spine are routed to the brain. These nerve fibers may be either myelinated or nonmyelinated.

The other side of the vertebra is the *anterior horn*, which includes gray matter and efferent nerve fibers that transmit signals from the brain to the muscle. These nerve fibers originate in the brain and pass through the spinal cord and ventral root to the peripheral nervous system's muscles. These nerve fibers may also be either myelinated or nonmyelinated. Reflex movements are faster than a voluntary movement because the signal does not have to travel to the brain for processing. The *parasympathetic and sympathetic nervous systems* supervise autonomic functions for organs. Many of these signals have a different pathway and travel to and from the brain via cranial nerves. 282 283 284 285

Figure 8.3: Vertebra (From bing.com/images)

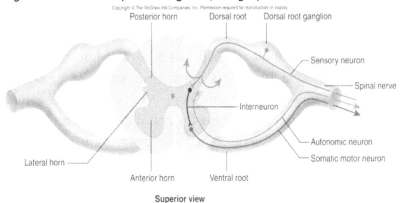

The *forebrain* is extensive and comprises the frontal lobe, motor cortex, somatosensory cortex, parietal lobe, and occipital lobe, which have the following functions (see Figure 8.4): The *frontal lobe* administers processing information for speaking, problem-solving, and movements. The *motor cortex* administers voluntary movements or those movements a person thinks about performing and gait, balance, and motor control. Neurotransmitters affecting muscle movements are controlled by the motor cortex and are attenuated during the aging process. These neurotransmitters are dopamine, serotonin, acetylcholine (ACh), norepinephrine, gamma-aminobutyric acid (GABA), and glutamate. The *somatosensory cortex* administers some sensory functions such as smell and taste. The *parietal lobe* administers other sensory functions such as touch, temperature, and pain. The *occipital lobe* administers vision function. The *temporal lobe* administers hearing function. [286]

The midbrain, pons, and medulla comprise the *brainstem*, which administers autonomic functions. The *medulla* controls cardio, respiratory, and digestive functions, as well as autonomic functions like breathing, heart rate, blood pressure, swallowing, coughing, and reflex activities. The midbrain supervises temperature regulation, sleep cycles, and alertness. Most information processed by the brain must transverse the brainstem (and the pons) since almost all of the cranial nerves and the spinal cord nerves terminate at the brainstem. The *hindbrain* houses the cerebellum and is responsible for the refinement of skeletal muscle movement, including coordination and balance. The *cerebellum* does not control muscle power and contraction force, but cerebellum dysfunction may result in loss of muscular power due to clumsy and uncoordinated movements. [287] [288]

Figure 8.4: The Brain (From bing.com/images)

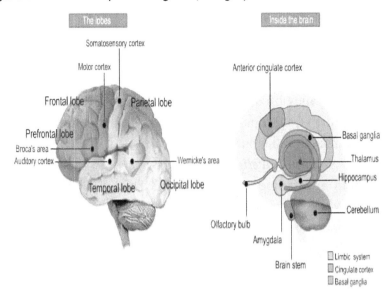

The Sensory Nervous System [289] [290] [291] [292]

The nerves controlling body function may be sensory, motor, or autonomic. ***Sensory systems*** may function consciously or unconsciously and are administered by four receptor systems in the peripheral nerves: (1) the ***exteroceptor system*** regulates stimuli from the external environment such as temperature, hearing, touch, vision, smell, and taste; (2) the ***proprioceptor system*** oversees balance and body posture by monitoring the tension in muscles, tendons, and joints; (3) the ***nociceptor system*** manages pain sensations; and (4) the ***interoceptive system*** unconsciously controls information about internal organs. For example, unconscious interoceptive or visceral sensations are controlled by cranial nerves III, VII, IX, and

X, and they regulate hunger, blood pressure, heart rate, sex drive, nausea, and pain.

Sensory nerves place the individual in relationship to the environment. *Sensory nerve endings* are found throughout the body, in particular on the skin and in membranes of organs. Sensory nerves are more abundant on the fingertips, tongue, lips, and genitals and less abundant on the buttock and trunk.

Small unmyelinated sensory nerves (Type IV) regulate pain and temperature sensation. Thin myelinated sensory nerves can vary in size and control touch, pressure, and temperature sensation. Thick myelinated sensory nerves control most bodily functions, including body coordination. *Large myelinated sensory nerve fibers* (Type I) may conduct at velocities up to 100 meters per second (m/s), and small unmyelinated nerve fibers may conduct at speeds as slow as 1 m/s. Most neuropathies affect both small and large nerve fibers, but some disorders may only affect large or small fibers.

Sensory symptoms may be either positive or negative. Positive symptoms enhance senses, such as feeling more pain or paresthesia. Negative symptoms diminish senses, such as those to feel or touch. The sensory exam is considered the most difficult, tedious, subjective, and least useful part of the patient exam and may explain why so many neurologists give little credence to sensory symptoms.

Chapter 8 covers my sensory symptoms, which may or may not be associated with neurological disorders. I am certainly not suggesting all of the symptoms outlined in this chapter or the next two chapters are related to my neurological disorder, but they must be analyzed along with other plausible causes of their occurrence. This process is essential for diagnosing any disorder.

My Sensory Symptoms

Sensory Symptom Phenomenon

Sensory symptom phenomenon is a term I coined to explain the sensory symptoms that one may feel, but others cannot see or verify. All sensory symptoms felt by a patient cannot be verified by others and include pain, loss of sensation, and loss of taste and smell. I communicate with people who suffer from peripheral nerve disorders, and one of their biggest complaints, other than not enough is being done to help people suffering from these disorders, is that friends and family do not believe what they are feeling is real. There is evidence that social support fosters the best environment for resiliency and mental toughness to fight illness. [293]

People with PNH or neuropathy go to work, exercise, take care of their children, and do their best to function in society. This behavior gives friends and family a false impression that they must be doing okay if they are able to work and exercise. Why do people who are suffering from chronic pain go on with life? The answer is simple; they have no other choice (other than to go on the disability payroll). There are no cures for most neurological disorders, and research is very limited. Therefore, those inflicted with neurological disorders have a choice: They can be a couch potato, or they can try to live their life the best they can. Most people with PNH or other chronic neurological disorders are probably a couch potato most of the day while at the same time being as productive possible during fewer hours of the day.

Unfortunately, the success of people coping with chronic pain is directly related to if families and friends believe that their pain is real and not just a figment of their imaginations. [294] Norman Latov summarized the sensory symptom phenomenon when he wrote, "People may think that you are depressed or hysterical, or that you are exaggerating your symptoms. They may not provide much support. People with painful neuropathy often feel alone and with no one to talk to who understands their difficulties." [295] Furthermore, Latov opines, "We don't allow torture, but the pain of neuropathy can feel the same." One last important point by Latov, "Depression and anxiety are common consequences of the disease, causing further problems .... [creating a] vicious cycle that can make neuropathy such a debilitating disease." [296]

In the age of social media, everyone is seeking approval from others. It is human nature to want others to value our experiences. People may have hundreds of friends on social media, but finding true friendships is rare. True friends remain supportive regardless of the situation. Those inflicted with chronic pain and neurological disorders need to identify their true friends and disregard others. It is impossible to please everyone and, therefore, people with illnesses must be able to carry on with fewer friends. That is the bad news, but the good news is that those inflicted with nerve disorders will discover new friends experiencing similar adversity.

Failure to convince others of our hardships is an unfortunate part of life. When people see me competing in cycling at a fairly high level, nonetheless, there is no way they would ever think I have some debilitating neurological disorder. However, most people do not see me spending 12 to 16 hours confined to the couch or bed suffering from fatigue and pain. Why do people find it difficult to believe the sensory symptoms of others? One reason is that many sensory symptoms are conflicting. For example, onlookers may deduce that it is implausible to feel both pain and numbness in the same location at the same time. Unfortunately, with nerve damage, it is possible to feel both sensations simultaneously. [297]

Furthermore, I have found that one of the best ways to advocate for oneself is to write about my disorder and to discuss it with others openly. I am open about my disorder and like to discuss it or write about it for several reasons. First, the success of people coping with chronic pain and neurological disorders is directly related to if families and friends believe that their pain is real and not just a figment of their imaginations. [298] Thus, social behavior is necessary when trying to find new friends experiencing similar trials and tribulations when our current friends are ignoring us. Second, I find it therapeutic to write and talk about my condition even if people are not listening or reading my work. It feels good to get my concerns and worries out of my system to alleviate stress. Of course, mitigating stress works to reduce symptoms and pain. At a minimum, I truly believe that some people may benefit from writing a journal, especially if their disorder is being downplayed by family and friends. [299]

Touch and Vibration Sensation

Sense of touch or proprioceptive sensations is tested using a tuning fork. A gradual loss of sensation down the leg to the foot and toes generally fits a peripheral neuropathy manifestation (this fits my symptoms). Of course, loss of sensation distally could also be age-related, but a 57-year-old male should not have severely compromised sensation in his hands and feet. If the loss of sensation were equal down the leg to the feet and toes, then that would indicate some form of radiculopathy which is a compression of a nerve root at the spinal cord. Cerebellum involvement in sensory loss is identifiable through various tests such as stereognosis, graphesthesia, autotopagnosia, two-point, and sensory extinction. *Stereognosis* is the inability to recognize and identify common objects by touch. *Graphesthesia* is the inability to recognize letters and numbers written on the skin with a finger. *Autotopagnosia* is the inability to properly orient different parts of the body. *A two-point test* identifies the inability to distinguish the difference between two close and simultaneous pinpricks. Similarly, *sensory extinction* identifies the inability to distinguish between two pinpricks on opposite sides of the body. Thankfully, I do not have any cerebellum involvement in my sensory loss. [300]

Temperature Sensation [301]

Temperature sensation involvement from neurological disease involves several key processes. *Polyneuropathy* and many neurological symptoms originate from exteroceptive receptors or problems sensing stimulus coming from the environment. Sensory symptoms from neurological conditions are primarily confined in distal locations and could result in cold hands and feet. Sensory symptoms from neurological conditions affect both hot and cold temperature sensations equally. Furthermore, temperature and pain sensitivities are affected equally in neurological conditions because they are regulated by the same Type IV sensory nerve fibers. I certainly seem to have some type of Type IV sensory nerve fiber involvement in my case resulting in cold hands and feet and thermal regulation issues.

Taste and Smell [302]

Taste and smell are innervated by cranial nerves VII and IX. An impairment in smell always leads to an impairment in taste. Smell and taste can be affected in many ways. In the thalamus, smell may be affected by alcohol, tumors, epilepsy, and inflammation. In the nose, smell may be affected by genetic defects in chemical receptors, toxins, trauma, hypothyroidism, and certain drugs. Alterations in the sense of touch may be affected by any level of the nervous system, while a decrease in smell and taste (hyposmia) is only produced by inflammation of the nasal mucosa or some trauma to the olfactory cranial nerve.

Both smell and taste may be affected by age. Taste may be affected by genetic defects, radiation, medications (cocaine, penicillin, antibiotics, and anesthetics), diabetes, aldosterone deficiency, nerve lesions, epilepsy, and tumors. Some toxins that may affect smell (olfaction) are smoking, alcohol, lead, cadmium, cyanide, and chlorine compounds. Cadmium is a carcinogen and may also cause unfavorable methyl epigenetic changes. [303] People with serious neurodegenerative disorders such as Alzheimer's,

Parkinson's disease, and Huntington's disease may also have compromised senses of smell and taste. Impaired senses of smell and taste include many medications, including antibiotics.

Since I do not have any cranial nerve involvement in my disorder, there must be another reason for the lack of smell and taste. Age and prolong use of antibiotics are the more logical explanations for my slight decrease in smell and taste. My smell may also be affected by my never-ending amounts of mucous coming from environmental allergies and food sensitivities. [304]

Pulsatile Tinnitus [305] [306]

An unusual sensory symptom that I experience is called pulsatile tinnitus. I have had both hearing loss and a constant ringing (tinnitus) in my left ear since I was a youth. To others, tinnitus may sound like a swishing, roaring, buzzing, blowing, or whistling sound that affects sleep habits in most people afflicted with the disorder. Tinnitus is also related to hearing loss, and another symptom I have and will be discussed later - lightheadedness. I believe the root cause of my tinnitus stems from a staph infection I had on my eardrum when I was around ten years old (more on this later). Hearing loss and or tinnitus may be brought about by many factors, including exposure to high decibel noise and trauma as well as various infections such as the mumps, herpes, measles, MS, anemia, Epstein-Barr, and HIV. Hearing loss may also be associated with polyneuropathies such as a hereditary version called Charcot–Marie–Tooth disease (CMTD).

Once I began training more vigorously, the tinnitus turned into pulsatile tinnitus. ***Pulsatile tinnitus*** means, at times, I can actually hear or feel my heart rate pulsating in my left ear, and the condition is exacerbated following a high-exertion training session. Pulsatile tinnitus is produced by a pulsating blood vessel near the petrous bone, which protects the cochlea that translates sound into brain signals. Pulsatile tinnitus is rare and can result from serious conditions such as tumors, hardening of the arteries, infections, hypertension, and other reasons such as cranial nerve VIII demyelination damage. That said, pulsatile tinnitus can occur simply because there is more blood flow from a strenuous workout, or it can be an indication of the onset of peripheral neurological disease. [307] Is there a broader relationship between pulsatile tinnitus and any neurological manifestations that I may be experiencing? My guess is that pulsatile tinnitus is unrelated to my condition.

Swallowing and the Globus Sensation [308] [309]

Swallowing is controlled by many cranial nerves, including V, VII, IX, X, and XII and the entire process is under autonomic control. Another sensory condition or symptom that I have from time to time is a globus sensation. A *globus sensation* is the feeling of having something lodged in the throat that does not really exist. It is my belief that this feeling arises from an acid reflux condition (GERD – discussed later) and is unrelated to my neurological condition.

Balance

Both motor and sensory symptoms can affect balance. Balance is affected directly by the sensory system, but motor deficits such as weakness, atrophy, and paresthesia play an indirect role in balance dysfunction. [310] When the motor system functions abnormally, it is not difficult to imagine that the end result may be a loss of coordination or balance.

Sensory symptoms directly affecting balance is a function of the proprioceptor system. ***Proprioceptor sensory nerves*** are primarily located in the spindle muscle fibers but may also be found in muscles, tendons, and joints. Proprioceptor nerves are responsible for the balance and coordination of muscles with reference to the rest of the body. Since I have absent Achilles tendon reflexes, it is conceivable that proprioceptor sensory nerve dysfunction in the spindle muscle fibers is attributing to my balance dysfunction. [311]

During my first year at the Huntsman games, I was examined at the balance exhibit. One perk for paying the high registration fees is that they have a very extensive medical exhibit studying the effects of exercise on aging adults. The result suggested that my balance was in the lower third for my age group. I was mystified by this finding because I was leading 5.10+ rock climbs and wrestling in old-timer events just one year earlier. Knowing balance is also important for cycling; I dedicated training exercises to improve my balance. The last time I was tested for balance at the Huntsman exhibit, the findings suggested I was better than the 95th percentile. So, yes, it is possible to improve your balance despite weird sensations, absent reflexes, and motor and sensory nerve dysfunction. Are balance symptoms the direct result of my neurological condition? The verdict is mixed. Some of my balance issues are a direct result of the sensory symptoms, but motor symptoms may also have an indirect effect on balance.

Depression

Depression is believed to be brought about by deficient amounts of serotonin and norepinephrine at the nerve endings, which inhibit the production, transport, and reception of these chemicals in the brain. For instance, darkness may inhibit serotonin while producing melatonin. Darkness explains why people living in dark northern regions of the world or in rainy climates are more inclined to have depression. [312] Depression is also related to a disruption of good bacteria in the gut. [313] Depression, like stress, increases the aging process. [314]

I would be lying if I did not admit that the unknown nature of my neurological condition does not cause some level of stress and depression. If my level of depression was excessive, then I would lose interest in training and competing, and that has not happened.

Fear

A large percentage of people with PNH or other neurological disorders live in constant fear and, therefore, find it difficult to move on with their lives. The reason for fear is that many patients believe they have something more sinister such as ALS or MS. [315] After all, many symptoms of PNH disorders are onset symptoms for ALS and MS. Therefore, most PNH patients have brain MRI and EMG testing–to rule out MS and ALS. According to one source, "Patients with neurological complaints are often apprehensive about having some dreadful disease, such as a brain tumor, ALS, MS, or muscular dystrophy." [316] No evidence exists suggesting that anyone diagnosed with a PNH or some other neurological disorder has a greater probability of contracting ALS or MS than a person without PNH. That said, there have been a few papers written on the subject that strikes fear into everyone with some peripheral nerve disorder. [317] [318] However, for every paper suggesting potential doom and gloom, there are many more papers and studies that suggest the opposite. [319] The bottom line, fasciculations, and cramping in the absence of muscle wasting or atrophy is benign. [320] When I talk in terms of "benign", I am indicating the condition is not life-threatening. This by no means suggests that the condition is not debilitating, creating real and painful symptoms. [321]

How is fear realized and sustained in neurological patients? Imagine going into a neurologist office, and he or she says we got to examine you for amyotrophic lateral sclerosis (ALS) and multiple sclerosis (MS). Unfortunately, symptoms such as fasciculations are a common feature of motor neuron disease. Then, in the follow-up appointment to discuss the test results, the neurologist says everything is fine, you probably have benign fasciculation syndrome (BFS), and that is "no big deal." He or she offers you no advice or potential remedies that may alleviate the symptoms. He or she spends five minutes with you and sends you on your way. The neurologist's dismissive attitude raises more questions, leading to fear and depression:

- How is it possible that your symptoms are bad enough to warrant an extensive examination, yet he or she insists that there is nothing wrong with you?
- Why are not your motor or sensory symptoms severe enough to warrant any remedy recommendations?

- Why is BFS considered no big deal when you are having difficulties doing activities you used to do?
- To an educated person, the entire process is illogical, leading to fearful questions such as. Will ALS appear later, or have I been misdiagnosed since my symptoms feel like a big deal? In other words, the medical profession did nothing to alleviate concerns before or after the examination checking for ALS and MS.

It is not necessary to live in fear. If patients with PNH have a greater probability of acquiring ALS or MS, then why is the medical community ignoring these patients instead of studying them? After all, if they had a better chance to acquire ALS, then they could hold the key to understanding and curing ALS. Generally, patients with benign fasciculations can feel muscle activity, while those patients with ALS cannot feel muscle activity. It is very rare for people with ALS to only present with fasciculation symptoms during the initial diagnosis process.

ALS patients generally show signs of upper motor neuron disease that do not appear in lower motor neuron disorders such as PNH and neuropathy. ALS patient symptoms of weakness and atrophy are focal or asymmetrical during the onset of the disease, while those patients with other neurological conditions usually do not have atrophy, and symptom onset is symmetrical. [322] Furthermore, the epidemiology study presented in Appendix 1 proves that many people experience the same challenges, which should reassure PNH patients that they are not alone. Thus, PNH is common and progresses slowly; whereas, ALS is rare and progresses quickly; thus,

PNH patients with symptoms for years do not have ALS. From my personal interaction with PNH patients, women are more likely to live in fear. However, men are more likely to acquire ALS by a 3 to 1 or even a 4 to 1 ratio.

Bravery means to persevere in the presence of fear. People routinely tell me they are not very strong or brave in the face of adversity, and that is why they are fearful or unable to cope with pain. Nevertheless, strength and bravery can be enhanced and learned through personal training and experiences. Most people are not naturally born as brave individuals. I wouldn't call myself brave. Instead, I have had personal experiences that help me cope with fear and pain. Therefore, I purposely place myself into fearful situations such as suffering on bike, rock climbing, or mountaineering. This has helped me adapt to fearful life situations.

People with PNH are fearful for many reasons. First, I postulated the personality theory as one reason for fear. One example of personality types is *Type A and Type B personality theory*. According to this theory, driven, demanding, and achievement-oriented people are classified as Type A, while easy-going, relaxed individuals are designated as Type B. In my contact with dozens of patients, over 95% have a Type A personality. Type A personality commonly describes people who are "outgoing, ambitious, rigidly organized, highly status-conscious, sensitive, impatient, anxious, proactive, and concerned with time management." People with Type A personalities are often high-achieving "workaholics." [323] This would go a long way to explain their stress and anxiety, which exacerbates symptoms.

Those with a Type A personality are more likely to be an extravert, pursuing and thriving with more stimulation. These individuals often express intense passion in their work and just about anything else they undertake. The best attribute of passionate behavior is that people improve at their work and hobbies, but the downside is that their behavior can become obsessive. Individuals who are obsessive about work or some hobby probably rarely change their behavior unless there is a decline in their mental and physical health, burnout, injury, or death. Therefore, a Type A personality is more likely to stress about certain life experiences and, therefore, be more likely to have a *generalized anxiety disorder (GAD)* or even *obsessive-compulsive disorder (OCD)*. [324]

People with GAD are more likely to have persistent worries about life events, and these worries can even manifest stress symptoms into depression. OCD is characterized by irrational thoughts and actions that can produce severe distress. OCD is time-consuming and gets in the way of normal everyday functions such as relationships, work, and family. The bottom line, without any symptom relief, Type A personality PNH patients are likely to obsess over their health situation with continuous thoughts of believing there is something more sinister at work. [325] A Type A personality may link, for instance, stress and exercise as triggers for PNH. High achievers place a great deal of unwanted stress on their lives, and the same individuals may not use exercise to relax but to train rigorously for competitions placing more stress on their lives. Hence, it may not necessarily be the exercise triggering PNH symptoms, but the stress to achieve athletically that is triggering the PNH symptoms.

It is possible that Type B personalities acquire peripheral nerve disorders at just as high a rate as Type A personalities, but only those who stress out about their diagnosis contact me. If a Type B personality is more accepting and relaxed about their diagnosis, then they may do a better job controlling their symptom frequency and intensity instead of exacerbating symptoms with unnecessary stress and anxiety.

Second, another hypothesis I formulated is that many patients with PNH disorders often have difficulty distinguishing between muscle fatigue, muscle weakness, and muscle atrophy. I call this the *Fatigue Theory*. Fatigue is the feeling of tiredness, but weakness is a loss of strength. Fatigue and weakness are two completely different issues, yet many people think the terms are synonymous. That said, some confusion about weakness and fatigue may stem from the fact that some patients may reveal functional weakness during a physical examination but appear normal participating in everyday activities. [326]

Furthermore, there is a distinct difference between muscle weakness and muscle atrophy associated with ALS. Muscle atrophy related to ALS will result in dramatic wasting. ALS moves quickly, while peripheral nerve disorders may progress, but they generally do so very slowly. Furthermore, PNH patients may experience atrophy from exercise intolerance and avoiding painful exercise and not from any sinister neurological disease.

My final theory for PNH patients having fear and depression is because many PNH patients have been misdiagnosed. I call this the ***Misdiagnosis Theory***. Patients with chronic and multiple symptoms probably have CFS and not BFS. Doctors may be ignoring or discarding sensory symptoms of PNH patients leading to the misdiagnosis. I do not know if patients were diagnosed properly, it would eliminate the fear factor, but misdiagnosing someone with something they claim is no big deal only facilitates more stress, fear, and depression. I have data to support this conclusion in Appendix 1.

Cycling helps me cope with fear not only because it is a distraction, but it proves without a shred of doubt that my neurological symptoms are not sinister or something that will kill me. After all, a person with ALS could not ride to the top of Cottonwood Pass. Sure, there has been some atrophy in my feet, hands, and calves, but part of the reason for this is because I do not use these muscles as much when I cycle than in my previous activities. There is truth to the statement, "If you do not use it, you lose it," because muscles will atrophy as gene expression is changed. [327] To be sure, if I had ALS, I would not make it out of my driveway on a bike. It is also important to remember that atrophy may be associated with other less sinister disorders. The bottom line, when fear sets in, humans lose their deductive and rational based problem-solving skills. We do not always have to assume the worst.

Pain [328 329 330 331]

Pain is "an unpleasant sensory and emotional experience associated with actual or potential tissue damage or described in terms of such damage." Furthermore, "Adaptive responses to pain and avoidance learning may occur in the absence of conscience, but pain experience cannot." [332] Regardless, "Identification of effective therapeutic interventions [for pain] have been hampered by the realization that the [pain] system is far more complex than ever imagined." [333] Therapies and remedies for pain are elusive because the pain system, from the molecular level all the way to the nervous system, is vast and complex. [334] [335] The bottom line, pain treatment costs about 635 billion dollars annually in the United States. [336]

There are four different classifications of pain: Acute, traumatic, inflammatory, and neuropathic. *Acute pain* is a short-term soft tissue injury such as a sprained knee or paper cut. *Traumatic pain* is the outcome of a traumatic experience, which can include post-traumatic stress disorder (PTSD) and pain associated with witnessing horrific events. *Neuropathic pain* is the result of damage to the peripheral nerves or to the central nervous system that produces unique types of pain and symptoms. *Inflammatory pain* is associated with neurological pain, which can be an outcome of some neurological disease, disorder, or syndrome.

The perception of pain is triggered by a stimulus, which is detected by sensory neurons called nociceptors. *Nociceptors* are pain receptors that detect stimuli and respond to chemical, mechanical, and thermal stimulation. Nociceptors that are myelinated nerve fibers allow for fast transmission of sharp localized pain, while nociceptors that are unmyelinated nerve fibers allow for the slow transmission of burning and aching pains.

The *pain threshold* is the point at which pain is perceived, and this does not vary much among people. *Pain tolerance* is the duration of time and intensity of pain an individual endures before the initiation of pain response, and this varies significantly among people. Cognitive expectations may intensify the pain. For instance, if a person has an expectation that their pain will be relieved, it may not feel as bad as when they may know there is no relief for their pain. Neurotransmitter chemicals can elicit or inhibit pain. Gamma-aminobutyric acid (GABA) and glycine are pain inhibitors. Chemicals that may elicit a pain response are bradykinin, substance P, interleukins, and ATP. Interestingly, GABA may be deficient in people who had neglectful mothers, increasing their stress and pain levels into adolescence. GABA deficiency is also related to reduced good bacteria in the gut. [337]

Pain may also be exacerbated by the *hyperexcitation* or constant firing of cell membranes found in PNH and neuropathy disorders. This process might result from voltage-gated sodium channels (Nav1.8) promoting increased current flowing into the cell, while voltage-gated potassium channels (Kv4.2) promote reduced current flowing out of the cell. [338] [339] The COMT gene is known as the "warrior–worrier" gene. About 16% of people with one variant of the gene are worriers, and about 36% of people with another variant are warriors. The warrior variant allows people to tolerate higher pain levels because the frontal cortex of the brain receives less dopamine. [340]

The vast number of channels and body chemicals involved in pain makes it very difficult to not only diagnose neurological disorders but the source of pain. Pain can divert body resources and affect "clotting time, wound healing, immune function, muscle tone, cardiovascular stability, sleep, gastrointestinal motility, and our emotions." [341] Pain is addressed by the somatosensory cortexes in our brains. When pain is addressed in these cortexes, it is common for the pain to feel sharp, drilling, prickling, tingling, throbbing, itching, hot, or cold. However, the realization that pain may be long-lived due to a neurological condition or traumatic injury, pain sensation is described by affected adjectives such as fearful, frightful, cruel, vicious, suffocating, sickening, and frustrating. When pain evolves into the affected adjective stage it is being addressed in the anterior cingulate cortex (ACC) region of the brain responsible for modulating sensory pain to more serious pain from stress and emotional distress. [342] Most people reading this text are probably at the affected adjective level of pain (from the ACC), thinking the pain is chronic without much hope of future relief.

The bottom line, the correct response to fear, stress, adversity, and pain should be motivation and not long-term depression. Remember, pain is essential for life to exist. Without pain, humans could not survive. Motivation mitigates stress, fear, and pain whereas, depression exacerbates stress, fear, and pain. Finally, the difference between anxiety and stress is anxiety is an overactive stress response and may be caused by fear. [343] Hence, fear is the connection between anxiety and stress.

Lessons in Pain Management

The following points are my lessons learned about coping with pain that helps reduce fear and depression.

Acceptance: When coping with an illness, disorder, and disease, acceptance is the most important factor in reducing chronic pain. Deborah Barrett said this of acceptance, "This does not mean you like the situation or will stop trying to improve. On the contrary, acceptance is about acknowledging what *is*, rather than tormenting yourself with what *could be*. Through acceptance, you can move forward with your life, better equipped to care for yourself, adapt, and improve." [344]

Advocating for oneself: If the medical profession is failing to provide useful solutions, then advocate for oneself to find help. Search for a better doctor and research your condition to find potential remedies that you may try on a trial and error approach. In particular, I used a trial and error approach to understand my limitations in cycling, such as my 1.5-hour training limit and the need to have extra rest time in the afternoons.

Avoiding depression: Nonacceptance leads to the biggest consequence of chronic pain plaguing millions of Americans: Depression. Nonacceptance means obsessing about issues beyond our control that sets in motion a vicious cycle of events, including depression. Case in point, obsessing about ineffective or incorrect treatments, the horribly convoluted diagnosis process, the lack of support, and all those looks from others that think you are crazy will lead to depression. *Depression* leads to sleep deprivation, which further exacerbates pain. [345] A normal process of coping with neurological disorders encompasses five steps and the length to get through all the steps is dependent on the person. The steps include *denial*, *anger*, *bargaining*, *depression*, and *acceptance*. [346] If both depression and pain become chronic, then disability will follow.

Build confidence: *Confidence* may be the single most important variable to success because, without confidence, motivation, a positive attitude, and perseverance are impossible. Despite the need for mental toughness, most people only train for the physical aspects of competition. Mental toughness is synonymous with resiliency. Forgoing mental training is an unfortunate oversight by many cyclists. Mental toughness is "unshakeable perseverance and conviction toward some goal despite pressure and adversity." Professional athletes often relate mental toughness with winning at all costs. That said, like success, winning can have a different meaning for different people. Winning and success can be whatever we want it to be. It can mean winning, finishing, a personal best, or it can just mean enjoying another day without a wheelchair. [347] The adversity I face coping with a neurological disorder helps me build mental toughness.

Most athletes are motivated by desires such as winning, building friendships, maintaining health, or competition. On the contrary, I am motivated by the dire nature of my neurological disease to fight disability and live longer. Since cycling slows the progression of my disorder, it easy to endure the pain from training and competition because the pain is literally saving my life. Obviously, symptoms such as pain and fatigue can impair cycling performance. In fact, any illness will have a negative effect on cycling performance because it disrupts focus by inhibiting cognitive function. [348]

It may sound odd, but since I face pain and fatigue daily, my confidence is very high when I compete. One way to build confidence is to endure adversity in a training plan. Confidence is having the ability to adapt to situations beyond a person's control, such as the weather or having a bad day. For example, a cyclist willing to train in heavy winds and other adverse weather conditions helps them build confidence for any conditions they may face on race day. Similarly, even if I do not sleep well or have enhanced symptoms on race day, I am fairly confident I can fight through it since I fight through pain and fatigue every day. I have confidence because my neurological adversity prepares me for anything I may face in a race, making it easy to adapt and push forward. For example, when other cyclists do not feel well and are having a bad day, their effort during the race may diminish as they become discouraged. I know I am not going to have a good day, and I know I am going to have to fight every second during a race. Even if I am having a really bad day, I never stop fighting in a race. I never get discouraged and I never give up. I think this attitude explains why I am a consistent rider.

Coaching: A good coach can facilitate pain avoidance. A cycling coach can be a mental consultant at a much-reduced rate than a psychologist. My first coach had more faith in my abilities than I did. When my attitude became self-defeating, my coach lifted my spirits. Having someone raise your spirits helps, especially when coping with pain. My second coach is not so much a cheerleader, but his background is in biomedical engineering so, he understands how the body functions. He understands my condition and built a plan around my limitations, so I do not endure needless pain. In other words, he designed a plan, especially for me and my success. [349]

Diet: A healthy diet prevents pain by promoting proper bodily function. The following are some important facts about diet and preventing pain: [350] Do not overindulge in processed foods, trans-fats, and excess carbohydrates. Remember, when carbohydrates are processed, they turn into sugar. Sugar and carbohydrates are a leading cause of obesity, which leads to diabetes and heart disease. Carbohydrates stimulate insulin, and excess insulin prevents the body from burning off carbohydrates. Excess carbohydrates result in increased body fat, high cholesterol, fluid retention, dry skin, brittle fingernails, concentration concerns, fatigue, pain, headaches, irritability, and sleep disruptions. Anti-nutrient foods include whole grains, wheat, barley, rye, oats, spelt, brown rice, corn, quinoa, lentils, red beans, black beans, pinto beans, white rice, flour, bread, cereal, crackers, cookies, pasta, sugar, and soda. [351] Quinoa and beans are also a great source of protein. The human digestive system not only has difficulty processing the above-mentioned foods; they are low-performance foods. There are plenty of natural sources for carbohydrates found in meat, fruit, and vegetables.

I have mentioned many times, the gut has both good and bad bacteria. Bad foods promote bad bacteria, and good foods promote good bacteria. When the gut has too many bad bacteria, the body must use immunoglobulin A (IgA) to fight a leaky gut. Unfortunately, a bad diet may result in an IgA deficiency leaving the gut unable to fight a leaky gut. Acid-reflux medications decrease stomach acid, and that may make it hard for the gut to process proteins. Avoid foods that may produce allergic or intolerant reactions. Specifically, avoid foods that result in a negative reaction such as gas, bloating, runny nose, and dry mouth. Intolerant and allergic foods decrease immune system efficiency and initiate pain. It is best to get all the essential nutrients and vitamins from food. However, when that is not possible, then supplements are necessary. A healthy diet starts with the brain. If the brain is sidetracked coping with stress and anxiety, for instance, then the gut will fail to digest food properly. Thus, it is imperative to relax during and after each meal for optimal digestion benefits. [352]

Distractions: Distractions are the best to cope with pain. Put another way, it is possible to trick the mind to cope with pain. When people are active such as working, playing, exercising, and socializing, pain takes a back seat. Besides, being involved in an activity, even if it is painful, may help people cope with both anxiety and pain, especially if it is an activity, a person may be more likely to succeed. This phenomenon is referred to as the peak-end effect. The *peak-end effect* occurs when people tend to prefer painful experiences that end well, "even if they last longer and are objectively worse than mildly painful experiences that end badly." [353]

Eliminating anxiety: Anxiety tends to make people focus on their pain, making it worse. One reason for this behavior is because anxiety, and "suffering comes from uncertainty" or the unknown. [354] [355] This is so true; we tend to worry about issues we cannot control, and this ultimately leads to more stress and anxiety, causing more pain and suffering. One way to manage stress is to make lifestyle changes that eliminate issues that may annoy us or cause us to complain. Such changes are easier said than done, but doing so may be easy such as finding better friends or challenging like making a career change. Like most people with neurological conditions, I like to worry. Obviously, this behavior is very counterproductive. However, I made many difficult lifestyle changes, such as moving out of the city and changing jobs. It is difficult enough to sleep at night with a neurological disorder, but adding stress and anxiety into the equation only compounds the problem.

Eliminating excuses: The biggest obstacle to overcome for exercising is just starting. Once this hurdle is cleared, then it is all downhill. Comic Woody Allen once said, "Eighty percent of life is just showing up." [356] This is so true. After I begin a training session, it only takes about two minutes before I am committed to my training for that day.   **Enhancing the senses**: Enhance or stimulate one's senses of smell, taste, sight, touch, and hearing with enjoyable experiences to keep the mind off the symptoms and pain. [357] For instance, I generally listen to mellow music to calm me before sleep. I like classic rock, but that only gets me riled up. If I have a race coming up, I may visualize myself doing well in a race and mentally acquaint myself with the course. There is nothing wrong with some positive feedback and dreaming. So long as visualization remains positive, it can train the subconscious mind to realize race and training goals. [358] Humor stimulates the senses in a positive manner. I find it helpful not to take myself too seriously and to laugh at my shortcomings. There is nothing wrong with making fun of yourself so long as it is done in a positive manner. I eat fairly healthy, but I do like to indulge in some sinful desserts. Sweets always bring a smile to my face, but the healthier I eat, the less dry mouth and heartburn I have in the evenings.

Evolving: "Living with chronic pain is a continual process of learning and adapting." [359] I like to call it evolving. After all, without a neurological disorder and chronic pain, I would have never competed in cycling. I evolved to cycling when other activities were simply too difficult in terms of safety and pain. As I quickly learned, "Not all activity is helpful, and too much of it causes setbacks." [360] Adapting and evolving indicates finding those activities that work best and those that do not, even if it means giving up activities we love. Most people with chronic pain tend to be overcautious and rest too much. Very few sufferers of chronic pain try to do too much. [361] I actually do both: I do too much, and I do too little. I do too much in the morning and then do very little most afternoons to make up for my overactive mornings. It is not uncommon for people to feel okay while exercising but to suffer in agony later in the day. [362] Evolving does not mean for people to give up on activities in fear of those inevitable flare-ups for doing too much. Evolving means changing activities or doing less. [363]

Exercise: Exercising rigorously with pain is definitely possible. The key is to build up exercise capacity and pain tolerance slowly. There will be setbacks, and there will be pain, so the key is to take baby steps. [364] Finally, understand your limitations. Case in point, I do not have any long training rides because I fatigue quickly. Conversely, rest days are also vital because sometimes, to gain speed and strength, you must go slower. [365] This is particularly important for elderly individuals whose muscles need extra time to recover (even those who do not have any neurological disease).

Goal-setting: Competition helps me achieve numerous outcomes. [366] A competition sets clear goals that can be broken down into three categories. *"A" goals* should be challenging, realistic, and specific. *"B" goals* include training specific goals and specific event goals. *"Immediate" goals* are technique-oriented. A competition sets deadlines to meet those goals (structure or focus). *Focus* is monitoring those outcomes that a person can control. In fact, we can only control those aspects within oneself. Thus, it makes very little sense to worry about the competition and what they are doing for training and races.

Good pain versus bad pain: Pain from exercise is more desirable than neurological pain. Hence, strenuous workouts that mask neurological pain is not a bad thing. My philosophy is that if I am going to be in pain, I may as well be in good pain instead of bad pain. This philosophy makes motivation for training, especially at a high intensity, easier. Strenuous workouts also have the added advantage of making it easier to sleep on those evenings that, in turn, can also effectively treat pain.

Gratitude: Focus on what you can accomplish and not on your limitations. In other words, being grateful for what we have and never obsessing over what we do not have, like a pain-free body, is a key ingredient to cope with pain. [367] Being grateful will go a long way to help people cope with pain and finally come to accept their condition. [368] What does being grateful suggest: *Gratitude* signifies not wanting or wishing to change our destiny. I do not want to change my fate or anything that happened to me. I would not change my neurological disorder, nor would I change the abuse I faced as a child. That sounds strange, but I emerged from these experiences a stronger person. Gratitude indicates accepting your disorder, and not wishing your condition would go away or could be given to someone else. I certainly would not want someone else to have my disorder. Gratitude denotes having a good attitude to cope with adversity. After all, it is how we cope with *adversity* that shapes our personality. Said differently, our personality is less defined with how we may cope with success. Obviously, it is easier to cope with success. With that in mind, many people may let success or power get the best of them when they are no longer humbled by their fortunate circumstances. Hence, success can affect people in a negative manner too. That said, it is much easier to let adversity affect us in a negative manner than success. The bottom line, gratitude conveys an understanding that the situation can always be worse.

Knowing when to stop: Regardless if I exercise or not, pain and fatigue are a daily part of my life. Both pain and fatigue from a disorder and exercise make it difficult to gauge the warning signs indicating when it is time to quit and rest? That said, however, since I fatigue faster than a normal person, and if I were to stop exercising every time I had too much fatigue, I would never get enough effective training. The key for people with normal muscle function is to "know when to say when" and eliminate or scale back workouts when heart rate and power data indicate excessive fatigue or overtraining. The end result, since fatigue is part of my daily life, excessive fatigue is going to be part of my training and racing plans. [369] In fact, I have had some of my best results training or racing on days that I felt very fatigued. Doing well while feeling fatigued is a strange phenomenon and happens because I am prepared to handle any suffering and pain that I may face.

Medications: I take carbamazepine twice per day to cope with some symptoms, including pain. Carbamazepine is an antiseizure medication that has many applications in neurology. I experimented with several antiseizure medications, such as Lyrica and gabapentin, before settling on carbamazepine. Carbamazepine slightly improves pain, cramping, and those annoying buzzing or vibration sensations in my legs. Over time and experimentation, I decreased my dosage to 800 mg per day instead of my initial prescribed dosage of 1200 mg per day. Carbamazepine has many side effects, and dry mouth is the worst culprit.

Mental training: *Mental training* is an important attribute for success in both competitive cycling and coping with a chronic disorder, including pain. In fact, I see little difference between competitive cycling and battling my neurological condition for the following reasons. Although the circumstances are vastly different, both competitive cycling and my neurological condition bring about fear, pain, and stress. Furthermore, both cycling and my neurological disorder require a positive attitude, confidence, motivation, and perseverance to succeed and overcome both fear and pain. In cycling, it is generally the person who is most mentally prepared that wins. Conversely, the person with a strong mental attitude is best equipped to handle their neurological condition.

Manage expectations: Perfect days are rare for most people, and because of my illness, I will never have a perfect day. This means that athletes must constantly adapt to maximize their results. The best technique for adapting is to divide races and training sessions into sections. If one section of a race or training session did not go as expected, do not dwell on missing your goal, and instead, look forward to the next section. This means to focus and concentrate on adopting to the intrinsic and extrinsic factors to find improvement in the next section. [370] My disorder enables me to cope with training pain. This is a huge advantage in races because other competitors spend little time understanding and coping with pain. Of course, excessive pain tolerance makes it difficult to differentiate performance pain from other types of warning pain. Tolerating pain is an advantage in a competition, but if something is really wrong–that I am doing physical harm to my body–I may not realize it. [371] One cycling reference claims that time trialing is 10% aerodynamics, 10% the brain, and 80% the body. The brain aspect consists of pacing strategies or having the ability to set an even pace for the length of the race. While I agree that pacing is important, it is not as important as being mentally prepared to endure pain. I would estimate time trialing is 20% aerodynamics, 5% the brain for pacing strategies, 25% mental acuity to push through pain as well as intrinsic and extrinsic factors, and 50% the body. [372]

Mental attitude: Coping with pain takes the right mental state and attitude. For instance, "being in pain" is a different mental thought process than "having pain." In other words, "Negativity transforms pain into suffering." [373] In particular, I consider my pain and suffering as God's message to change my current path. [374] Having a good mental attitude is a good first step to cope with pain. Remember, regardless of how bad you may think your pain or suffering are, there are always others experiencing much more adversity and pain. If you see yourself as being lucky that you do not have ALS, cancer, or something more sinister, then that will go a long way to help your mental state and attitude moving forward.

Pain management and pain tolerance: Pain management is critical for anyone coping with some sort of chronic pain. Most references about pain management call for the patient to understand their limits and to never overdo it. In particular, one book suggests activities to avoid are "staying in one position for a long period of time, performing repetitive movements, and exercising too much." That said, it is important to evolve and cope with pain how we want to deal with it and not rely on what a book or doctor suggests. References are only guideposts. [375] Obviously, intense cycling training and racing violate most recommendations on how to cope with chronic pain. However, that is not to say I completely ignore the above advice. I stopped doing other physical activities because the pain was not as manageable as it was to cycle. In my opinion, the advice given by most books and professionals is not ideal. The best way to increase pain tolerance is to push the envelope, similar to overload theories, in athletic training. Pain and neurological symptoms are unpredictable and vary greatly hour to hour between those good times and those very painful flare-ups. Hence, managing pain can be complicated and is a never-ending process. [376]

    Practice focus, control, and motivation: *Focus* and *control* also means having the fortitude to acknowledge and learn from our mistakes. Focus is about being even-keel and not berating or congratulating oneself. Focus during a race and training can be difficult, especially during periods of intense pain. During these difficult times, I focus or think about others I know suffering from cancer to push through my pain. Many pro athletes will maintain focus by counting or repeating phrases. Focus also means having a positive attitude because of the way a person thinks directly affects how they train and race. Negative thoughts are counterproductive to meeting deadlines and goals.

Competition eliminates procrastination from a schedule and plan. Competition achieves a purpose or mission, which provides motivation. There are two types of motivations: Extrinsic and intrinsic. *Extrinsic motivation* means that athletes are motivated by money, fame, and awards. *Intrinsic or personal motivation* includes a passion for sport, personal improvement, and the challenge. I find that extrinsic motivation can make athletes complacent. For that reason, I routinely discard my awards, including both work and athletic honors. I do not want to be satisfied with the past; I want to be hungry about achieving new goals in the present and future. Every award I won before the age of 50 has been discarded. In fact, most professional athletes have short memories about winning races because they too want to remain hungry for future successes. All of the above reasons are effective treatments for neurological pain, which is not only masked by the training and racing pain but because motivation and focus shift from pain to another constructive goal. Professional cyclist George Hincapie said, "You can't do cycling half-arsed; you have to be all in, or it is not worth it. The pain is too much." [377]

Putting pain in perspective: It is easy to exaggerate the effects of pain. We tend to believe that others have it easier because there was an injustice placed on us.

Nevertheless, let's face facts: "We cannot know other people's experiences simply by observing them, just as our internal strife remains largely invisible to onlookers." [378] Besides, people may choose to be in pain: Giving birth, training, and climbing Everest without oxygen. Hence, pain is not necessarily a bad thing. Pain is a way to understand limitations and to populate the world. In other words, pain is a necessity for life. In fact, most people who have a genetic mutation that prevents them from feeling pain tend to die young. [379] My favorite saying is, "You only live once." This phrase means making the most of life instead of choosing to live in misery and self-pity. Deborah Barrett said it well: "At times, you may decide it is worthwhile to accomplish something, even if it guarantees additional pain." [380]

Sleep and rest: Sleep and rest are essential to cope with chronic neurological symptoms and pain. It is not always easy to get the daily recommended amount of sleep. I need assistance sleeping and take an antidepressant (amitriptyline) to try to shut off my brain from worrying about issues outside my control and zolpidem for sleep. They help some, but when I have to get up to urinate several times a night, this diminishes the effect of the drugs. Amitriptyline has an added benefit in that it can also be used to treat chronic pain. Amitriptyline has many side effects, but the only side effect I exhibit is a dry mouth. [381] Remember, even a partial night's rest reduces the effectiveness of the immune system. I do not sleep well the night before competitions, but that is fairly common and is called *anticipatory sleep disruptions*. Anticipatory sleep disruptions occur because people worry about if they thought of everything they need for the next day's activities. [382] Naps may be an effective way to make up for lost sleep, but when I nap, I never sleep well that evening. Hence, naps may be counterproductive and may not ultimately help with overall sleep and rest. There are many different types of sleep insomnia that I suffer from to varying degrees: (1) *sleep onset insomnia* is having trouble getting to sleep; (2) *maintenance insomnia* is getting up several times during the night; (3) *early a.m. insomnia* is getting up early and being unable to return to sleep; and (4) *compulsive urination insomnia* is having to wake up throughout the night to urinate. [383]

Stimulate endorphins: Pain management books do not recommend competition and pushing beyond your capabilities. That said, doctors and pain management books usually leave it up to the patient to determine what pain level is acceptable [384] Remember, "Cardiovascular exercise releases endorphins and other chemicals with morphine-like properties into your bloodstream that relieve pain and elevate the mood." [385] Although the high is short-lived, it is possible to push through exercise pain. However, chronic pain becomes difficult to tolerate when the body produces fewer endorphins to counteract the pain. [386]

Taming emotions and expectations: Humans can condition the mind to cope with pain by taming emotions and expectations for pain relief. For instance, patients may find pain relief from a placebo treatment because it provides hope or some expectation of pain relief. If pain is not expected to go away, then the pain gets worse and vice versa. The following excerpt on emotions and pain is insightful: "Negative emotions generally increase clinical pain, particularly pain unpleasantness, and are consistent predictors of pain behaviors, and disability". Furthermore, "Emotions that are pain-related or directed toward the self, appear to have the most deleterious effect." [387] The bottom line is that emotions can turn pain into suffering. Why do emotions and expectations play such a dramatic role in pain management? The answer to this is simple: the brain has two opposing forces for any body function. Like feeling happy or sad. In the brain, cholecystokinin (CCK) is a chemical initiating the feeling of pain.

However, the CCK antagonist, proglumide, can counter CCK and inhibit pain. [388] In other words, controlling our emotions and expectations for pain treatment can alleviate pain symptoms by signaling the brain to inhibit pain. Emotions, fear conditioning, spatial learning, memory, and cognitive or rational thinking are controlled by the hippocampus portion of the brain. Unfortunately, over the age of 55, the hippocampus and other important parts of the brain begin to atrophy at a rate of 1-2% per year on account of increased apoptosis, decreased proliferation, and degeneration of nerve cells. Thus, pain may be enhanced in aging adults. [389] The best way to counteract emotions and the effects of aging on pain is through gene expression alterations by manipulating emotions, thought, and memories which can create new neural connections (neural plasticity). [390]

Training the brain: Many individuals coping with pain have heard the expression, "It hurts me just as much as before, but it no longer bothers me." This actually happens and can be "reflected in extensive training of the limbic system in functional brain imaging activations as well as in neuroanatomical connectivity." [391] Hence, similar to the previous point, it is essential to exercise our brain limbic and connectivity system for effective pain treatment. The easiest way to accomplish this is by exercising the brain with new information every day, daily exercise, sleep, intermittent fasting, and eating right. In essence, patients can teach both the conscience and reality-self to cope with pain.

Therapeutic methods: Hot and cold applications can treat pain. Cold treatments are the best way to heal sore muscles. However, the cold makes me stiff and enhances other uncomfortable symptoms such as pain. Hence, I rely on hot baths with Epsom salts. [392] Besides, some evidence suggests that sauna applications can enhance time trial performance by as much as 2%. The reasoning behind time trial improvement happens as the core temperature of the body is elevated; it initiates a parasympathetic response, including increased heart rate simulating a training workout. There is also some evidence that flotation tanks with Epsom salt decrease cortisol that may impair training and exercise. Most training recovery plans include a cool-down period of light exercise to rid the body of lactate. Recovery plans may also include compression clothing, massage, water immersion, and electrical stimulation. That said, water immersion, compression clothing, and massage are said to have the most impact, but access and expense for water immersion treatments and massage do not necessarily make them the best options. Furthermore, some studies indicate that massage may impair lactate removal. [393] Moreover, since I train in cool weather (generally under 60 degrees), hot baths have the added benefit to prepare me for races in hot and humid climates. The bottom line, I have fewer symptoms and pain following a bath, and it also provides a comfortable atmosphere to relax.

Patrick Bohan

Chapter 9: My Motor Symptoms

Motor nerves direct muscle movements. The *descending motor pathway* encompasses the **upper motor neuron system (UMNS)** located from the brain to the spine and the **lower motor neuron system (LMNS)** located from the spine to the motor units. *Motor units* are comprised of peripheral nerves, neuromuscular junction, and muscle fibers. My motor symptoms encompass muscle fasciculations, muscle cramps, paresthesia, numbness, muscle weakness, muscle atrophy, muscle stiffness, muscle heaviness, muscle contraction concerns, diminished reflexes, and feet swelling. Before discussing my symptoms, I elaborate on the science of ions and ion channels because they play a big role in motor and other bodily functions.

The Science of Ions and Ion Channels

Ions [394 395 396 397 398 399]

Ions are charged molecules and the most common ones are sodium (Na+), potassium (K+), chlorine (Cl-), hydrogen (H+), hydroxyl (OH-), phosphate, (HPO_4-), bicarbonate (HCO_3-), magnesium (Mg++), and calcium (Ca++). Ion imbalance is prevalent among athletes, who may lose critical nutrients when they perspire. An *ion* is an element or molecule that has a positive or negative charge. Ions with a positive charge have lost an electron or, in the case of calcium, lost two electrons. Conversely, a negative charge signifies the ion gained an electron. *Ion levels* are measured in the blood or the extracellular serum fluid. If, for example, serum sodium (Na+) is deficient, then cellular concentrations of sodium are generally abundant—and vice versa. Ions are also commonly referred to as electrolytes. *K+ ions* commonly appear within a cell, whereas Na+, Ca++, and Cl- are more commonly found outside the cell in the extracellular fluid.

A *cell membrane* comprises lipids, and water-soluble elements do not pass through a cell membrane. Water-soluble molecules are salts such as sodium chloride (NaCl–table salt), potassium chloride (KCl), and calcium-chloride (Ca_2Cl). When these salts diffuse in water, it leaves behind charged particles called ions: K+, Na+, Ca++, and Cl-. Since these ions do not naturally pass through cellular membranes, they need the assistance of voltage-gated ion channels, or ion pumps, to accomplish the task.

An *ion deficiency or surplus* is the most common reason for muscle dysfunction and paresthesia sensations. Thus, ion level blood work is the first step in the diagnosis process of PNH type symptoms.

Hyponatremia is a low concentration of sodium (Na+) in the extracellular space. The outcome of hyponatremia results in both water and sodium diffusing into the cellular space leading to cellular swelling and death. Symptoms for *hypochloremia*, or low concentrations of chlorine, mimic hyponatremia.

Hypernatremia is a surplus concentration of sodium (Na+) in the extracellular space. Hypernatremia also indicates that both water and sodium will diffuse into the extracellular space leading to dehydration, muscle weakness, muscle twitching, muscle cramping, and muscle fatigue. Peripheral nerve hyperexcitation (PNH) disorders mimic less severe hypernatremia symptoms. More severe symptoms of high sodium levels include weight loss, fever, and coma. Symptoms for ***hyperchloremia***, or surplus levels of chlorine, mimic hypernatremia.

Hypokalemia is a low concentration of potassium (K+) ions in the extracellular space. Losses of ions such as potassium and sodium usually happen after strenuous exercise or from gastrointestinal distress such as diarrhea. Hypokalemia symptoms include decreased neuromuscular excitation or the opposite of what happens in PNH disorders. Both hyperkalemia and hypokalemia may result from hereditary mutations discussed later. [400] Hypokalemia can be brought about by the consumption of alcohol and high carbohydrate meals. [401]

Hyperkalemia results from an increase in extracellular potassium (K+). High levels of extracellular potassium mean that the muscle cell membrane potential is more positive, which can result in muscle excitability since cells depolarize more easily. The topic of membrane potential and polarization will be discussed in the section on ion channels. Hyperkalemia also results in a change in the cell membrane permeability leading to several problems, including hypoxia, acidosis (low PH levels), and insulin deficiency. Therefore, it is easy to understand why people with diabetes have peripheral neuropathy and or PNH symptoms. Permeability is the process at which ions, chemicals, and water flow between inter and extracellular fluids. Depending on the level that potassium surges in extracellular serum, hyperkalemia symptoms may vary. However, some of the symptoms can include elevated neuromuscular activity, distal tingling, intestinal cramping, diarrhea, muscle weakness, numbness, hyperactive muscle reflexes, loss of muscle tone, and periodic paralysis.

Hyperkalemia can result from fasting, high potassium intake, and cold temperatures. An increase in calcium concentrations in the intracellular fluid may override the effects of hyperkalemia.

The following equation shows the relationship between calcium (Ca++), potassium (K+), and phosphate (HPO$_4$-) ions: [402] (Ca++) * (HPO$_4$-) = K+.

Hence, an increase in calcium ions leads to a decrease in phosphate ions and vice versa. The regulation of calcium and phosphate ions is administered by endocrine system chemicals such as parathyroid hormone (PTH), calcitriol hormone, calcitonin hormone, and vitamin D. When Ca++ ions diminish, PTH, vitamin D, and calcitriol initiate the reabsorption of Ca++. Conversely, when Ca++ ions are abundant, calcitonin activation inhibits the absorption of Ca++ ions.

Hypocalcemia, or deficient serum calcium, may arise from the overproduction of calcitonin. Chronic hypocalcemia leads to escalated muscular activity, tingling, paresthesia, muscle spasms, tetany, and hyperactive bowels.

Hypercalcemia, or a calcium surplus, might result from the overproduction of PTH. Chronic hypercalcemia can lead to calcified kidneys, fatigue, weakness, depression, calcium deposits (calcinosis), and constipation.

Hypophosphatemia, or phosphate deficiency, leads to deranged nerve and muscle function from insufficient ATP or energy production, in addition to clotting impairments, a greater risk of infection, confusion, numbness, and irritability.

Hyperphosphatemia, or a phosphate surplus, results in symptoms similar to hypocalcemia.

Hypomagnesemia, or magnesium deficiency, leads to muscle cramps, behavioral changes, irritability, tetany, and ataxia. *Tetany* is a condition characterized by muscle spasms, and *ataxia* is a condition characterized by repeated deviations in normal muscle movement patterns.

Hypermagnesemia, or a magnesium over-production, results in the movement of potassium out of the cellular plasma. Hypermagnesemia leads to depressed muscle contractions and nerve function, muscle weakness, drowsiness, lethargy, and nausea. PTH also regulates magnesium.

PH [403 404 405 406 407 408]

PH (acid-base regulation), or hydron ion regulation, is vital for homeostasis. Even slight changes in cellular PH can negatively alter tissue and organ function and the basics are as follows: (1) Water is neutral and has a PH of 7; (2) PH can range between 1 and 14; (3) a PH between 1 and 7 is acidic, and a PH between 7 and 14 is basic; (4) normal cellular PH is between 7.35 to 7.4, which is slightly basic; (5) when the PH drops below 7.35, it forms a condition called acidosis, and when the PH is above 7.4, it forms a condition called alkalosis; (6) since the human body has more OH- ions than H+, the consequence is a more basic or alkaline PH of around 7.4; and (7) cellular ions are routinely exchanged to maintain PH homeostasis. For instance, to prevent acidosis when potassium leaves the cell, hydrogen ion uptake compensates for cellular metabolic changes. The opposite is true for preventing alkalosis. *Uptake* is a term used to describe the movement of ions or molecules from the extracellular fluid into the intercellular fluid.

Alkalosis, or elevated PH, causes muscle weakness, paresthesia, muscle excitability, including seizures, cardiac arrhythmia, and muscle cramps catalyzed by electrolyte losses in the intracellular fluid, including ions such as calcium, potassium, bicarbonate, and chlorine. Alkalosis may also promote the formation of lactic acid and cell division.

Acidosis inhibits the function of potassium channels, chloride channels, Na-K (sodium-potassium) ion pumps, intercellular connections, and cell division. On the other hand, acidosis stimulates the function of Na-H (sodium-hydrogen) ion pumps leading to an uptake in cellular sodium. An uptake of sodium leads to cellular swelling and necrosis. Acidosis is associated with autoimmune disorders such as diabetes and inflammation. In a state of acidosis and inflammation, various proteins and cytokines, such as interleukins (IL-2, IL-6, and IL-12), are elevated.

The critical point to remember from this section is that when ion homeostasis is upset either in the inter or extracellular spaces, the result can lead to many problems, including those found in many neurological disorders (although they are not necessarily related). Thus, the first step in the diagnosis of muscle cramping and fasciculations (muscle twitching) symptoms are blood tests to check ion levels. Mineral supplements are commonly used to treat ion depletion.

The depolarization process of a nerve cell membrane is complex (see Figure 9.1). [409] First, a resting nerve cell membrane has a potential of -70mV, which denotes that the inside of the membrane is -70mV, as compared to the outside of the membrane. ***Depolarization*** is the process of changing the polarity of the cell membrane voltage from negative to positive. ***Repolarization*** is the process of changing the cell membrane voltage polarity back to its equilibrium state of -70mV. Second, when a signal arrives at the cell nerve membrane, the voltage-gated ion channels start the depolarization process resulting in sodium ions flowing into the cell, increasing the membrane potential. When the membrane potential increases by 10mV or 15mV to -60mV or -55mV (reaches a depolarization threshold voltage), the membrane rapidly depolarizes to a value of +30 to +50mV. This change in the membrane potential of about 100 to 120mV from its resting value. Finally, the impulse produced by cellular depolarization travels the length of the neuron (nerve) cell. The cell membrane potential is repolarized, returning to its resting potential of -70mV once the membrane stimulus ceases. Repolarization happens when voltage-gated potassium channels open to allow an outflow of potassium from the cell.

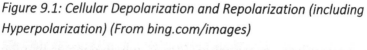

Figure 9.1: Cellular Depolarization and Repolarization (including Hyperpolarization) (From bing.com/images)

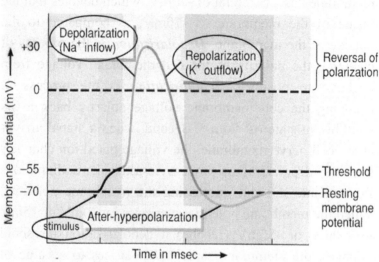

One important thing to understand from this section is that it does not take a substantial metabolic change in cellular ion concentrations to result in muscle excitability. If a cell membrane potential is changed from an average resting value of -70mV to, say, -65mV, then a muscle may twitch more readily because it is easier for it to reach the -60mV threshold voltage to depolarize. Thus, there is less margin of error between the resting membrane voltage and the threshold voltage (5mV instead of 10mV). If the cellular resting membrane potential elevates to a value above the threshold voltage, say, for example -58mV, then the muscle may be paralyzed since it would become stuck in a depolarized state.

Urinary System [410]

The kidneys control the urinary system and its function include: First, regulating mineral-rich urine, they are critical to regulating electrolytes such as potassium, magnesium, calcium, chlorine, sodium, hydrogen, and other ions. Thus, the kidneys are critical for maintaining pH homeostasis. Second, controlling and regulating other molecules such as glucose, proteins, amino acids, and lactate.

When the kidneys fail (*renal failure*), survival is not possible without dialysis. When electrolyte or ion concentrations are no longer in a state of homeostasis, numerous issues may arise. Examples include hyponatremia (low sodium), hypernatremia (high sodium), hypokalemia (low potassium), hyperkalemia (high potassium), hypocalcemia (low levels of calcium), hypercalcemia (high calcium), hypomagnesemia (low magnesium), or hypermagnesemia (high magnesium). Disruptions in ion levels can lead to heart arrhythmia, renal failure, cardiac failure, cirrhosis of the liver, muscle weakness, and temporary muscle paralysis.

My Motor Symptoms
Fasciculations, Cramps, and Exercise Intolerance

My muscle fasciculations (twitching) occur everywhere, but most notably in the calves. My twitching symptoms generally include the following muscles of the calves: *gastrocnemius, soleus, peroneus longus, flexor hallucis longus*, and it even looks as if the Achilles tendon twitches. Muscle fiber activity in the calves also correlates to where I feel the most pain, followed by the hands, feet, and quads. [411]

Fasciculation is a medical term given to muscle twitching and comes from the word fasciculus. A fasciculus is a bundle of muscle fibers. Some fasciculi contain as many as 200 muscle fibers. Fasciculi are combined to form a muscle. [412] Muscle twitching is the most common symptom for peripheral nerve disorders like BFS, CFS, and IS. Muscle twitching usually starts in the calves, but fasciculations can happen in any muscle. Every human being on the planet will have fasciculations from time to time. However, in some PNH patients, the fasciculations are chronic because the twitching never stops. [413 414 415]

I postulate fasciculation activity is partly to blame for muscle cramping. There are some misconceptions about cramping only occurring due to dehydration. That statement is only partially true. While cramping and dehydration are related, cramps can start anytime when the muscles are fatigued, even before they are dehydrated. It is easy to surmise that patients with a PNH disorder have muscles that fatigue quicker on account of their constant muscle fiber activity, and henceforth, they are more prone to painful cramping.

Exercise intolerance is an indirect or secondary symptom occurring from the primary symptoms of PNH. For instance, muscle cramping, stiffness, pain, and fatigue result in exercise intolerance. Thus, a vast majority of people with PNH symptoms will not exercise, and even fewer people will exercise intensely since it is just too painful. Of course, when people fail to use their muscles, weakness and atrophy will follow, only leading to more fear that their illness is more sinister.

Paresthesia: Numbness, Pins and Needles, Tingling, and Vibration [416]

Paresthesia symptoms are quite common in the hands and feet for peripheral neuropathy. A medical term given to the symptoms of numbness, tingling, and pins and needles is called paresthesia. *Paresthesia* is the sensation that happens when the hands and or feet go to sleep. Paresthesia symptoms are generally defined as only having motor involvement. In fact, PNH disorders are generally only considered a disorder of the motor nerves. However, I hypothesize that paresthesia has both motor and sensory involvement because motor symptoms also seem responsible for dulling the sense of touch. Case in point, I struggle to open and to close certain types of food containers, pick up a coin, or button or unbutton a shirt due to both a lack of motor and sensory nerve function. One reference on peripheral nerve disorders suggests, "Nonspecific complaints of numbness and paresthesia, may represent either an associated peripheral neuropathy or an analogous overactivity of sensory nerves." [417] The preceding statement suggests that paresthesia can also be a sensory symptom.

What does a vibration sensation feel like? It is as if the muscles in my legs are a guitar string, and when at rest, the guitar string remains active, and vibrations will go up and down the length of the muscle. Fortunately, carbamazepine medication helps to diminish those annoying vibration feelings, cramping, and some pain produced by the muscle stiffness. [418] Carbamazepine does not eliminate these symptoms, but it can lessen its impact.

Without question, motor-sensory symptoms have had a huge effect on my life, especially my physical activities. These symptoms forced me to give up rock climbing and wrestling. With both weakness and diminished sensations in my hands and feet, it was undoubtedly a safety concern to continue these activities. Since cycling can increase the effects of paresthesia in the hands from holding the handlebars for long periods of time, I migrated toward becoming a time trial specialist. Time trials have several advantages in minimizing paresthesia symptoms and they are outlined below.

Cyclists use aero bars in time trial events, which allow them to apply little to no pressure on the hands, so paresthesia symptoms are not exacerbated. I am actually a terrible cyclist. I believe a vast majority of people cycle better than me in terms of bike handling skills. My only true asset is that I am faster on a bike than most people. My subpar bike handling skills primarily arise from a lack of confidence brought about by the motor-sensory symptoms. That said, bike handling skills are not as important in time trials as they are in other mass-start cycling events such as road races and criteriums for the following reasons. First, mass start events generally have many more turns to navigate. Mass start races require cycling in close proximity with other cyclists. As mentioned earlier, in time trials, riders are sent off individually in 30-second intervals. Time trials are individual events, and therefore, no drafting is allowed. Conversely, in mass start races, riders are shoulder to shoulder navigating difficult and fast turns while other riders are drafting 1 inch off the back wheel of a competitor who is doing the same to the racer in front of them. Road races can have high-speed downhill segments (over 50 mph) requiring solid bike handling skills. Time trial races are generally much shorter than road races. Bad motor-sensory symptoms at the start of a race are bad enough but deteriorating hand and feet sensation in long races is even more concerning.

Weakness and Atrophy

My hands and feet are a big concern when it comes to muscle pain, weakness, and atrophy, and it may be partly explained by several symptoms. For example, *Dupuytren's contracture* may be associated with sensory and motor symptoms such as paresthesia, numbness, and Raynaud's syndrome. Dupuytren's contracture describes fingers permanently stuck in a contracted position; movement is impossible without surgery or medical treatment. [419] More specifically, Dupuytren's contracture is the result of a buildup of collagen in the palm. [430]

Not surprisingly, I have also had a keloid scar from a deep wound. *Keloid scars* are uncharacteristically large scars caused by an excess amount of collagen and elastin utilized in the wound healing process. Keloid scarring is an adverse side effect of a prolonged inflammation process. Prolonged inflammation also means the activation time of growth hormones that respond with collagen and elastin is lengthened. Hence, it may be postulated that prolonged hand inflammation from a neurological condition may activate growth hormones, which respond with collagen creating problems such as Dupuytren's contracture.

To avoid more contractures, it is recommended to stretch the fingers as well as use personal hand massages to break up the collagen deposits. Contractures that happen from a neurological disease usually originate from prolonged muscle spasms, resulting in rigidity and contractures. [421] My Dupuytren's contracture was not a result of any prolonged muscle spasm.

Bloodwork is conclusive that I do not have arthritis, but nonetheless, I have painful bone spurs on my knuckles. These bone spurs are not the outcome of elevated calcium levels but may be more readily explained by *osteoarthritis (OA)*. OA is a joint disease that is disabling and usually inflicts older individuals. OA is characterized by damaged or lost cartilage, new bone formations, bone changes, and thickening joint capsules. OA was originally considered a noninflammatory disorder, but that changed since inflammatory interleukins may be involved. Symptoms of OA include pain, stiffness, swelling, tenderness, and deformity of the joints. In the fingers, these deformities are called Heberden and Bouchard nodes. OA has no specific etiology. [422]

A medical exhibit at the Huntsman Games is to test participants' grip strength. I take this test every year, and the past seven years, my grip strength in both my right and left hands have gone from one standard deviation above average to one standard deviation below average. That is a very sharp decline in strength. It is also important to note that many articles indicate there is a correlation between grip strength, heart health, mortality, and longevity. [423] I have hypothesized that there is a link between my OA, declining grip strength, and Dupuytren's contractures to my neurological condition.

Swelling

Whenever I am standing or walking for over an hour, I become very stiff, and my feet and ankles start to swell. The swelling is never severe, but nonetheless, it is painful, and I need to sit. Swelling is common in other types of disorders associated with chronic pain, such as fibromyalgia. *Swelling* is the consequence of an accumulation of lymph fluid. When the lymph node system becomes constricted due to muscle stiffness, constipation, or other irregular body functions brought about by dysfunctional sensory, motor, or autonomic nerves, lymph fluid fails to flow through the body properly, and it may pool in various locations. [424] For example, since I endure both muscle stiffness and bowel motility dysfunction, these malfunctions may explain the swelling in the feet or the inability of the lymph fluid to flow through its proper channels.

Heaviness [425]

Another common motor symptom is a heavy feeling in the legs (fatigue), and in particular, the quads. *"Heavy legs"* is a common symptom of cyclists, especially after intense workouts. Of course, cycling places considerable stress on the quads since these muscles account for over 80% of the power generated. Studies indicate a cyclist's legs vary between a normal and heavy feeling during the course of training and competition. [426] At the same time, regardless of my level of rest, my legs feel heavy all the time.

My *creatine kinase (CK)* is generally two or three times over the maximum specification. As we learned, CK is an indication of muscle damage. For instance, a heart attack patient's CK would be 100 times higher than the max specification due to massive muscle damage. Even moderate exercise can elevate CK because of muscle damage. That said, my high CK may be explained by both vigorous exercise and the chronic denervation process in the quad muscles, possibly resulting in constant "heavy legs".

I learned that my energy crossover point started very early in the stress test, but the test also revealed that my resting lactate levels were also very high before I was under stress. Normal resting lactate is between 0.5 to 1.0 mmol/L. My resting lactate was about 2.0 mmol/L, and the measurement was taken after two rest days. Thus, it may be hypothesized my resting lactate could be slightly higher the day after intense training. Unsurprisingly, these elevated lactate levels correlate with the high CK levels. Hence, it should come as no surprise that lactate is also a measure of muscle tissue damage. [427] The word "elevated" denotes the readings are high but still within an acceptable range, while "high" suggests the readings are out of specification. An overproduction of lactate is sometimes called **hyperlactatemia**, and symptoms for this condition include unexplained tiredness, fatigue, cold hands and feet, and heavy legs in cyclists. My heavy leg phenomenon worsens later in the day and after a vigorous workout. The heavy leg phenomenon persists on rest days, but it is a little less extreme. Elevated lactate and high CK may be a byproduct of the chronic denervation process happing in my quads, and it may also explain why I lay down for well over 12 hours each day.

The good news is that my training plan was changed to optimize my fat and carbohydrate energy systems (change my crossover point from 50% to over 75% of max heart rate). The bad news is that the source of the denervation process leading to elevated lactate and high CK remains unknown. It is unknown if these abnormal results are from neuropathy, CFS, or some other unidentified reason.

The denervation process in my quads is the biggest mystery of my disorder. ***Denervation*** is the process where muscle motoneuron and motor unit function is lost, which is definitely a source of muscle damage. Fewer motoneurons and functional motor units in the quad muscles correspond to less power in cycling. Initially, during exercise, muscles compensate by recruiting healthy motor units to replace diseased or denervated motor units, but since there are fewer healthy motor units, muscles fatigue faster, and this can certainly be a plausible explanation for the heavy legs feeling.

Muscle Contraction

Most muscle abnormalities associated with PNH disorders encompass muscle firing problems such as twitching or fasciculations. However, people with CFS also have contraction dysfunction that results in muscle cramping. People with IS may have cramping as well as a delayed relaxation from a contracted state (myotonia). It is estimated, by one neurologist, that my quad muscles may contract up to twelve times slower than a normal muscle. The delayed muscle relaxation from a contracted state is limited to my upper leg, and the symptoms are symmetrical. In particular, the contraction malfunction affects three of the four quadriceps muscles: *Vastus lateralis*, *rectus femoris*, and *vastus medialis*.

Isaac syndrome is considered a myotonia disorder. Since my first two EMGs and nerve conduction studies were negative, the assumption that the contraction malfunction was myotonia was logical because myotonic discharges may or may not be present on an EMG. To determine the root cause of the delayed relaxation from a contracted state, I was tested for a variety of hereditary and acquired muscle diseases, including myotonic dystrophy type 2, rippling muscle disease, stiff person syndrome, and small fiber neuropathy (a skin biopsy). After these tests came back negative, it was presumed I had a myotonia condition such as IS. However, a third EMG (five years later) came back positive for denervation in the quad muscles. Hence, the myotonia presumption was incorrect, and the cause of the denervation process remains unknown.

Diminished Reflexes

Tendons are strong, stiff, dense regular collagenous connective tissue. Tendons are comprised of collagen and fibroblast cells and are responsible for transferring muscle forces to the bone. Deep tendon reflex testing is probably the most important test of a neurological exam because diminished reflexes are sometimes the earliest sign of neurological dysfunction. *Reflexes* are important because they help individuals maintain an upright position to stand and walk. Reflexes also serve as a protective function. For instance, reflexes protect against any unexpected forces while walking and standing. Remember, spindle muscles or tendons sense muscle tension, and they are important for coordination and balance. Generally, reflexes are graded on a 0 to 4 scale with a 0 indicating absent reflexes, a one representing slightly diminished but normal reflexes, a 2 denoting normal reflexes, a 3 signifying slightly hyperactive but normal reflexes, and a 4 indicating abnormally hyperactive reflexes. Individuals with normal reflexes still may present with a neuromuscular or muscular disorder. Individuals with decreased or absent reflexes generally present with a peripheral nerve disorder. Conversely, individuals with increased reflexes generally present with a disorder of the upper neuron system located in the spinal cord or the brain of the central nervous system. My deep tendon reflexes vary from absent (Achilles) to slightly hyperactive. Reduced or absent reflexes will impact balance and coordination as well as negatively impact muscle power generation. [428]

Superficial reflexes refer to reflexes of the skin and mucous membrane. Superficial reflexes are different from deep tendon reflexes in that they respond slowly to stimulus, fatigue easier, and are not always present. In lower motor neuron diseases, superficial reflexes are generally normal but can be decreased or absent in conditions such as peripheral neuropathy. In upper motor neuron diseases, superficial reflexes may be decreased, normal, or increased. [429] *Pathological reflexes* are reflexes not found in "normal" people. *Associated movements* are unintentional or involuntary movements. Both pathological reflexes and associated movement conditions are not found in people with lower motor neuron disorders of the peripheral nerves, muscles, and neuromuscular junction, such as peripheral neuropathy. However, pathological reflexes may present in some upper motor disorders of the central nervous system. [430]

We previously learned subconscious or involuntary movements are those the body completes without human control like autonomic organ functions, including digestion, heart rate, respiration, and temperature regulation. Subconscious movements also include many reflex actions. There are dozens of reflex actions activated to prevent injury, including shivering, coughing, yawning, changing of pupil size to different stimuli, or various tendon reflexes such as knee jerk or ankle jerk (Achilles). The most important *deep tendon reflexes* are for the triceps, biceps, brachioradialis, patellar (knee), Achilles, and plantar reflex tests. A *stretch reflex* refers to the involuntary contraction of a muscle in response to an unexpected increase in its length. The muscle quickly reverts back to its normal resting state. [431] [432]

Muscle Stiffness

I theorize, muscle stiffness, like exercise intolerance, balance, and heaviness, is the outcome of other primary symptoms such as diminished reflexes, fasciculations, cramps, paresthesia, and denervation. Said differently, some symptoms, such as muscle stiffness, are a sub symptom that results from the primary symptoms of the neurological disorder.

Chapter 10: My Autonomic Symptoms

The Science of the Autonomic Nervous System [433] [434]

As we learned earlier, *Autonomic nerves* supervise unconscious functions, including blood pressure, heart rate, sweating, sexual drive, and bowel motility. The *autonomic nervous system* comprises a sympathetic nervous system and a parasympathetic nervous system. The sympathetic system's nerves originate from the thoracic and lumbar regions of the spine (T1 to T12 and L1 to L3). See Figure 8.1 for clarity and Table 10.1 for specific nerve functions. The parasympathetic system nerves originate from the cranial nerves (CN III, VII, IX, and X) or the sacral region of the spine (S2 to S4). See Figure 8.1 for clarity and Table 10.1 for specific nerve functions.

The *sympathetic nervous system* (SNS) is responsible for the stress response to a stimulus. It is sometimes referred to as the *"fight or flight" system*, and the parasympathetic nervous system is responsible for restorative functions such as rest and digestion. The sympathetic nervous system controls the opposite functions of the parasympathetic nervous system. It dilates pupils, increases saliva production, enhances bronchial dilation, and increases heart rate. It also elevates blood pressure and increases sweating, and escalates sphincter contractions, while decreasing intestinal motility. The SNS may be activated by emotions (stress), decreased blood pressure, pain, exercise, numerous prescription drugs, and hypoglycemia. SNS failure is associated with autonomic system failure or hypotension, as well as diabetes, alcoholism, or autoimmune disease. [435] [436] The *parasympathetic nervous system (PNS)* controls the opposite function of the SNS, including decreasing pupil dilation, limiting sweating, minimizing contractions of the stomach, gut, bladder, and bronchi muscles. It also decreases the secretion of tears and saliva, increases the gastrointestinal system's motility, and promotes glycogen synthesis and impotence. [437] [438]

Since most nerves do not innervate muscles and organs directly, electrical signals must be converted into chemical signals, called neurotransmitters, at the nerve ending (see Figure 10.1). Nerve endings and organs or muscles are separated by what is called a *synapse or synaptic cleft*. A synapse or synaptic cleft is a narrow gap filled with extracellular fluid. The objective of *neurotransmitters* is to transverse the synaptic cleft to deliver the signal to the muscle or organ cells. For muscles, the junction comprising of the nerve ending, synaptic cleft, and a muscle cell is called the *neuromuscular junction*. The primary neurotransmitters in the autonomic nervous system are acetylcholine (ACh) and noradrenaline, which activate nicotinic receptors at the neuromuscular junction or organ membrane. Neurotransmitters cross the synapse and bind with nicotinic receptors located on muscle or organ cells. Neurotransmitter chemical signals are converted back to electrical signals once ACh or noradrenaline initiate muscle or organ cells to depolarize voltage-gated ion channels.

Figure 10.1: The Neuromuscular Junction (From bing.com/images)

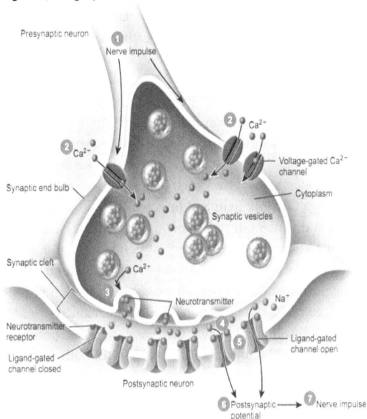

Information between the sympathetic and parasympathetic nervous systems is processed in the hypothalamus whose objective is to maintain homeostasis. More specifically, "The hypothalamus is a small gland in the brain. It regulates eating, drinking, and sexual urges. It also regulates the autonomic nervous system, which controls many autonomic functions of the body. These functions include the rate at which your heart beats, digestion, and how widely your blood vessels dilate at any given time." During autonomic regulation, the hypothalamus signals the pituitary gland, which, in turn, signals the adrenal glands. These glands are a pair of tiny glands located on the top of the kidneys. The adrenal glands produce adrenalin and cortisol under times of stress to regulate the autonomic nerves. The entire autonomic system may dysfunction from an autoimmune disease. Furthermore, autoimmune disease and atrophy can be brought about by the many symptoms described in this chapter, such as hyperhidrosis, temperature regulation, and changes in the skin, hair, and fingernails. [439]

Most disorders of the autonomic nervous system affect both the cardio and respiratory systems such as multiple system atrophy (MSA), dysautonomia (dysfunction of both parasympathetic and sympathetic systems), Guillen-Barré syndrome (GBS), disorders of the hypothalamus, disorders of the neuromuscular junction, and various peripheral neuropathies. It's rare, albeit possible, when both the cardio and respiratory systems are spared from autonomic disease. For instance, Table 10.1 illustrates how cranial nerve X (the vagus nerve, CN X) administers many functions within the parasympathetic nervous system. Thus, any damage to CN X usually results in the autonomic dysfunction of many organs. [440]

Table 10.1: Innervation of the Autonomic Nervous System [441]

Organ or Gland	Parasympathetic	Sympathetic
Eye	CN III	T1
Salivatory Glands	CN VII	T1

Parotid Gland	CN IX	T1
Heart	CN X	T1–T4
Lungs	CN X	T4
Stomach	CN X	T5–T11
Small Intestines	CN X	T5–T11
Suprarenal Glands	CN X	T5–T11
Kidney	CN X	T12
Large Intestines, Colon, Rectum	CN X, S2–S4	T5–T11, L1–L2
Bladder	S2–S4	L1
Sex Organs	S2–S4	L2

My Autonomic Symptoms

My autonomic symptoms associated with the neurological disease are vast and encompass lightheadedness, cold hands and feet, dry mouth, hyperhidrosis, bladder dysfunction, hair loss, changes to skin and fingernails, digestive dysfunction, high blood pressure, headaches, and inability to detect low blood sugar. This section analyzes each of the symptoms and attempts to determine which ones are best explained by my neurological condition.

Dry Mouth

Nerves responsible for saliva production are cranial nerves V, VII, and IX. Dry mouth is from the limited production of saliva. As people age or become stressed, the number of acinar cells decreases, which inhibits saliva production. [442] Dry mouth is more troublesome than it sounds, and it produces three problems. It interferes with sleep. Humidifiers do not help, and mouth moisturizers only help for short periods of time. I have been on a mission the past few years to condition myself to sleep with my mouth closed, and that has worked with some success. Dry mouth also is problematic when riding a bike in a dry climate, especially since I am a mouth-breather. When competing, I cannot get enough oxygen into my system by breathing solely through my nose, causing dry mouth. Since time trial races are short, I do not intake any water or food during competitions. Besides, it is difficult to consume fluids when you are out of breath. My solution is to put a slow dissolve energy food source called a "Shot Block" under my tongue. It is not ideal, but it keeps my mouth moisturized. Lastly, dry mouth is the primary culprit leading to a dull, but a very annoying daily headache.

Chronic dry mouth may be associated with an autoimmune disorder called Sjögren's syndrome. [443] Neuropathy symptoms can appear in up to 22% of patients with Sjögren's syndrome. Besides dry mouth, Sjögren's syndrome symptoms may include sensory tingling and numbness in the limbs as well. [444] However, it is most likely that my dry mouth is not from Sjögren's syndrome or any neurological disorder, but instead, a side effect of medications, from increasing age, elevated blood pressure, or from a hypersensitive reaction to certain foods. Reducing dosages of my medications to a bare minimum and healthy eating helps to alleviate some dry mouth symptoms.

Sweating or Hyperhidrosis and Temperature Regulation

Profuse sweating can also be related to neurological disorders. Profuse sweating or *hyperhidrosis* is a symptom of PNH when it affects the central nervous system or the cranial nerves. Usually, when Isaac syndrome progresses in such a fashion, the syndrome is no longer called Isaac syndrome, but it is called Morvan's syndrome. [445] Hyperhidrosis is also common for neuropathy patients. I do not have hyperhidrosis, but excessive sweating that is better controlled by moving to a cooler and dryer climate.

Profuse sweating or hyperhidrosis is a concern for many reasons. First, it causes heat intolerance. [446] *Heat intolerance* is the inability to tolerate hot temperatures. Second, as anyone knows, sleeping is almost impossible if one becomes too hot and sweaty. Third, temperature regulation initiates many problems when cycling, especially racing. During time trial races, competitors do not have the luxury to add or take off clothes since races are too short. If competitors are not dressed properly, they must live with the consequences of being too hot or too cold or lose significant time by changing clothing. Finally, irregular sweating is common for people with hyperhidrosis. For example, my sweating is unique in that it is very heavy on my upper body, but not so much for my legs. This may be partly explained because sweat gland density is greater in the trunk then the legs. In fact, there are over 2.5 million eccrine glands, and most are located on the back and chest. [447]

There are numerous causes, functions, and characteristics of sweating and temperature regulation. For instance, when the parasympathetic nervous system is active, it results in lower core temperatures, respiration, heart rate, and blood pressure. As sympathetic nervous system activity increases, the opposite is true, and core body temperatures increases. Sweating is also initiated by the sympathetic nervous system that supervises eccrine glands. Sweating cools the core body temperature when it is evaporated. At slow rates of sweating, sodium and chloride ions may be reabsorbed, but these important electrolytes are lost when sweating is profuse such as in warmer climates, more humid climates, and under strenuous exercise. Moreover, loss of electrolytes leads to an acidic pH and that may trigger the central nervous system (CNS) to cool the body or begin a heat ventilation process. [448] [449]

One major function of the hypothalamus is to act as the body's thermostat to regulate the core body temperature at 98.6 degrees Fahrenheit via Type IV sensory nerve fibers found in the skin, internal organs, and spinal cord. Body temperatures fluctuate about one degree per day, and humans generally have a lower temperature in the mornings and a higher temperature in the evenings. My average body temperature is lower than the normal person creating a larger gradient between the body and outside temperature. Hence, on warmer days, my cooler body temperature may initiate the sweating process very quickly. [450] [451]

Hyperthermia is the warming of the core body temperature, while *hypothermia* is the cooling of the body temperature. Body heat is produced by any chemical reaction, such as generating ATP for muscle contractions, as every cellular activity produces heat. Heat gains are primarily regulated through the skin in the form of sweat, radiation, convection, and conduction. ***Radiation*** is the most common form, which is heat loss to the surrounding air. Excessive cellular activity may explain why some PNH patients suffer from extensive sweating or hyperhidrosis. For instance, many people with PNH have continuous small muscle fiber activity, primarily in the form of fasciculations; therefore, the body is generating excess heat 24 / 7. Hence, it is plausible that some PNH patients may compensate for the excess heat generation with increased sweating. [452] [453]

I suffer from cold hands and feet daily, and it may or may not be associated with the temperature regulation system. During intense exercise, I sweat profusely, but my hands, feet, lower arms, and lower legs may remain cold. Something that I learned from personal experience is that pain, muscle stiffness, and cold sensation are directly related. Case in point, if my feet are cold, then they are also most likely stiff and in pain. Cold hands and feet are the signature symptom of acute stress and the autoimmune dysfunction called Raynaud's syndrome. ***Raynaud's syndrome*** occurs from excessive constriction of peripheral arterioles in the hands and feet in response to cold temperatures. The constriction of blood vessels leads to less blood flow and oxygen in the hands and feet, and henceforth, temperature regulation is compromised. [454] Raynaud's syndrome is associated with many diseases, such as peripheral neuropathy. [455] My cold hands and feet symptoms are possibly a result of my neurological condition, but I do not believe there is any link to Raynaud's syndrome.

Skin

I have had many skin disorders including *Grover's disease* which is a benign skin condition characterized by itchy red bumps. While the link between Grover's disease and sweating is only a theory, it makes sense since sweat seems to exacerbate the condition. Grover's disease usually appears on the trunk of men in their 50s. [456] Furthermore, while Grover's disease is considered a temporary condition, it has persisted in my case for several years and shows no sign of remission. *Staphylococcus aureus infections (staph)* can result in skin abscesses.

Pityriasis rosea (PR) usually occurs in children or young adults, so it is no surprise it appeared when I was 23. PR symptoms include skin rashes that can look similar to those coming from syphilis or psoriasis. PR is thought to be brought about by human herpesvirus 6 and 7, and the rashes clear up in about three months without any treatment. *Folliculitis* is a staph infection of the hair follicles. To make matters worse, I was on two antibiotics for several years to fight the infection: Minocycline and tetracycline. Of course, in the previous chapters, we learned that a major cause for an autoimmune disease might be the prolonged use of antibiotics. There is something called *minocycline induced autoimmune syndrome* where the excessive use of the antibiotic minocycline can introduce an autoimmune disease. [457] The folliculitis cleared up after a move to a cooler and drier climate because it minimized my excessive sweating problems. This result is unsurprising since prolonged skin moisture is one known reason to exacerbate the symptoms of folliculitis.

Squamous cell carcinoma (SCC) is most likely brought about by exposure to the sun, especially for fair skin individuals. However, SCC can also be a consequence of immunosuppression. The squamous cell carcinoma was removed using micrographic surgery (MOHS), and I have not had another recurrence in over 13 years. [458] *Eczema*, which is a side effect of IVIg treatments, is extensive and wide spread. Apparently, the new immunoglobulins from IVIg were removing antibodies protecting me from eczema. One byproduct of neurological symptoms in the hands has possibly been a change in the texture of my fingernails. In particular, my fingernails have developed vertical ridges. There are other plausible causes for texture changes in fingernails such as age, but other conditions such as iron (Fe) deficiency (anemia), Fe overproduction, diabetes, or thyroid concerns have been dismissed. [459]

Many skin gene variations can identify how well this barrier protects individuals from hypersensitive autoimmune reactions. Protection from air toxins and pollution (EPHX1 and NQO1), antioxidant capacity (NQO1, SOD2, EPHX1, and CAT), inflammation (IL18, IL6, IFNG, ADADL, and IL10), sensitivity to the sun (NTM, TYR, ASIP, and LOC10537487), and overall sensitivity (IL18, ADAD1, and EPHX1) can be evaluated as part of the human genome. [460] Unsurprisingly, my overall skin genome is unfavorable and subject to poor genetic outcomes for the above genes.

Urination Symptoms

My bladder dysfunction is called *nocturia* and describes multiple nightly sleep interruptions to urinate. Bladder dysfunction or urinary manifestations are a symptom of Isaac's syndrome and many neurological disorders. [461] Nocturia is primarily problematic because it interrupts sleep. I have been told I am too young (57) to be having this problem, and medications such as Flomax are not prescribed until men reach 60. The autonomic function of the urinary system is regulated by both S2–S4 of the sacral spine (parasympathetic) and T12 to L2 of the thoracic and lumbar spine (sympathetic). The sphincters of the bladder are controlled by the pudendal nerve, which originates from S2–S4. My neurological condition seems to be one possible explanation for my nocturia symptoms since there is no evidence of any radiculopathy or mechanical compression affecting the nerve roots of the pudendal nerve. [462]

That said, the most plausible reason for nocturia symptoms is not my neurological condition but a condition called *benign prostate hyperplasia (BPH)* that inflicts men between the ages of 45 and 75. BPH results from an enlarged prostate that can restrict the flow of urine from the bladder. I have many of the symptoms associated with BPH, such as interrupted sleep to urinate, difficulty beginning to urinate, sensations of an unemptied bladder, and low flow. [463]

The Digestive System [464]

About 70% of the immune system is in the gastrointestinal tract. Since most pathogens are ingested, having a large part of the immune system in the gut is not surprising. As alluded to earlier, the immune system within the gastrointestinal tract is called the *gut-associated lymphoid tissue (GALT)*. The gut comprises good bacteria, which boosts the digestion process. Therefore, it is imperative that immune cells, such as dendritic cells, be able to recognize the difference between good and bad bacteria. Dendritic and other immune cells accomplish this task through a process called tolerance. Tolerance is a process administered to immune cells as they grow and mature in the GALT. See Figure 10.2 for more detailed information on the digestive system.

The digestive system is controlled by the parasympathetic and sympathetic autonomic nervous system (See Table 10.1). Both of these nervous systems combine to form the enteric nervous system (ENS) or the "mini-brain" of the gut. The bottom line, the parasympathetic nervous system is responsible for promoting digestion, whereas the sympathetic nervous system is responsible for inhibiting digestion. Digestion motility and homeostasis are promoted by both the nerve and hormonal systems (endocrine system).

Saliva [465] [466]

Saliva production is the first step in the digestion process and was discussed earlier in this chapter. Saliva is produced by the transport of ions and water into the saliva duct. This activity is accomplished primarily by ion pumps and hormones. More specifically, saliva contains mostly water along with mucus, sodium, bicarbonate, chloride, and potassium; it also contains ***ptyalin***, which initiates the digestion of carbohydrates. The chemical agent ***atropine*** inhibits salvation, and saliva contains mucin and IgA to prevent infection. The overall effect of the sympathetic nervous system is to reduce saliva production. Conversely, the parasympathetic nervous system stimulates the saliva glands. Except for swallowing and defecation, the functions of the gastrointestinal tract are controlled by autonomic nerves and intestinal hormones (including saliva). The salivary glands include the submandibular, sublingual, and parotid glands. Overproduction of saliva may lead to drooling, which is a symptom of some neurological diseases.

Esophagus and Stomach [467] [468]

The esophagus has two sphincters. The *upper esophageal sphincter* is the *cricopharyngeal muscle* that prevents the entry of air during respiration. The *lower esophageal sphincter* is the *cardiac sphincter* that prevents gastric acid from the stomach flowing into the esophagus. The *esophagus* is a muscle that propels food to the stomach via contractions.

The primary function of the stomach is to breakdown food and absorb minerals. *Parietal cells* manufacture gastric or hydrochloric acid to breakdown foods. *Gastric acid* production is stimulated by the vagus nerve (cranial nerve X), neurotransmitters such as acetylcholine (ACh), and hormones such as gastrin and histamine. Hormones such as secretin and cholecystokinin inhibit gastric acid production and motility. Gastric acid, when combined with stomach muscle contractions, promotes the mixing of food for digestion. The mixture of undigested foods in the stomach is called *chyme*. The stomach has three different types of muscles to churn and mix food: *Circular*, *longitudinal*, and *obliquely arranged*. *Circular* stomach contractions also promote the absorption of nutrients, while *longitudinal* contractions promote motility. Gastric acid has a pH of 1.5. A pH of 1.5 which is very acidic and stimulates not only digestion but the killing of any harmful pathogens that may be ingested.

The acidic pH of the stomach also fosters the absorption of vitamins and minerals. Good bacteria are tolerant of acidic acid; bad bacteria are not. The function of antacids and proton pumps is to reduce gastric acid and elevate PH. Therefore, one dire consequence of antacids and proton inhibitors is to allow the stomach to tolerate bad bacteria.

People use antacids like Tums or Rolaids and proton ion inhibitors like Omeprazole primarily to prevent heartburn, although not all cases of heartburn are brought about by gastric acid burning esophagus tissue. Most cases of heartburn may be explained by gastric acid burning the stomach wall after the protective stomach lining has been damaged. This condition is called *gastritis*. However, when the stomach lining is damaged, the stomach actually produces less gastric acid, not more. Less gastric acid is produced because the parietal cells are damaged. Hence, the consequence of decreasing gastric acid from antacids and proton ion inhibitors could exacerbate symptoms from gastritis and heartburn.

Small Intestines [469] [470] [471]

The primary function of the *small intestines* is to absorb vital minerals, vitamins, and nutrients from the chyme with the help of various enzymes. The absorption process includes the conversion of proteins to amino acids, the reduction of complex sugars into simple sugars, and the conversion of fats into simple molecules. The small intestines comprise three sections: The duodenum, the jejunum, and the ileum. The ***duodenum*** is responsible for absorbing calcium, magnesium, and iron, as well as producing acid-neutralizing agents to combat the low pH of the chyme coming from the stomach. Acid neutralizing agents, such as bile and pancreatic juice, are pumped into the duodenum to advance the digestion process started in the stomach. The ***jejunum*** is responsible for absorbing carbohydrates, vitamins, alcohol, sodium, potassium, fats, and amino acids. The ***ileum*** is responsible for absorbing vitamin B12, sodium, and potassium, as well as bile. The process of absorption happens when vitamins and minerals diffuse through the small intestines lining with the help of surface absorptive cells (SAC) and a transporter molecule such as sodium. In the ileum, motility is fostered or inhibited by the hormones gastrin and cholecystokinin, respectively.

A complete list of other vitamins and minerals absorbed in the small intestines includes A, D, E, K, B1, B2, B6, B12, C, folic acid, nicotinic acid, biotin, and pantothenic acid which are essential for life. Motility and absorption are both advanced by *circular* and *longitudinal* muscle contractions and the swaying of ***villa*** located on the intestinal walls. Villa movement is facilitated by muscle contractions. Villa assists mineral absorption primarily because they increase the surface area of intestinal walls by a factor of 600. An aging person's intestinal surface area declines, making the absorption of minerals and vitamins more difficult. Furthermore, there is also decreased absorption of bile acids in aging adults.

Large Intestines / Colon [472]

The large intestines also use *circular* muscle contraction to advance motility. The sympathetic nervous system facilitates pain, fullness, and constricts blood vessels within the digestive system. The parasympathetic nervous system facilitates relaxation once the rectum is full. Since the large intestines play a role in water absorption (1400 ml per day), the chyme passing through becomes dehydrated and is formed into solid waste.

Sodium, potassium, chloride, and bicarbonate ions are absorbed or excreted by the large intestines. Absorption during digestion transports minerals and ions into the bloodstream or the lymph fluid system. The intestines secrete **immunoglobulin A (IgA)** to fight microorganisms. Acidic environments in the stomach and duodenum inhibit most bacteria's survival. Hence, the millions of good bacteria that make up the flora of the gut are mostly located in the large intestines, colon, and in the lower small intestines (ileum). Population and diversity of good bacteria may be dictated by several environmental factors such as diet, environment, drugs, personal hygiene, vaccination, infection, and antibiotics. These factors may change flora populations and diversity for better or for worse. Good bacteria play no role in the absorption process but help metabolize fats, carbohydrates, and drugs. Good bacteria can destroy toxins and enhance the function of neurotransmitters, hormones, and the immune system to fight infection and trigger an inflammatory response.

The colon delivers the final mixing and propulsion contractions also via *circular* and *longitudinal* muscles. These contractions move fecal material to the rectum leading to an urge to defecate. [473] Finally, hemorrhoids may inhibit defecation reflexes.

Pancreas / Liver / Gallbladder [474] [475]

The liver, gallbladder, and pancreas secrete substances critical for the digestion of chyme. The *pancreas* produces enzymes to digest carbohydrates, proteins, and fats from *pancreatic juice*. The pancreas produces about 1200 ml of juice each day. Enzyme production is stimulated by the neurotransmitter ACh and hormones such as cholecystokinin. The pancreas produces alkaline fluid to neutralize the acid produced in the stomach. *Alkaline fluid* enables both enzymes and good bacteria to flourish in a less severe environment. The *parasympathetic nervous system* stimulates pancreatic hormone and enzyme secretion, while the *sympathetic nervous system* inhibits the secretion of these important hormones and enzymes. The pancreas is regulated by both the ENS as well as chemical regulators such as cholecystokinin, gastrin, acetylcholine, substance P, secretin, insulin, and somatostatin. The most important hormone regulated by the pancreas is insulin, which regulates cellular glucose and protein synthesis for muscle cells.

The pancreas has alpha cells, beta cells, delta cells, gamma cells, and F cells. Alpha cells produce glucagon, which is secreted inversely proportional to glucose. Glucagon production results in the glycolysis of glycogen to escalate glucose in the bloodstream. Beta cells synthesize insulin, which regulates glucose and metabolizes proteins, fats, and carbohydrates. Beta cells also regulate amylin, which stimulates insulin secretion, inhibits glucagon, and delays gastric emptying. Delta cells help fabricate somatostatin, which inhibits insulin and glucagon. Somatostatin, as discussed earlier, is a growth-inhibiting hormone. Gamma cells are stimulated after fasting, exercise, or protein-rich meals that lower blood sugar concentrations. F-cells promote gastric secretion.

The *liver* metabolizes or synthesizes the nutrients received by the small intestines. These nutrients are released into the bloodstream or stored for later use. Digested and absorbed substances from the small intestines flow to the liver via the hepatic portal vein. The liver metabolizes proteins like actin and myosin, both necessary for muscle contraction. The immune system of the liver comprises Kupffer cells--macrophages, stellate cells, and natural killer cells. These cells fight bacteria and infection and play a role in repairing liver damage. The liver fosters digestion by secreting bile, which digests and absorbs fats. Bile is injected into the duodenum, and then bile salts are reabsorbed at the ileum and returned to the liver for reuse. [476] The liver's primary function in the immune system is to filter the blood of any toxins. Toxins are transported to the liver, where they are removed from the bloodstream. Liver enzymes transform the toxins into non-toxic molecules excreted via urine or in the bile of stool. [477] The liver is also responsible for carbohydrate metabolism and storage (glycogen), protein metabolism, fat metabolism, iron storage, and vitamin A, D, and B12 storage. The liver regulates cholesterol, which is important to synthesize steroid hormones. *Low-density lipoproteins (LDLs)* carry cholesterol to tissues. *High-density lipoproteins (HDLs)* transport cholesterol to the liver where it is removed from the system in the bile. When there is excessive cholesterol exported for waste, the result may be a collection of plaque on blood vessel walls or gallstones.[478]

The *gallbladder* stores bile not immediately required for digestion. The gallbladder boosts the process of forcing or moving bile from the liver to the small intestines. The process of forcing or the movement of bile to the small intestines is accomplished by contractions stimulated by the hormone cholecystokinin (CCK). Bile's primary function is to digest fat and to eliminate cholesterol. [479]

IBS

The most common gastrointestinal concerns for people with neurological disorders are constipation and diarrhea. Constipation can be brought about by diet, medications, or neurological conditions such as Parkinson's disease or multiple sclerosis (MS). When neural pathways and neurotransmitters become diseased or degenerated, then constipation may occur. Indicators of *constipation* comprise of straining during defecation, hard stools, a sensation of incomplete evacuation, and fewer than three bowel movements in a week. *Diarrhea* may be of three varieties: Osmotic, secretory, and motility. *Motility diarrhea* may result from neuropathy, while *secretory diarrhea* may be prompted by inflammation as a result of increased smooth muscle contractions.

The lower portion of the gastrointestinal autonomic function is regulated by the same nerve roots and nerves as the bladder. Thus, the gastrointestinal autonomic function is managed by both S2–S4 of the sacral spine (parasympathetic) and T12 to L2 of the thoracic and lumbar spine (sympathetic). The anal canal and rectum sphincter are also controlled by the pudendal nerve that originates from S2–S4, and there is no evidence of any radiculopathy or mechanical compression of the nerve to produce any digestive concerns. The upper part of the gastrointestinal system is supervised by cranial nerve X (the vagus nerve) for parasympathetic function and by T1 to T11 of the thoracic spine for sympathetic function. [480]

IBS is one of the most common causes of digestive motility abnormalities. However, before discussing IBS, there are many disorders that disrupt the motility of the gastrointestinal system that need to be recognized. [481] [482] A common reason for motility problems is *gastroesophageal reflux disease (GERD).* GERD refers to gastric juices burning the lining walls of the esophagus and may have the following etiology and symptoms: [483] (1) GERD may result from the lack of a certain bacteria in the gut called *helicobacter pylori.* [484] (2) Hypomotility that results from GERD may be precipitated by a lack of saliva production during sleep. (3) GERD can be a side effect of neurological disorders such as neuropathy since damaged nerves can weaken the sphincter muscle between the stomach and the esophagus. [485] (4) GERD may result from a decreased pressure on the lower esophagus sphincter, which protects the esophagus from dangerous stomach acid. Decreased sphincter pressure may result from fatty foods, changes in the level of gastric juices, or an increase in various hormones such as cholecystokinin (CCK). [486] (5) GERD may originate from increased pressure in the stomach, caused by deficient acid levels, which has real consequences, including the dysfunctional signaling of enzymes to break down food and the inability to bring the nutritional vitamins and minerals from the food to the cells.

[487] (6) One common cause of GERD is a *hiatal hernia*, and the most common hiatal hernia is called a *sliding hiatal hernia*. A sliding hiatal hernia may be brought about by excessive vagus nerve stimulation or a weakening of the diaphragm muscle at the stomach–esophagus junction.

GERD leads to inflammation, ulcers, fibrosis (scarring), and thickening tissue that may result in more serious ailments such as *Barrett's esophagus* and esophageal cancer. GERD may be exacerbated by lying down, coughing, or straining during defecation. GERD and Barrett's may be treated with proton pump inhibitor (PPI) medications such as Nexium and omeprazole, which reduce gastric acid production. However, PPI usage may result in diarrhea and constipation, and long-term effects can precipitate hypomagnesemia, low absorption of vitamin B12, and other serious ailments outlined earlier.

GERD can be the result of an unhealthy gut. Conditions such as an overgrowth of bacteria and the malabsorption of carbohydrates can lead to acid reflux. IBS is associated with low stomach acid and conditions such as GERD, flatulence, constipation, diarrhea, and food sensitives. [488] I have both GERD and Barrett's esophagus, so it unsurprising that I have been taking omeprazole for a long time. Since individual reactions to omeprazole are widely varied and dependent on our genetic makeup, it could be a logical source of my digestive problems. [489]

Gastritis can alter digestive motility and is defined as inflammation of the gastric lining or membrane of the stomach or intestines. Note that: (1) Common erosive or hemorrhagic gastritis can lead to ulcers. (2) Alcoholism can be a major contributing factor to gastritis. (3) Chronic gastritis can result from any disorder that elevates gastric acid production. (4) Health problems, such as gastritis and ulcers, led me to quit drinking alcohol. [490]

Anismus is a condition that causes the pelvic floor to contract instead of relaxing during defecation, resulting in constipation. Anismus is common for women who were abused as children, individuals with Parkinson's disease, or those with other neurological disorders such as polyneuropathy. Keep in mind that certain medications, such as opioids, are also a common reason for constipation. Food allergies and sensitivities may also alter intestinal bacteria and digestive motility. Additionally, psychological factors, including stress and early life trauma, may modify the autonomic nervous system, gut microbiota, the inflammatory response, and the pain response contributing to motility dysfunction. [491]

Figure 10.2: The Digestive System (From bing.com/images)

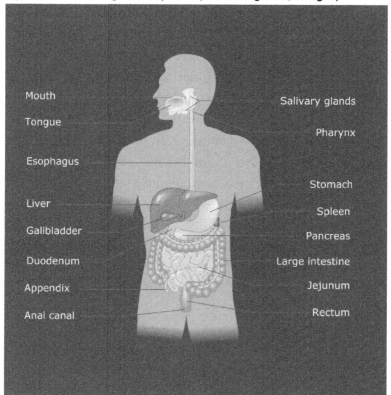

Irritable bowel syndrome (IBS) is the most common disorder that can lead to motility abnormalities. IBS is the inability of the large intestines to move chyme at the proper speed: Too slow leads to constipation, while too fast leads to diarrhea. IBS symptoms are characterized by abdominal discomfort, urgency, bloating, fullness, gas, diarrhea, and constipation. Digestive symptoms are coupled with fatigue, decreased energy level, impaired sleep, depression, and anxiety. IBS is associated with myopathy, neurological conditions, cancer, and phycological conditions. [492 493 494]

IBS usually precipitates constipation, diarrhea, or both. IBS has a higher prevalence among aging and female populations but is fairly common and may inflict up to one in every seven people—and half of the cases involve alternating between diarrhea and constipation. IBS may be brought about by alterations to immune cells, acute gastroenteritis, inflammatory bowel disease, alterations in normal gut flora, stress, and responses to prolonged antibiotic or probiotic treatments. [495] [496] [497]

There are many theories about the causation of IBS. IBS may be provoked by the inability of the gut to absorb sugars or bile acids to break down fats and rid the body of wastes. This theory explains why foods and drinks rich in carbohydrates trigger the most extreme cases of IBS. Spicy foods, fatty foods, caffeine, and alcohol may also contribute to IBS symptoms. IBS may be triggered by food allergies and minor food sensitivities (Type I hypersensitivity reaction). Further, it may be precipitated by a breakdown in communication between the brain and gut. When there is a breakdown in the signals between the brain and gut, the consequence is abnormal small and large intestines function.   IBS may be linked to psychological stress such as panic disorders, anxiety, depression, and other stress disorders. In particular, IBS is more likely to happen in those who have been physically abused. Finally, IBS may be initiated by bacterial infections or genetics. However, the reason for this is unclear. [498] [499]

Imbalances of gut bacteria may trigger IBS symptoms or even an autoimmune disease. One example of an imbalance of bacteria is a condition called dysbiosis. *Dysbiosis* means having too few good bacteria. There are five types of dysbiosis: First, when there is an unidentified reason for insufficient levels of good bacteria, for instance, there may be several environmental reasons triggering dysbiosis such as antacids, antibiotics, alcohol, stress, proton ion inhibitors, and a bad diet. Second, small intestinal bacterial overgrowth (SIBO) happens when good bacteria growth occurs in the wrong place, for example, in the small intestines instead of the colon. Third, immunosuppressive dysbiosis occurs from toxins, resulting in a reduction of good bacteria. Fourth, inflammatory dysbiosis often results from an autoimmune disease. Finally, when a parasite results in a good bacteria reduction. The bottom line, any disruption of good bacteria will negatively alter vitamin reabsorption and metabolizing bile, reduce the ability to detox the body of foreign chemicals, make it difficult to convert the bacteria populations back to normal, and inhibit the digestion fiber and complex sugars. A disruption of good bacteria refers to a decrease in diversity, stability, and resiliency of the bacteria. Diversity denotes there are a wide variety and abundance of good bacteria to prevent illness. Stability signifies maintaining the same bacterial composition, so bacteria are more resilient to prevent illness. [500]

The best ways to maintain and improve gut bacteria are to: Reduce animal fat intake; avoid eating when stressed, angry, or sad; practice occasional fasting; eating more probiotics and fermented foods; eating organic vegetables (free of pesticides) and grass-fed organic meats (free of steroids and antibiotics) and; eating vegetables and natural foods over mass-produced and processed foods. [501]

People with a diet high in animal fat can generate intestinal inflammation, resulting in a disruption of gut bacteria leading to a leaky gut. A leaky gut refers to undigested molecules released into the bloodstream, activating an unwanted immune system or cytokine response. One explanation for the above outcome is obesity. Obesity from a diet high in fat interrupts the gut-brain communication cycle by disrupting bacteria flora and removing toll-like receptors. The hypothalamus is responsible for signaling the gut when it has eaten enough calories. However, when the gut bacteria and toll-like receptors are disturbed, sensing functions of the hypothalamus are shut off, and people overeat. Further complicating matters is that fatty and sugary comfort foods initially help most people cope with stress. However, in the long run, a poor diet makes stress worse if a leaky gut and obesity are the end result. [502]

According to Silbernagle, "Despite its high prevalence, and considerable burden of illness, treatment of IBS remains unsatisfactory." IBS-like symptoms are probably the one condition that makes exercise and competing very difficult. I refer to my symptoms as IBS-like because I have not been officially diagnosed with IBS. My IBS-like symptoms may have been triggered by: Stress and anxiety, childhood trauma and abuse, gastritis (I was diagnosed with this when I was 36, but it has since cleared up), an autoimmune or neurological disorder, prolong use of an antibiotic for folliculitis, and prolong use of a proton pump inhibitor (omeprazole) to treat Barrett's esophagus

When a good day is a day you have diarrhea, you know something has gone terribly wrong with your digestive system. I can go up to five days without a normal size bowel movement and then can go days or weeks with diarrhea. It is important to distinguish the difference between diarrhea from an illness, like the flu, and diarrhea from IBS-like symptoms. When I am sick, diarrhea episodes occur multiple times a day; however, diarrhea from IBS-like symptoms never results in more than one or two bowel movements per day. In other words, IBS-like diarrhea is not as chronic, but the end result is similar: A yucky feeling. Since diarrhea is the more desirable result, I eat over two pounds of vegetables and fruit each day, so it is difficult to imagine why I have any issue with constipation. For me, chronic constipation has led to other medical problems like hemorrhoids and, eventually, a hemorrhoidectomy to alleviate the problem. Irritable bowels produce hemorrhoids because of the strain from trying to force a bowel movement when feeling constipated and bloated. Forcing a bowel movement also has another downside, in that it may produce acid reflux, which can burn the esophagus. The bottom line, constipation, and IBS-like symptoms give rise to a vicious cycle of events. The bottom line, it is estimated that IBS costs the United States 20 billion dollars annually from impaired workforce productivity. [503]

Detection of Low Blood Sugar

My hypoglycemic workouts have fostered a tolerance to low serum blood sugar, and this is not necessarily a good thing. There are many master cycling events around the country. As I mentioned before, one such event is the Huntsman World Senior Games in Saint George, Utah. One morning after fasting and getting a workout in, I got my blood sugar tested at the Huntsman Senior Games. They performed the test twice and then brought over medical professionals to check in on me. They said most people could not walk around with blood sugar levels that low. So, the question that needs to be asked is my tolerance to low blood sugar due to my training, the neurological disorder, or a combination of both? It is difficult to answer this definitively, but it more than likely a result of the training and not the neurological condition.

Blood Pressure [504] [505]

The autoimmune system regulates heart rate and blood pressure. My blood pressure has been slightly elevated for as long as I can remember, and the condition is serious enough to warrant a small amount of medication. Blood pressure concerns (mostly high) can precipitate the following problems: General fatigue, energy changes, waking up tired, insomnia, inability to focus, mental confusion, blurred vision, headaches, weakness in the legs, dry mouth, weight gain, mood swings, cravings for sugar and carbohydrates, constant hunger, compulsive eating, loss of drive, loss of appetite, and rapid heart rate.

Since I don't believe my cardiovascular system has been harmed from my neurological condition, then there must be some unknown explanation for my high blood pressure. I do not have hypertension, only elevated blood pressure, medically called *prehypertension*. The following are some causes of high blood pressure. [506] First, strenuous exercise may elevate blood pressure. That said, I only tax my cardio system about eight hours a week, and about one or two hours of that time is intense exercise. To put that in perspective, eight hours is less than 5% of the week, and only about 1% of the week is engaged in intense training. Second, some people who have high salt intake may have elevated blood pressure if they cannot regulate the increased intake. Third, serious ailments such as kidney failure, which has been ruled out in my case, may result in high blood pressure. Finally, a few better explanations for my high blood pressure are stress, elevated blood viscosity on account of a higher red blood cell count from living at altitude, and vasoconstriction, which refers to a narrowing of the blood vessels impeding blood flow. Vasoconstriction is a possible explanation for cold hands and feet and Raynaud's similar symptoms.

Hair Loss

It is difficult to ascertain if my hair loss condition is hereditary, being brought about by a neurological disorder, or being exacerbated by some other ailment. Male hair loss is common in our family history, but my hair loss is much more extreme than any other family member. Thus, I am not sure where hair my loss fits, but a plausible explanation for my hair loss is folliculitis. I was diagnosed with chronic folliculitis a few decades back. Folliculitis can produce both temporary and permanent hair loss.

Folliculitis is a bacterial infection (inflammation) around the hair follicles and is similar to acne and can occur anywhere on the body, but in my case, it was isolated to the scalp region. Profuse sweating can exacerbate folliculitis, and my symptoms went away once I moved to a drier and cooler climate. To treat the folliculitis, I was prescribed the antibiotics minocycline and then tetracycline over the course of nearly a decade. I stopped using the medications altogether once I learned about the many ill effects of being on an antibiotic for long periods of time. Antibiotics may kill the bad bacteria causing the infection, but antibiotics can also kill good bacteria, especially in the gut. One book on chronic pain suggests, "Neither antibiotics nor steroids are to be given routinely" to patients because of the adverse side effects. [507] Needless to say, hair loss, folliculitis, and antibiotic use raise many more questions than answers about my health. For instance, is there any relationship between antibiotic use and irritable bowels? Did the antibiotic use create any other adverse side effects? The bottom line is that the most plausible explanation for my hair loss is a combination of being a hereditary condition that was exacerbated by a long bout with folliculitis.

Sleep

Sleep may be the most important variable when it comes to athletic performance. It should come as no surprise that lack of sleep not only affects performance but increases the chances of an accident while training. Napping and caffeine have been proven to combat lack of sleep, but both will disrupt my ability to sleep and caffeine exacerbates my PNH symptoms. [508]

The primary gland and hormone responsible for sleep are the pineal gland, which produces melatonin. Sleep is divided into *rapid eye movement (REM)* and *non-rapid eye movement (NREM)* segments. During NREM sleep, there is no dreaming and restorative, reparative, and growth processes occur. During REM sleep, there is dreaming and rest. Hence, sleep is disrupted if either the REM or NREM sleep cycles are bothered. There are many sleep disorders associated with neurological dysfunction. However, in my situation, I believe sleep is inhibited not necessarily by the neurological disorder itself, but by the primary symptoms that originate from the disorder. I take several medications to help me sleep, such as zolpidem and an antidepressant called amitriptyline. However, they do not help much if sleep is being constantly interrupted on account of an overactive bladder or increased muscle activity.

Sleep is the most important factor related to recovery for training and competition. Without sleep, the body becomes fatigued and overtraining syndrome may occur. Athletes rank lack of sleep as the most important reason for fatigue. That said, most instances of sleep disturbances do not necessarily lead to reduced endurance for workouts. Instead, lack of sleep leads to an illusion that people think they are going faster than what they can actually accomplish. Additionally, some evidence supports that lack of sleep will compromise the immune and endocrine systems making people more susceptible to illness, especially after a challenging race or training day. [509]

Most people with peripheral nerve hyperexcitation (PNH) claim their symptoms of constant muscle fiber movement contribute to their sleep disruptions. The constant muscle fiber activity is usually fasciculations and fibrillations or muscle twitching. The difference between fasciculations and fibrillations is that fasciculations can be visually confirmed. This type of unwarranted muscle activity is called *agrypnia excitata* and describes constant muscle hyperexcitation that leads to sleep disruption and disturbances. Hyperexcited muscles are particularly troublesome because they can affect any stage of the sleep process, ranging from trying to fall asleep to waking. Most sleep disorders affect particular stages of sleep, such as trying to fall asleep, early sleep, mid-sleep, or late sleep. [510] However, sleep disorders may be present in neurological conditions for other reasons. For example, Isaac syndrome (IS) and Morvan's syndrome (MoS) sleep disorders result from a hormone deficiency of melatonin or an overabundance of norepinephrine. Insomnia from MoS could be a contributing factor in the death of up to 20% of those inflicted. Other autoimmune disorders, such as Guillen-Barré Syndrome (GBS), can present with deficient concentrations of hypocretin, which disrupts sleep. Hypocretin is also associated with sleep disorders such as narcolepsy. Another autoimmune disorder, myasthenia gravis (MG), is associated with sleep disruptions as a result of respiratory dysfunction. Patients with MG may have a normal respiratory function during the day, but on account of the slow release of pyridostigmine at night, MG patients may have respiratory dysfunction at night. Pyridostigmine is a chemical involved in nerve impulses and muscle movement, and it can affect many muscles, not just those involved in respiration. [511] [512]

Lack of sleep increases anxiety and stress, which initiates a vicious cycle of events leading to even less sleep. Both lack of sleep and anxiety are directly related to increases in steroids (adrenalin) and hormones epinephrine, norepinephrine, and cortisol that stimulate the sympathetic nervous system. The overall effect of the above-mentioned steroids and hormones is to dampen the immune system, in particular, a decrease in natural killer cells, one of the first immune cells to fight any pathogen. [513] Lack of sleep has also been correlated to the increased production of another hormone called ghrelin, which may also result in a larger appetite and weight gain. [514]

Lightheadedness

My lightheadedness happens when I sit up, and it is exacerbated in a hot environment. Lightheadedness may also be associated with symptoms such as tinnitus, discussed earlier. [515] That said, there is no evidence that lightheadedness is related to any of my neurological symptoms.

One plausible explanation for lightheadedness is a fairly common condition called ***benign paroxysmal positional vertigo (BPPV)***. BPPV attacks last only a few seconds and are generally related to the position or movement of the head. BPPV attacks are medically explained by the movement of loose or free-floating debris in the ear canal. [516]

Another plausible explanation for lightheadedness is that I have a forward-leaning head. I have to do specific exercises to try to minimize the lean of my head. A forward-leaning head puts significant pressure on the neck muscles and spinal cord discs, affects overall posture, affects breathing, and affects the blood supply to the head and could, therefore, give rise to my lightheadedness symptoms. [517] The forward-leaning head situation is exacerbated by sleeping on my back using two or more pillows to lessen acid reflux. In other words, sleeping with the head propped up allows the neck muscles to move or shift permanently into a forward-leaning position. Said differently, many symptoms are probably not the direct result of the neurological disorder but instead the outcome of the treatment. This is a common theme seen throughout this chapter. [518]

Headaches

Most headaches are benign and do not have any sinister etiology, including the most common benign headache called a *tension headache*. My headache symptoms do not compare to a tension headache because the pain is mild, they do not worsen with exertion, and there is no nausea. I generally wake up with headaches probably brought about by an excessively dry mouth, but the symptoms are, for the most part, manageable. I exercise intensely and compete with headaches so they cannot be too severe, but they are an annoyance. The bottom line is that my headaches are not the result of stress, anxiety, or a neurological condition, but instead of medications producing a dry mouth that may promote a headache. In fact, proton inhibitor medications, such as omeprazole, are directly associated with headaches. [519]

Chapter 11: Environmental Factors: What Causes PNH and Other Neurological Disorders?

An environmental cause or trigger for autoimmune disease may happen in two ways. First, individuals may have a genetic predisposition for a particular disorder, and it may only be triggered by some environmental factors. Second, individuals may not have a genetic predisposition. However, exposure to some environmental factors may initiate a mutation or expression change in their genetic DNA code triggering the disorder. In fact, our genetic makeup or expression is a culmination of all our life experiences and the experiences of our parents, and we pass this on to our children. [520] In some circles, these genetic predispositions are called evolutionary mismatches that cause disease mismatches. When our evolutionary genetic code is incompatible or mismatches with environmental conditions, then disease may be the outcome. In fact, many of the disorders and diseases discussed in this book might result from a genetic predisposition or evolutionary mismatches such as GERD, depression, chronic pain, and irritable bowel syndrome (IBS), to name a few. The problem of mismatch diseases is exacerbated when the *symptoms* are treated instead of treating *curable diseases*. For instance, many cases of diabetes can be cured with both diet and exercise instead of using drugs to treat symptoms. Ultimately, these diabetic hardships will be passed on to the next generation. [521]

There are many potential environmental factors that result in peripheral neuropathy, PNH, and other neurological disorders. Symptoms may originate from a virus, infection, illness, prescription drugs, exposure to toxins such as organophosphates and heavy metals, hereditary gene mutations, Lyme disease, kidney disease, benign tumors, pregnancy, vaccinations, alcohol and drug dependency, malabsorption conditions such as Celiac's disease or some food allergies, deficiencies of vitamins B and E, carpal tunnel syndrome, anxiety and stress, cancer, and thyroid conditions. [522] [523]

In this chapter, the focus is on specific underlying environmental factors that may have had an impact on my disorder. My health history revealed a vast number of environmental factors that were possibly involved in the manifestation of my neurological condition. The vast number of environmental triggers may explain why my neurological disorder is a mystery. For example, it is possible that multiple triggers initiated not only new disorders but also exacerbated current symptoms. That said, the removal of many of these environmental factors from my lifestyle should result in the improvement of symptoms or at least the halting of the progressive nature of the symptoms. Since that has not happened, it is difficult to suspect that alcohol, toxins, or other factors are involved. Nonetheless, all these environmental factors are important to any medical history and require a thorough investigation.

Alcohol

One potential cause, trigger, or source to initiate autoimmune disease or exacerbate symptoms of any neurological disorder is alcoholism. I abused alcohol from age 15 to age 37. I come from a family of alcoholics. In fact, I had several cousins die from alcoholism. I was, for the most part, a functional alcoholic: By age 37, I received a high school diploma, graduated from Penn State with an electrical engineering degree, I was employed in the same job for fifteen years, and I was married for eight years. I only drank beer, and I did not drink every day. However, the type of alcoholic beverage and frequency of consumption does not define all the parameters of alcoholism. My situation was either I had no beers, or I had 20 beers; I could never just drink one beer.

After having some stomach and esophagus discomfort, I was diagnosed with Barrett's syndrome at age 37. Alcohol is widely known to exacerbate Barrett's symptoms. [524] **Barrett's syndrome** results from GERD (acid reflux) burning the tissue of the esophagus. Barrett's generally does not go away, and it can develop into cancer. To avoid GERD, I go to bed on an empty stomach, and I also prop my head up on several pillows, so gravity works against the source. These techniques, no alcohol consumption, and a small dosage of omeprazole have kept my Barrett's syndrome under control. Omeprazole also has another function because it is often used as a magnesium supplement. Magnesium is a common treatment for motor neuropathy symptoms. I do not think omeprazole has worked to alleviate my motor neuropathy symptoms, but I also do not think that it has hurt. GERD was discussed in previous chapter in the section covering IBS.

When my doctor revealed Barrett's is a very serious condition, and it could develop into esophageal cancer, he got my attention. He told me one lifestyle change that will improve the disorder is to quit drinking. Alcohol abuse is destructive and is associated with other disorders besides GERD, including: (1) cancers of the oral cavity, larynx, and esophagus; (2) higher HDL cholesterol, lower LDL cholesterol, increased coronary blood flow, low blood pressure, and a reduction in platelet aggression; and (3) fibrosis and or cirrhosis of the liver. [525]

Chronic alcoholism can damage a liver in three stages. [526] First, it creates dysfunction in ATP production. Second, it increases reactive oxygen species (ROS) and free radicals coupled with fewer antioxidants. This dangerous combination leads to ROS destroying healthy cells. The third way is by damage and inflammation produced by Kupffer cells, T-cells, and macrophages, which are called into action to fight damaged cells from ROS and the lack of ATP production. This process induces the activation of growth cells that generate matrix and collagen (scar tissue). Essentially, cirrhosis of the liver is a liver damaged with scar tissue.

Sensory peripheral neuropathy symptoms are defined by numbness, paresthesia, and burning pain-causing sensory symptoms in both the lower and upper limbs of the body. Neuropathy brought about by alcoholism is progressive, and sometimes it can resemble ***Guillain-Barré syndrome (GBS)***. [526] Alcoholism may lead to a vitamin deficiency of B1 and B6, which may also mimic symptoms of peripheral neuropathy. Other types of vitamin deficiencies that may produce neuropathy symptoms from alcoholism include B12, E, and Copper. [527] An overproduction of copper is called Wilson's disease. Wilson's disease is brought about when copper (Cu) ATP pumps fail to maintain homeostasis. Symptoms from Wilson's disease include neuropathy, tremors, rigidity, and dysphagia. [528]

I quit alcohol cold-turkey and have not had a drink in 20 years. I do not know if alcohol caused or exacerbated my neurological symptoms, but it certainly cannot be ignored.

Digestive Problems [529]

Irritable bowel syndrome (IBS) may be diagnosed if a patient has one or more of the following: (1) stomach discomfort for at least three out of the last six months and the discomfort is relieved by a bowel movement; (2) a change in frequency of bowel movements; or (3) a change in the consistency or appearance of a bowel movement. [530]

As mentioned in the previous chapter, one condition potentially causing IBS is called *small intestinal bacterial overgrowth (SIBO)*. The colon and intestines contain trillions of bacteria. However, even having too much good bacteria (SIBO) can be a bad thing, usually defined as having more than 100,000 bacteria per milliliter of fluid. SIBO initiates a process called fermentation and is brought on by eating an abundance of carbohydrates such as foods made from flour and sugars. [531]

Another condition causing IBS-like symptoms is a *leaky gut*. As we already learned, when the brain is not communicating with the digestive system properly, or there is some kind of stomach dysfunction such as a leaky gut, the digestive system will malfunction. Consider the following about a leaky gut: A leaky gut happens when the lining of the intestines is compromised, allowing undigested food, bacteria, and toxins into the bloodstream. When this happens, the body is unable to prevent the triggering or exacerbation of food sensitivities and autoimmune disorders. Since 70% of the immune system is in our digestive system, an immune response to a leaky gut is the normal protocol and, therefore, the propensity for autoimmune disorders to originate from the condition. Conditions that may result in intestinal permeability that lead to a leaky gut are stress, inflammation, alcohol, prolong use of antibiotics, low stomach acid, high-intensity exercise, gastrointestinal infections (food poisoning), gluten or other food sensitivities, and toxins. Autoimmune dysfunction from a leaky gut includes acne, allergies, arthritis, attention deficit disorder, autoimmune conditions, bloating, cancer, canker sores, celiac disease, chronic fatigue syndrome, depression, edema, and epilepsy.

IBS-like symptoms may also be a consequence of the digestive system struggling to digest certain foods for several reasons, including food sensitivities. A healthy small intestine breaks food down into small proteins or amino acids. The proteins and amino acids can pass through the small intestine lining and into the bloodstream to repair muscles and tissues. However, when the small intestines are filled with foods not easily broken down, such as many bad carbohydrates or gluten, two things may happen. First, nutrients cannot be released into the bloodstream, and second, undigested foods in the intestines are seen as "invaders," and the immune system works to fight these invaders.

When the digestive system has SIBO, a leaky gut, or undigestible foods, the following immune response may occur. [532] [533] In defense of SIBO, a leaky gut, and undigested foods, the body will send an immune response to the parts of the body invaded by the toxins. At this point, the body may attack itself, which may initiate an autoimmune condition. The immune response is mediated by the release of cytokines to warn white blood cells to fight harmful pathogens. The immune response encompasses antioxidants to cleanse the body of harmful pathogens. The bottom line, when the body is fighting non-harmful inflammatory conditions such as undigested foods, SIBO, or a leaky gut, the body's immune system is compromised to fight other harmful inflammatory conditions.

My IBS-like symptoms have led me to believe that my condition is both associated with a leaky-gut (possibly from SIBO) and a neurological disorder. It is impossible to know if the two are related or if the leaky gut precipitated the neurological disorder or vice versa. Nevertheless, I changed my diet to eliminate many potential food sensitivities or foods that may be difficult to digest.

Bacterial Infection

The first possible trigger of my neurological condition was due to an illness as a child. Between 8 and 10 years of age, I contracted skin staph infections (boils or abscesses). Most prominently, the infections would show up in my nose, but I could get them anywhere. Most books on neuropathy and other neurological conditions only list human immune deficiency (HIV), hepatitis C, diphtheria, and leprosy as infectious causes. [534] [535] Although staph is not included as a reason for neuropathy, its presence validates a weakened immune system, and a weakened immune system is a prerequisite to trigger autoimmune disease.

Thinking back on my medical history, trying to remember what could have triggered my neurological condition, I completely forgot about my staph infections as a child. Then that horrid repressed memory of unimaginable pain from an earache came back. One night, when I was 10, I was screaming in agony the entire night. The pain was unbearable. Then, finally, the morning came, and my parents rushed me to our doctor. He looked into my ear and said I had a boil or staph infection on my eardrum. At that point, our doctor personally escorted me to the hospital, where I would stay for what seemed to be a week or two before he diagnosed me with a gamma globulin deficiency. This is called hypogammaglobulinemia. Each week, for about one or two years, I would receive a painful gamma globulin shot in the rear-end. Gamma globulin is synonymous with present-day terminology of immunoglobulins and IVIg treatments.

Back in the early 70s, the medical profession operated much differently. Patients were not passed on to one specialist after another to uncover and resolve diseases. I was fortunate to have a doctor who worked tirelessly to find out what was wrong. Thinking back, I believe if I were passed from one specialist to another, I would have probably died. My doctor saved my life because my immune system was seriously compromised. At the time, I was unaware of being in any danger. I do not even think my parents understood how harmful this condition was to my wellbeing.

Hypogammaglobulinemia is not only challenging to diagnose, but it is a serious condition: "Early detection and treatment of hypogammaglobulinemia are known to reduce rates of morbidity and the chance of long-term pulmonary complications. Evidence shows that there is an association between achieving higher IgG levels and reduced infection frequency. If hypogammaglobulinemia remains undetected and untreated, outcomes are generally poor, especially if chronic lung damage or bronchiectasis has occurred. Unfortunately, the diagnosis of it is often significantly delayed." [536] Hypogammaglobulinemia is not easily detected because it has a broad range of symptoms, and it affects each person in seemingly unique ways. For instance, hypogammaglobulinemia can result in skin infections, but hypogammaglobulinemia is not considered a leading reason for causing skin infections. [537]

Similar to how gamma globulin treatments cured me of a chronic staph infection problem, present-day *intravenous immunoglobulin treatment (IVIg)* may also cure immune deficiencies and autoimmune disorders such as autoimmune neuropathies. [538] According to the National Institute of Health for rare neurological disorders, IVIg and plasmapheresis are common treatments for Isaac syndrome and many neurological conditions triggered by an autoimmune attack. The problem with plasmapheresis and IVIg is not only are the procedures expensive but that the relief is generally temporary, and the treatment must be repeated with maintenance dosages every few weeks or months. Over time the effectiveness of IVIg and plasmapheresis may also decrease significantly.

Thinking back on those childhood years, it was apparent that I repressed those memories. However, some of my behaviors as a child are beginning to make sense. In particular, I remember having some weird tingling sensations beginning around the time of my staph infections as well as problems with cramping when I was active. In response to these sensations, I was hyperactive, and even to this day, I cannot sit still. I now postulate my fidgeting behavior was an unconscious defense mechanism because it prevented me from feeling any motor or sensory symptoms so long as I was continuously in motion. Of course, the cramping may have been exacerbated by my constant need to move.

From the information in the above paragraph, it is safe to assume that I had *attention deficit hyperactivity disorder (ADHD)* as a youth. Persons with ADHD have a difficult time to focusing, they get distracted easily, and they are fidgety. ADHD is very common, and it may be influenced by a mutation with gene DRD4 that results in fewer of one type of dopamine receptor. Thus, individuals with ADHD have less dopamine. With that said, there is a relationship between ADHD, exercise, and dopamine genes since people with this DRD4 mutation are freaks of nature when it comes to endurance training and this may partly explain both my ADHD and endurance training ability. [539]

My theory for my immune deficiency issues probably started at birth for two reasons. First, my mother had a C-section and second, I was not breast fed. My mother said that when she tried to breast feed me, it was not enough food to keep me satisfied and quiet. Thus, I was put on an oatmeal and formula diet at only a few days old. Unsurprisingly, by the time I was a year old I weighed over 30 pounds. Several references suggest that both a C-section and the lack of breast milk can lead to both an underdeveloped immune system and gut microbe. To compound issues, my mother was a germaphobe, and that too may have also been another childhood factor that led to an underdeveloped immune system. The bottom line, a combination of a C-section, lack of breast milk, and a germaphobe environment prevented my gut microbe and immune system to fully develop. [540]

Viruses [541]

Neurological disorders may also result from viruses. One common virus that results in neurological disorders is **Epstein-Barr (EBV).** The host body usually fights viruses such as EBV via natural killer T-cells and macrophages. EBV is more commonly called *mononucleosis* (the kissing disease). About 90% of all people have the antibodies for EBV, which generally infects B-cells via a receptor on C3 complement, and the virus can remain dormant within these cells. EBV can lead to more serious ailments, including cancer. For example, EBV has been associated with thymoma (as well as lymphoma), which have also been associated with peripheral nerve disorders such as Isaac syndrome. EBV may be the most common virus associated with autoimmune disorders. "Associated" denotes the medical industry is unsure if EBV causes the autoimmune disorder or if EBV exacerbates symptoms after the autoimmune disorder has been contracted. Alternatively, possibly, EBV can trigger both an autoimmune attack and exacerbate symptoms depending on the individual. Nevertheless, there are links between EBV and many autoimmune disorders such as multiple sclerosis, lupus, rheumatoid arthritis, Sjögren's syndrome, and Hashimoto's thyroiditis. [542] I had EBV when I was a sophomore in college, though I have no evidence that EBV has any ties to my lifelong neurological situation.

Toxins

One potential environmental culprit for my neurological condition may be the drinking water in Colorado. [543] For example, high levels of lead can alter intercellular concentrations of calcium by inhibiting Na-K ion pumps. Lead exposure is linked to both neurological and immune system disorders. [544] I drink much water, about 120 ounces daily, due to a heavy training load. I choose water over other sport drink options because I elect to eat my calories and not drink them. The human body needs water to survive, which is not surprising since 65% of the body is comprised of water. Water serves numerous critical functions in the body and water with toxins can create a plethora of issues. [545] (1) Water is essential to eliminate toxins and waste. (2) Water is the earth's natural healing power to prevent arthritis, kidney stones, constipation, obesity, glaucoma, cataracts, diabetes, hypoglycemia, headaches, muscle aches, and fatigue. (3) Unfortunately, today, there are not many clean sources of drinking water–distilled water is the closest option. (3) At least one paper attributes peripheral nerve hyperexcitation (PNH) to high levels of lead and silver. [546]

According to one reference, the faucet water is full of harmful chemicals. Although this reference is old, concerns about drinking water have not improved primarily because utility companies struggle to keep pace with population increases. For instance, Peter Ward, who wrote *Lamarck's Revenge,* claims the drinking water at his work (University of Washington) is too toxic to drink. There are numerous documented controversies about faucet water. Consider the following: [547]

- Parkinson's disease may be tied to environmental toxins consumed in drinking water.
- More than 20,000 cases of giardiasis, caused by an intestinal parasite in drinking water, have been reported in the United States.
- Over one-third of all community water systems have been cited for failing to meet minimum EPA standards.
- Pesticides contaminate water supplies, especially in rural areas dominated by agriculture.
- More than 700 contaminants have been uncovered in water supplies nationwide, and 200 are classified as toxic chemicals. The EPA monitors fewer than 50 toxic chemicals.
- In 1987, 36,000 public water supplies were in violation of federal standards.
- One in six Americans is exposed to dangerous levels of lead. Lead may lead to liver, kidney, cardiovascular, immune, and gastrointestinal dysfunction.
- In 2014, there was a crisis emanating from lead exposure in drinking water. [548]
- Other references on pain management are wary of water and its contents, suggesting other toxins like pesticides, industrial chemicals, and synthetic compounds are in unfiltered drinking water. [549]

Remember those Coors commercials bragging about brewing beer from snowmelt water found in crystal clear rivers and creeks in the Rocky Mountains? They leave the impression that the water in Colorado is clean and pristine. Nevertheless, that is not necessarily true. States where drinking water is filtered by the ground may have better water supplies than States that have no natural filtration process in addition to their treatment facilities. Furthermore, Colorado is one of the biggest mining states in the United States, and therefore, the state has a high probability of heavy metals getting into the waterways. Most treatment plants do not expect heavy metals in the water, so filtration methodology is not effective.

One Colorado neurologist told me that their hospital diagnoses one person with ALS every week. He said when he worked for the Mayo Clinic in Minneapolis, they diagnosed a person with ALS, maybe every month or two. He said the amount of people in Colorado with neurological symptoms seems to be very high. No data exist to support this claim, but his observation should be alarming. I truly believe something is going on with the water in Colorado. We filter our water, but the damage may already be done, and it does not seem reversible. I have never been checked for high concentrations of heavy metals since I do not think these conditions exist anymore. If all of that is not bad enough, living in rural Colorado may also lead to the exposure of agricultural chemical toxins in the drinking water.

What type of heavy metals may be found in Colorado drinking water? The ones causing neuropathy symptoms are lead, mercury, arsenic, and gold. Lead may find its way into drinking water via old pipes. In other words, the treatment factory may eliminate lead, but it may be reintroduced when it travels to homes. The following points outline those neuropathy symptoms that come from heavy metal poisoning: [550] [551] (1) Symptoms for lead-induced neuropathy are primarily motor function such as weakness with no effect on the sensory nerves. (2) Symptoms for mercury neuropathy are paresthesia in the hands and feet along with possible gastrointestinal symptoms such as constipation. Mercury is also a leading cause of autoimmune diseases as well as other symptoms, including depression, gum disease, memory loss, fatigue, and sleep disorders. Studies have tied mercury to lupus, Graves' Disease (overactive thyroid), Hashimoto's thyroid (underactive thyroid), and multiple sclerosis. (3) Arsenic neuropathy results in severe sensory symptoms, including burning pains in the hands and feet. Severe illness or gastrointestinal symptoms are also common. Arsenic poisoning may also cause transverse white-lines on the fingernails called Mee lines. Symptoms from arsenic poisoning very closely resemble peripheral neuropathy. [552] (4) Symptoms for gold neuropathy encompasses paresthesia in the hands and feet along with mild weakness and fasciculations may be present. It may be difficult to determine the difference in symptoms brought about by rheumatoid arthritis and gold neuropathy.

Mercury and gold neuropathy-like symptoms correlate with my move to Colorado, such as experiencing more paresthesia and pain in the hands and feet, increased fasciculation activity, and more intense gastrointestinal dysfunction.

Toxins may be ingested or transmitted through touch. A list of toxins includes dry-cleaning solvents, gasoline, automobile fumes, tobacco smoke, glue, paint, stain remover, heavy metals, plastic chemicals, pesticides, and even toxins released by harmful bacteria. Heavy metal toxins such as mercury and aluminum can also be contracted via vaccinations. Mercury and aluminum are added to vaccines to improve the immune-stimulating response, so they are more effective. Guillain-Barré syndrome (GBS) was linked to influenza vaccinations in 1976. Other autoimmune disorders like lupus and rheumatoid arthritis have been linked to vaccinations for hepatitis B, scarlet fever, and typhoid. [553]

Toxins found in chemicals and pesticides can generate hormonal effects. Many chemicals affecting estrogen may explain why more women have autoimmune disorders. Since immune cells have estrogen receptors, chemicals that mimic estrogen result in the overproduction of antibodies. Since the liver metabolizes estrogen vastly different depending on the genetic makeup of the individual, it affects some more than others. The liver filters toxins that find their way into the bloodstream. However, the liver filtration system may malfunction after chronic exposure to toxins making it unable to eliminate toxins via bile or the urinary tract. [554]

One commonly overlooked toxin comes from prescription drugs. One study found that over 41 million Americans are exposed to dangerous prescription drugs. Moreover, most treatment facilities do not test for these types of toxins. [555]

One important antioxidant found in every human cell is called glutathione. *Glutathione* is important to protect the body from many toxins ranging from heavy metals to those found in pesticides and plastics. Glutathione fights any toxin that produces free radical oxygen molecules. Low production of glutathione can lead to autoimmune disorders. The body also has a *metal management system called metallothionein (MT)*. MT's are a family of sulfur molecules found within the cells that bind with heavy metals. The primary purpose of MT's is to regulate zinc and copper, but MT's can also bind with other metals preventing them from binding with other molecules within the cell. Low concentrations of MT's can lead to an autoimmune disorder brought about by heavy metals. [556]

Child Abuse

One environmental factor that cannot be ignored in causing or worsening neurological symptoms is child abuse. I have absolutely no idea how much these experiences played in my neurological disease, but childhood was a very traumatic and turbulent time that affected me both mentally and physically. My stepfather was an alcoholic who would usually take his anger out on my mother. I would get in the middle of those battles to protect my mother from both his physical and mental abuse. My stepfather's anger was, at times, directed toward my brothers and me. The unfortunate side effect of these battles was that it turned my mother against me. Yes, she wanted my protection, but she often objected to the ferocity at which I played my role as protector. She was angered because I would sometimes hurt my stepfather.

From my perspective, I had no choice. I had to be forceful because he was twice my size. I really thought that one day, it might come down to killing him or being killed, so I did not want to hesitate or be too lenient with my defense. Apparently, my aggressive actions reminded my mother of abusive experiences directed at her by her father when she was a child. My mother compared me with her father and said incredibly hurtful comments to me. For instance, she would remind me of how dumb I was compared to my older brother. Unfortunately, my relationship with my mother, over the years, never improved. It is one of my regrets in life. My mother died young, and I wish I could have helped her achieve a better life, but I only brought her grief. Needless to say, the relationship resulted in considerable mental anguish.

I had no idea how much these experiences affected me physically until I went through extensive testing to figure out why I had so many bone spurs. To make a long story short, the orthopedic doctor said I was either hit by a Mack truck or was abused as a child. He said that I had many fractures that were never treated, and therefore, they healed improperly, causing large bone spurs. In particular, I had a broken lower right leg and right elbow that were never medically treated. In other words, it was common for me to walk around my high school years with untreated broken bones. According to the doctor and books on physiology, most broken bones set properly will recover without any deformity.[557] I was perplexed by the orthopedics' findings because I still participated in sports and was not missing much time in school.

Traumatic experiences and injuries commonly have links to neurological symptoms and pain. For example, both physical and mental trauma can manufacture ailments, such as post-traumatic stress disorder (PTSD). Furthermore, child abuse is related to having an exaggerated digestive response to any type of stress or emotion, especially fear, anger, or sorrow. [558]

A couple of positive outcomes transpired from my years of abuse. First, I worked hard to succeed and to prove my mother wrong. Second, physical abuse taught me to cope with both future mental and physical pain. At the time, I never really thought I was suffering from any mental anguish or physical pain. After all, not one friend, student, teacher, or administrator ever asked if I was being abused. This is quite remarkable considering my junior and senior years of high school. I was the only student in the cafeteria, not eating lunch. No one ever offered me any food or money (not that I would have accepted). I doubt, today, that this type of situation would fail to raise red flags. That said, I learned to survive, and this experience helped me cope with adversity later in my life.

Although child abuse did not seem to create any bad epigenetic outcomes such as massive depression, hate, anger, and criminal behavior, it may be an explanation for some risk-taking behavior such as rock climbing, mountaineering, wrestling, or the need to go fast on a bike.

High Cholesterol

Another contributing factor to peripheral neuropathy or neurological symptoms is high cholesterol. There are studies indicating that not only does high cholesterol contribute to peripheral neuropathy [559], but so to do the statin medications used to treat the ailment. [560] [561] Statins can produce both motor or sensory neuropathy symptoms, including muscle cramping and high creatine kinase (CK). My total cholesterol readings are 1.5 times higher than the maximum specification. High cholesterol or *hypercholesteremia* can be induced by disorders of low-density lipoproteins (LDL) receptors causing the inability of LDLs to attach to the liver to be processed for removal. [562] My high total cholesterol led doctors to prescribe a statin called Pravachol. However, a decade later, I decided against using the medication because most of my total cholesterol was from HDLs (high-density lipoproteins). HDL is considered "good" cholesterol and having a low ratio between total cholesterol and HDL is what matters. Although my total cholesterol is high, it comprises a high percentage of HDL or good cholesterol. Getting off Pravachol was a good decision, and it correlated with less cramping and the lowering of my creatine kinase (CK). There is definitive proof that statin-induced neuropathy symptoms can be reversed by removing the medication from the patient's use.[563] Since this did not happen, it led me to believe it was not a source of my neurological condition.

As long as I continue to exercise and eat right, I should be able to control my cholesterol ratios. I believe doctors overreacted by placing me on Pravachol. Therefore, it is important to advocate for yourself and your health. After all, "It has been shown repeatedly that those who take charge of their own healthcare and reach out to others for advice, assistance, and support, are those who achieve the highest levels of health." [564] Thus, I am open about my neurological condition, and I am willing to talk to anyone who will listen. You never know who may offer insight information.

It should come as no surprise that there are many different types of medications (other than statins) that may induce peripheral neuropathy or neurological symptoms: medications to treat cancer, HIV, tuberculosis, arthritis, abnormal heart rate, bacterial infections, malaria, seizures, and vitamin B-6 deficiency. [565] For these reasons, it is imperative to take only medications that are absolutely necessary. Furthermore, all medications have side effects, and although they may correct the problem, they can also generate new symptoms. Thus, patients must decide what symptoms they would more likely want to live with: Those from their disorder or those from their medications.

Intense Exercise

Another form of *hypoxia (lack of oxygen)* occurs when muscles are starved of oxygen during intense anaerobic workouts. When the body consumes carbohydrate energy for rigorous exercise, it produces many toxins such as lactate. Vigorous workouts may also spawn free radicals such as reactive oxygen species (ROS). A free radical is any molecule that may contain an unpaired electron. When molecules with unpaired electrons react with other molecules, they, in turn, lose an electron, and this results in a chain reaction. The following are some characteristics of ROS molecules: [566] [567]

(1) ROS molecules are generated from normal mitochondrial respiration and energy generation and are formed from oxygen. ROS is a type of free radical. Types of free radicals include hydrogen peroxide, hydroxyl radicals, and nitric oxide. (2) Free radicals and oxidative stress can lead to both autoimmune and neurological disorders. (3) The following disorders have been linked to oxygen-derived free radicals: Aging, heart disease, Alzheimer's disease, cancer, diabetes, inflammatory

disorders, Parkinson's disease, amyotrophic lateral sclerosis (ALS), and Rheumatoid arthritis. ROS molecules' immune function is to damage the cell membrane of foreign pathogens. (4) There is a biological process to eliminate ROS molecules. However, when there are too many ROS molecules, or that process breaks down, it can wreak havoc like DNA damage, cellular death by apoptosis or necrosis, and the development of ALS.

Four factors may characterize cellular injury, resulting in cellular necrosis death from intense exercise: (1) the depletion of ATP; (2) a decreased level of oxygen but elevated levels of oxygen-derived free radicals (ROS); (3) an increased concentration of intercellular calcium; and (4) an increase in cellular membrane permeability defects.

Strenuous exercise certainly has many negative consequences. For me, the biggest consequences include pain and fatigue, requiring me to lay down for 12 to 15 hours each day. This is true even on days off from exercise, but it is not quite as extreme. My sources of muscle damage include denervation, constant muscle activity, intense exercise, and possibly other ailments that elevate lactate and CK. High lactate and CK are the primary causes of my muscle weakness, fatigue, and pain. [568] That said, *moderate exercise* is important to rid the body of toxins and lactate. Exercise is effective at keeping lymph fluid flowing to cleanse the body of dangerous toxins. However, moderate exercise and intense training are two distinct actions. *Intense exercise* can increase the toxins, including lactate and free radicals, while moderate exercise does not have the same effect. [569]

Lactate, CK, and ROS brought about by intense cycling workouts may be controlled to some degree by properly cooling down and stretching. [570] First, properly cooling down is achievable via a very light ride following a race or workout. Second, proper stretching is essential and encompasses three options. ***Dynamic stretching*** is accomplished by moving quickly from one stretching exercise to the next in a fluid motion. There is evidence that shows dynamic stretching works better than traditional static stretching to rid the body of lactate. ***Static stretching*** is holding a stretch or pose for a longer period of time than one would for dynamic stretching. If muscles are sore from stretching, they will manufacture more lactate and elevate CK. Results indicate that static stretching is more likely to produce sore muscles. It should be pointed out that there is no proof that either static or dynamic stretching foster any cycling preparation or recovery benefits. That said, there is no evidence it does not help, especially for someone with neurological symptoms. [571] Finally, foam rollers can eliminate toxins, such as free radicals, that may build up in the muscles. The roller frees the oxidative toxins from the muscles, and they may be excreted via the urine. Proper cool down methods, dynamic stretching, and foam roller techniques help but are not enough to combat my elevated levels of lactate and CK.

Altitude

My move to Colorado also had another reason to trigger neurological symptoms—living at 8,000 feet, where there is approximately 25% less oxygen than there is living at sea level. [572] Oxygen levels remain constant at any elevation, but reduced air pressure makes it more difficult for the body to uptake the oxygen. Hence, the body has less oxygen to function. [573] At 8,000 feet, even when completely acclimated to the low levels of oxygen uptake, the best pulse oximeter readings for human beings is between 95-98%. In other words, people will only function, at best, anywhere from 95 to 98% efficiently. [574] That said, I do not believe altitude produced my neurological symptoms or made them worse for many reasons. First, my pulse oximeter levels of 96 to 97% are not much different from people with 100% readings at lower elevations. Besides, many people have low pulse oximeter readings when they sleep (90 or less), and there is no evidence that this phenomenon triggers any neurological disease. Second, I can exercise strenuously without incident above 10,000 feet. Third, my symptoms do not improve when I return to sea-level. Hence, I am not convinced that altitude is a plausible explanation for my neurological disorder.

Altitude sickness is awful and can lead to death if the situation is not remedied. However, for me, the effects of high-altitude sickness are short-lived. The effects of altitude may certainly exacerbate symptoms of neurological disorders while people acclimate to a higher elevation, but it is less probable high altitude may precipitate long term symptoms in most healthy people. I suffered from altitude sickness in the past. Nevertheless, that was because I was not very smart and was climbing at high elevations without allowing myself proper time to acclimate. The best chance to introduce neurological symptoms from altitude may result after severe altitude sickness occurs (HACE–High Altitude Cerebral Edema). [575] [576]

Food Sensitivities and Allergies

I tested positive for the Celiac disease gene, but my IgA count was normal, indicating only a 10% chance that I have Celiac's disease. Since I have a predisposition for the disorder, I removed gluten from my diet, but I have not seen any improvement with my neurological symptoms. Although I do not have Celiac's disease, that does not imply I do not have a sensitivity to gluten. Celiac disease or gluten allergies are linked to a plethora of neurological and neuropathy disorders, and they are outlined throughout this text.

Part IV: The Diagnosis

Chapter 12: Initial Diagnosis Theories

Regardless as to whether or not I have Isaac syndrome (IS), differential diagnosis of similar disorders is necessary to make a correct diagnosis by verifying or nullifying the IS hypothesis. **Differential diagnosis** is a probability process that suggests evaluating different disorders in the order of their probability to be correct. For instance, it is more probabilistic that I have a disorder with a prevalence rate of 100 out of every 100,000 people than having a disorder with a prevalence rate of less than 5 in 100,000. Hence, in a probability process, the disorder with the highest prevalence is evaluated for differential diagnosis first. The most common reason for misdiagnosis is a premature closure of a case before all the facts are uncovered, which certainly seems to be the case in unraveling my diagnosis. Under most circumstances, the simplest diagnosis is most likely the solution, but that did not turn out to be the case for my diagnosis process. [577]

Why is it difficult to quickly and properly diagnose individuals with neurological conditions? One reason is that PNH and many neurological disorders are identified as syndromes and not diseases. The difference between diseases and syndromes is that "*diseases* have known causes and well-understood mechanisms for producing symptoms," whereas, "A *syndrome* is a specific set of signs and symptoms that occur together." Both diseases and syndromes may be life-threatening, have debilitating symptoms, and they may be progressive. Many times, progression may be due to some underlying condition that has not been addressed. [578] Thus, since syndrome causes, symptoms, and mechanisms are not very well-understood, diagnosis of the many neurological syndromes is difficult.

When muscles are affected in all four limbs, then there are generally four potential reasons: Myelopathy, myopathy, a neuromuscular junction disorder, and peripheral neuropathy: [579] (1) *Myelopathy or radiculopathy* is a compression of the spinal nerve roots or spinal cord and usually results in no fasciculations, increased reflexes, normal muscle tone, pain, some sensory involvement, and often digestive and bladder dysfunction. *(2) Myopathy* generally presents with proximal weakness and atrophy, normal reflexes, normal sensory function, no pain, and generally, the bulbar muscles are spared. The bulbar muscles are those controlled by cranial nerves, which include swallowing, vision, hearing, and speech. Myopathies are also characterized by a significant loss of muscle power despite minimal weakness and atrophy. One reason for power loss is because myopathies and myotonias present with pseudohypertrophy. *Pseudohypertrophy* means having larger muscles with reduced strength, increased fatigue, and are markedly slower. Pseudohypertrophy muscles grow simply because muscle mass is replaced with fat and collagen. Myopathies generally affect proximal muscles, while distal myopathies affecting the hands and feet are very rare. (3) Neuromuscular junction disorders generally present with proximal weakness, fatigue, normal muscle tone, sometimes fasciculations are present, spared sensory nerves, normal reflexes, no pain, and bulbar muscle involvement. (4) *Peripheral neuropathy* generally presents in distal muscles with weakness and atrophy, fasciculations may be present, reflexes diminish or are absent, pain, sensory loss, and bladder and digestive system are usually not affected.

Neurology defines four descending levels for motor signals originating from the brain and terminating at the motor unit of the muscles. The two levels above the spinal cord, affecting upper motor neurons, including the brain, are not included in the differential diagnosis because they include more severe symptoms such as rigidity and spastic movements, including ataxia. Instead, differential diagnosis of my disorder focuses on lower motor neuron dysfunction since my disorder is related to the two levels below the spinal cord or, more specifically, at the peripheral nerves, skeleton muscles, motor units, and the neuromuscular junction. Since my symptoms do not fit any general definition of any disorder, differential diagnosis is a difficult objective.

The above definitions are general because, for example, some neuropathies may present with proximal symptoms, and some myopathies may present with distal symptoms. Since diagnosis methods rely heavily on nerve conduction studies (ENG) and electromyography (EMG), the chapter opens with an explanation of these techniques.

Nerve Conduction Study and EMG Testing

Nerve conductions studies (ENG) and EMG tests are confusing, so it is best to try to clarify their function. *Nerve conduction studies or electroneurography (ENG)* check for *compound motor action potentials (CMAP)* and *sensory nerve action potentials (SNAP)*. There are three parameters evaluated for CMAP and SNAP, and they include amplitude, distal latency, and conduction velocity as a signal propagates from one muscle to another. Nerve conduction studies can determine the size of the nerve dysfunction as well as the type of nerve dysfunction. Nerve conduction study findings may be as follows. [580] [581] [582]

First, ENG amplitude information characterizes the integrity of axons and can identify neuropathies that involve dysfunctional axons. *Axon dysfunction* may be characterized by either increased or decreased amplitudes. For instance, a greater number of functional axons in a muscle yields a higher amplitude than a muscle with a reduced number of functional axons. Said differently, an ENG can identify the number of functional motoneurons or motor units. Axonal neuropathies generally show length-dependent symptoms. In other words, the nerves that travel the furthest from the spine to the muscles they control are affected first. Hence, symptoms begin in the feet, lower legs, and hands. Axonal neuropathies are generally the consequence of some type of toxin or an adverse side effect to certain medications.

Second, ENG conduction velocity information characterizes the integrity of myelin sheaths. *Demyelinating neuropathies* are brought about by nerves losing their myelin sheath or protective coating and are generally the result of an autoimmune disorder. Nerves that have demyelination damage are slower than nerves that are pristine and have no myelin damage. Normal conduction velocities are 40 to 60 (meters/second) in the lower limbs and 50 to 70 (m/s) in the upper limbs. Demyelinating neuropathies are non-length dependent, and therefore, symptoms may start in any location. If there is a non-uniform slowing of conduction velocities, then this phenomenon suggests acquired neuropathies such as *chronic inflammatory demyelinating polyneuropathy (CIDP)*. If there is a uniform slowing of conduction velocities within the affected nerves, then this may indicate a hereditary disorder such as *Charcot-Marie-Tooth disease (CMTD)*.

If SNAP findings are normal, but CMAP findings are abnormal for the same muscle, then this may indicate radiculopathy. However, abnormalities for specific nerve conduction tests such as H reflex or F wave tests may indicate GBS. *H reflex* and F wave tests measure nerves not accessible to direct stimulation, such as those in proximal locations. An *F wave* is a reflected wave. When an ENG stimulus is initiated on a nerve, the signal travels both ways on the nerve toward both the spinal cord and the peripheral muscles. The signal that travels to the spinal cord is reflected back to the muscle being tested. Thus, the reflected signal is delayed and with lower amplitude. A longer than usual reflected time may represent an adverse situation with the nerve roots.

An EMG is not as complicated as a nerve conduction study because the test only requires one needle inserted into a muscle (instead of two). EMG findings are divided into three categories: (1) *Insertional activity* when the needle is initially placed in the muscle; (2) *spontaneous activity* when the muscle is at rest; and (3) *voluntary activity* when a muscle is flexed. The following are some findings that can be determined with an EMG: [583] [584] [585]

During needle insertion, there may be some abnormal activity, but it should stop once the needle has been put in place. Activity may continue in a muscle that may have denervation or myotonia abnormalities. When an insertional activity is limited, it may represent unexcitable muscles possibly from disorders such as periodic paralysis and muscular dystrophy when muscle is replaced by fat and connective tissue (*pseudohypertrophy*).

Muscles at rest should be silent, but sometimes there is a spontaneous activity, which may be pathologic or benign, such as fasciculations.

Muscle dysfunction may be located in the nerves, the muscle, or the neuromuscular junction. An EMG uncovers the mystery of where a muscle dysfunction is specifically located. For instance, during voluntary movement tests, *motor unit action potentials (MUAP)* are evaluated for amplitude, duration, and phase. In muscle diseases, MUAP amplitude and duration are decreased, while in nerve diseases, MUAP amplitude and duration are increased. For example, during a denervating process, functional axons take over for unfunctional axons. When this process occurs, muscle unit action potentials (MUAPs) may have an increased amplitude, duration, and complicated phase. When MUAPs fire more readily to compensate for lost muscle fibers, a pattern called *early recruitment* is also observed on EMGs. Early recruitment of motor units happens so muscles can generate the proper force. Said differently, motor units are activated early to compensate for lost motor units to complete a muscle contraction with the proper force. Myopathies are characterized by a loss of muscle fibers and motoneurons, resulting in lower amplitudes and shorter durations on an EMG, while neuropathies are characterized by longer durations and higher amplitudes due to the early recruitment phenomenon. The EMG helps to distinguish between myopathies and those disorders "masquerading" as myopathies such as myasthenia gravis (MG) and CIDP.

Myotonia Disorders

Since it was originally theorized, I had a myotonia called Isaac syndrome (IS), the vast ocean of myotonia disorders had to be evaluated for differential diagnosis. In neurology, a contraction malfunction where the muscle is delayed relaxing is known as *myotonia*. Most myotonias are inherited, and the exact gene mutation is known. Myotonias affecting any peripheral nerve voltage-gated ion channel are known as *channelopathies*. More specifically, the type of myotonia that I was thought to have is called percussion myotonia. *Percussion myotonia* is one where the myotonia is produced by a tap on the muscles. Furthermore, the magnitude of percussion myotonia decreases with the increased exercise of the affected muscle. [586] [587] The following are myotonia epidemiology, symptoms, etiology, diagnosis methods, common myotonia disorders, test results, and diagnosis probability: [588] [589]

Epidemiology

Since many myotonias are hereditary, they have childhood-onset. But some myotonia diseases may have adulthood onset. Myotonia disorders may result in premature death.

Symptoms

Symptoms are vast including temporary paralysis, vision or hearing loss, an abnormal or unusual gait (walk or stride), psychiatric and mental dysfunction, skeleton deformities in the hands, feet, and back (*scoliosis*), attacks on vital organs such as the lungs and heart, muscle contractures, pseudohypertrophy, muscle contractions slow when the muscles are cold, elevated creatine kinase (CK), muscle contractions slow after prolonged exercise, muscle contractions initially improve during exercise with a repetitive warm-up, and muscle atrophy, stiffness, and weakness with some pain.

Specifically, *pseudohypertrophy* is when muscles seem as if they are larger, but it is due to fat and connective tissue not actual muscle tissue. Furthermore, a contracture occurs when the muscle involuntarily shortens as a result of dysfunctional calcium ion pumps. A pathologic contracture is a permanent muscle shortening brought about by muscle spasms or weakness. As explained earlier, a common type of hand contracture is called *Dupuytren's contracture,* but it is not the result of muscle spasms but instead excess collagen in the palms.

Etiology

Most myotonias are hereditary. *Inherited myotonia's or channelopathies* are mutations of the sodium, chloride, potassium, or calcium voltage-gated ion channels. Channelopathies are myotonia disorders affecting ion channels. There are two types of skeleton channelopathies: Myotonia with and without periodic paralysis. In channelopathies where muscle relaxation is delayed after a contraction, this is classified as myotonia. When the muscle becomes paralyzed for extremely long lengths of time between contraction and relaxation, this is called *periodic paralysis myotonia*.

Myotonias have been reproduced by removing extracellular chloride in the sarcolemma membrane, resulting in a higher membrane potential to stimulate a contraction. A chloride disruption also causes myotonia by disrupting in the influx of sodium intercellular uptake and the influx of potassium to the extracellular plasma. Membrane hyperexcitability can also be precipitated by abnormal levels of both inter and extracellular potassium, resulting from dysfunctional potassium voltage-gated ion channels.

Common Myotonia Disorders and Test Results [590][591][592][593][594]

I tested negative for all the gene mutations discussed in this section on various myotonia disorders.

Central core disease (CCD) involves mutations to the ryanodine receptor (RyRs) ion channels, causing a disruption to both inter and extracellular calcium, and its consequences lead to variable cellular membrane potentials. *Hypokalemic period paralysis* is inherited and can be brought about by a mutation of the SCN4A sodium channel gene as well as the CACNA1S calcium channel gene. The disorder is autosomal dominant (passed down by one parent) with childhood-onset and a higher prevalence in men. Symptoms include muscle weakness and paralysis, and it is generally triggered after the consumption of a large carbohydrate meal or physical activity. Episodes generally start in the legs and ascend to the trunk. Serum potassium levels are variable during attacks. Hypokalemic attacks usually last a few hours, and the frequency of episodes fluctuates greatly. EMG and CK analysis may be normal. The prognosis for those inflicted is good. Another potential reason for hypokalemic periodic paralysis results from abnormal levels of triiodothyronine (T3), a hormone that regulates potassium channel function.

Hyperkalemic periodic paralysis is inherited and can also result from a genetic mutation to the SCN4A gene affecting sodium ion channels. SCN4A mutations can be triggered by environmental factors, including alcohol, exercise, and diets, such as fasting or vigorous physical activity. This disorder is autosomal dominant (passed down from one parent) with onset in childhood. Symptoms include muscle weakness, and it is less severe than hypokalemic periodic paralysis.

There are two types of myotonia congenita. First, *Thomsen myotonia* is a genetic mutation involving the CLCN1 chloride channel gene, and the condition is autosomal dominant (from one parent). The onset of Thomsen's is in childhood with stable and nonprogressive myotonia symptoms. Sudden movements are difficult but become more fluid after repetition. There is no atrophy, and patients may have athletic builds due to pseudohypertrophy. Second, *Becker myotonia* is a genetic mutation also involving the CLCN1 chloride channel gene, and the condition is autosomal recessive (from both parents). The onset of Becker's is in childhood with stable and nonprogressive myotonia symptoms. It is more severe than Thomsen and can lead to atrophy or hypertrophy. Life expectancy is normal, and the condition can improve over time. Myotonic discharges are confirmed on an EMG.

Myotonia fluctuant involves a genetic mutation to the SCNA4 sodium channel gene, and the condition is autosomal dominant. The onset of the disorder is in childhood with stable and nonprogressive painful myotonia symptoms. Pseudohypertrophy is a common symptom. *Paramyotonia congenita* also involves a genetic mutation to the SCNA4 sodium channel gene, and the condition is autosomal dominant. The onset of the disorder is in childhood, with myotonias improving over time. Pseudohypertrophy is a common symptom. *Andersen-Tawil syndrome* involves a genetic mutation to the KCNJ2 potassium channel gene, and the condition is autosomal dominant. The onset of the disorder is in childhood with muscle weakness, periodic paralysis, and life-threatening ventricular arrhythmias.

Rippling muscle disease (RMD) blood test checks for mutations in the caveolin three protein (CAV3), which appears in the membrane of skeletal muscle cells.

Myotonic dystrophy type 2 (DM2) blood test checks for ATP2a1 gene mutations or dysfunction with the ATP energy source that supply certain calcium ion pumps. DM2 is referred to as Brody's disease, which is classified as a myopathy. DM2 is autosomal dominant (passed on by one parent) and characterized by proximal muscle atrophy and mild myotonia and weakness (mainly in the quadriceps muscles). Onset symptoms start in the third or fourth decades, and the genetic mutation is with the zinc finger protein. Cardiac arrhythmias and cataracts may also be present. Walking may be impaired in old age, and other symptoms may include baldness, low IgG, symptoms worsening at cold temperature, and dementia. [595]

Stiff person syndrome (SPS) blood test checks for anti-glutamic acid decarboxylase antibodies (GAD) responsible for forming gamma-aminobutyric acid (GAMA). GAMA is a neurotransmitter inhibitor found in the brain. GAD antibodies may also be found in other neurological disorders such as *Miller-Fisher syndrome* and epilepsy. When there is not enough GAMA, then muscles may become hyperexcitable since the neurotransmitter to inhibit hyperexcitability is deficient. It may be confusing that SPS is associated with hyperexcited muscles since stiff muscles do not sound as if they are hyperexcited. That is true; however, the consequence of some hyperexcited muscles is that they contract but fail to relax, resulting in a muscle that will become stiff or paralyzed. SPS includes painful muscle stiffness and rigidity, and it may be associated with a malignancy, sporadic autoimmune syndrome, or diabetes. Pseudohypertrophy is a common symptom. A positive EMG for SPS reveals continuous muscle activity.

Diagnosis Probability

The probability I have myotonia is very unlikely because three EMGs showed no signs of myotonia, and I have no hereditary family history of any myotonia disorders. Moreover, I tested negative for many genetic myotonia disorders including those that best resemble my symptoms (Isaac syndrome, stiff person syndrome, rippling muscle disease, and myotonic dystrophy type 2).

Neuromuscular Junction Disorders

Myasthenia Gravis (MG)

The following are the epidemiology facts, symptoms, etiology, diagnosis methods, treatment methods, test results, and diagnosis probability for *myasthenia gravis (MG)*: [596 597 598 599 600 601 602]

Epidemiology

MG is a neuromuscular junction disorder, which is classified as a post-synaptic disorder because the dysfunction happens on the muscular side of the junction. Pre-synaptic disorders, such as *Lambert–Eaton myasthenia syndrome (LEMS)*, occur when the dysfunction is on the nerve side of the junction (see Figure 3.1). MG usually affects women under 30 or men older than 60. Women are affected more than men by a 3:2 ratio. Two-thirds of women acquire MG before the age of 40. The prevalence of MG is about 2.5 cases for every 100,000 people. Under normal operation, cells manufacture a two to three-fold excess of acetylcholine (ACh) molecules. This safety margin in ACh production is to guarantee a successful muscle contraction.

Symptoms

Symptoms for disorders of the neuromuscular junction are sometimes exercise-induced. Muscle weakness and fatigue worsen with prolonged exercise, which is generally relieved with rest. The onset of symptoms is sudden, and remission may occur in forms of MG that only affect the eye muscles. In fact, many forms of MG are primarily characterized by weakness of the eye muscles. MG symptoms affect the bulbar muscles, including muscle fatigue and weakness, swallowing, choking, drooling, elevated CK levels, and respiratory problems. MG can also affect the lips, tongue, cheeks, and the gag reflex muscles. Initially, the muscles affected are those that carry out fine movements or those that have a small number of muscle fibers innervated by a motor unit such as the ocular (eye) muscles.

MG may also be characterized by dysarthria, dysphagia, and sometimes respiratory weakness. MG is most serious when it inhibits breathing. When the respiratory function is inhibited, it is called a *myasthenic crisis*, which can be triggered by stress or certain medications, including antibiotics. MG can present with diminished reflexes in severe cases, but usually, reflexes are normal. MG may affect gait and produce weakness in the muscles of the arms, hands, legs, and feet. Symptoms often improve in the cold.

Etiology or Causation

When the neuromuscular junction is disrupted, critical proteins such as actin, titin, and myosin cannot produce muscle movements, including contraction and rest. Anti-titin antibodies may appear in MG. Titin is necessary for muscle contractions along with proteins such as tropomyosin, actin, and myosin. [603] MG is most commonly the result of antibodies blocking, damaging, or destroying acetylcholine (ACh) receptors at the neuromuscular junction, preventing muscle contractions (Hypersensitive Reaction Type 5). Hence, the safety margins of ACh production does not matter when ACh receptors are blocked. The antibodies involved in MG are primarily IgG class 1 and class 3. The antibodies are usually directed against the myoid cells of the thymus, but during an immune response, these antibodies can be misdirected to ACh receptors.

A muscle-specific kinase (MuSK) is a form of MG and is characterized by an attack against the MuSK protein, which is carried out by the antibody IgG class 4.[604] MG may result when antibodies interfere with cellular membrane function. For instance, membrane dysfunction could lead to the leakage of potassium out of the cell and water into the cell. [605] MG can also be induced by the botulism virus, creating an autoimmune attack that may inhibit ACh release from nerve cells into the synapse. This version of the disorder is different from traditional MG since it is pre-synaptic. MG may result from thymoma, and it can be treated with thymectomy. Thymoma appears in about 15% of all cases. Hypo and Hyperthyroidism appear in about 10% of the cases of MG.

Diagnosis Methods

MG diagnoses can take years since there are numerous disorders causing muscle weakness. Antibodies may be absent, and the EMG may be normal for individuals with ocular myasthenia or MG that solely affects the eye muscles. The EMG shows a decline in signal amplitudes of affected muscles, and the amplitude will continue to decrease the more the muscles are exercised. About two-thirds of MG cases have antibodies against the ACh receptors, and another one-third of cases have antibodies against muscle-specific tyrosine kinase (MuSK). Those individuals with MuSK antibodies are more likely to be women, and they are more likely to have respiratory distress. Another antibody against low-density lipoprotein receptor-related protein (LRP4) appears in some MG cases.

Treatment Methods

Once diagnosed, MG is very treatable using various drugs as well as ***plasma exchange*** and ***intravenous Immunoglobulin (IVIg)*** treatments. One treatment medication includes a drug called pyridostigmine, which increases the number of ACh receptors at the neuromuscular junction. Thymectomy can be considered for all myasthenia patients, even those that do not present with a thymoma. Results indicate an improvement in symptoms for 80% of all patients who undergo the procedure.

Test Results

The following are the blood tests that I had for neuromuscular disorders, and they all came back negative: ***Paraneoplastic AB panel blood tests*** search for a variety of antibodies associated with tumors and neurological symptoms. For example, the paraneoplastic panel checks for VGKC antibodies found in Isaac syndrome (IS), ACh receptor antibodies found in myasthenia gravis (MG), calcium channel antibodies found in Lambert-Eaton myasthenia syndrome (LEMS), and other autoimmune neurological conditions that may be triggered by cancer. To elaborate further, the presence of VGKC or ACh antibodies may indicate a thymoma (cancer of the thymus) or, more rarely, small cell lung cancer. It is also important to note that, although I tested negative for VGKC antibodies, found in 40% of all IS patients, it obviously did not exclude me from having the disorder since 60% of individuals with IS do not have the VGKC antibodies.

Neuromuscular junction disorder blood tests check for many of the same antibodies in the paraneoplastic AB panel test completed six years prior. Both panels check for antibodies that result in MG, LEMS, and IS. The blood work was retaken because the neuromuscular junction disorder blood test also checks for leucine-rich glioma-inactivated-1 protein (LGI1) and contactin-associated protein-2 (CASPR-2) antibodies that may also be found in IS. I tested negative for these antibodies.

Diagnosis Probability

The probability that I have MG is very unlikely because I tested negative for the ACh receptor antibodies, and EMG diagnostic testing showed no signs of MG.

Lambert-Eaton Myasthenic Syndrome (LEMS)

One disorder fitting under the MG umbrella is *Lambert-Eaton myasthenic syndrome (LEMS)*. The following are the epidemiology facts, symptoms, etiology, diagnosis methods, treatment methods, and diagnosis probability for LEMS: [606 607 608 609 610]

Epidemiology

There are numerous variations of LEMS, but it affects males more than females by a 5:1 ratio, and onset is usually after 40 years of age. Sometimes, younger females are also affected by LEMS.

Symptoms

LEMS has many symptoms, including weakness, paresthesia, fatigue, and numerous autonomic neuropathy symptoms, including dry mouth, impotence, and dysfunction of the bladder, digestive system, and temperature regulation. LEMS, unlike other neuromuscular disorders, almost always presents with diminished or absent tendon reflexes. LEMS is also associated with slurred speech, double vision, it affects the central nervous system, and it is more likely to affect smokers. It is characterized by affecting lower proximal limbs as well as the hips, neck, and shoulder muscles. In response to exercise, weakness improves but prolong exercise exacerbates symptoms. Dysarthria, dysphagia, and respiratory weakness are rare.

Etiology or Causation

LEMS is a pre-synaptic disorder affecting the calcium channels at the nerve ending and may be associated with small-cell lung cancer in two-thirds to 75% of all patients. The condition progresses slowly, and some people can live normal lives while others may have shortened life expectancies. LEMS is usually brought about by an IgG attack against the voltage-gated calcium channels (VGCC) at the nerve ending of the neuromuscular junction. Reduced calcium flow from damaged VGCCs inhibits the release of ACh from the nerve into the synapse. Antibodies usually show up in about 20% of the cases. Additionally, LEMS may be associated with hypo and hyperthyroidism, MG, and Sjögren's syndrome. Only older men affected by LEMS are prone to carcinoma, not the younger women affected by LEMS.

Diagnosis Methods

EMG findings show an amplitude (CMAP) decrement, but amplitudes will increase with a higher frequency of exercise until premature fatigue results. Blood test checking for calcium channel (VGCC) antibodies.

Treatment Methods

LEMS may be treated using potassium channel blockers. Since LEMS is autoimmune, many cases respond positively to *IVIg* and *plasma exchange*.

Diagnosis Probability

The chance I have LEMS is unlikely since I tested negative for the voltage-gated calcium antibodies, EMG diagnostic testing was negative, and I do not have a carcinoma.

Initial PNH Theory

The original theory of my neurological disorder was some form of PNH, in particular, CFS or IS. In this section, I explain why IS was a logical initial diagnosis theory since all my symptoms fit into one bucket. For instance, Isaac syndrome is both myotonia and neuromuscular disorder with PNH like symptoms. That said, although IS was later ruled out as a diagnosis possibility, there is still a distinct chance that I have both the PNH disorder CFS coupled with some type of neuropathy.

Isaac's Syndrome (IS)

Acquired Isaac syndrome (IS) or hereditary neuromyotonia has the following epidemiology study, etiology, symptoms, diagnosis methods, and treatment methods: [611]

Epidemiology Study

IS is very rare, and there may only be a few hundred cases in the United States. Data also suggests that men are affected more frequently than women.

Symptoms

About 20% of IS patients have paresthesia symptoms suggesting both motor and sensory nerves are hyperexcitable. Typical IS symptoms include cramping, fasciculations, myotonia, muscle stiffness, and hyperhidrosis. IS originates in the motor neuron and not the muscle.

Diagnosis Methods

EMG analysis may be negative in IS patients, or it could reveal spontaneous and repetitive myotonic discharges. CFS is a milder form of IS and presents with a clean EMG. About 30 to 40% of IS patients test positive for low levels of VGKC antibodies. The VGKC antibody test is less robust than the antibody tests for myasthenia gravis (MG) or Lambert-Eaton myasthenia syndrome (LEMS), which include the ACh and VGCC antibodies, respectively. [612] Some cases of IS may be present with elevated IgG antibodies, and ACh antibodies also found in MG. [613]

Treatment Methods

IVIg or ***plasma exchange*** treatment work best to alleviate or slow the progression of symptoms, especially for those patients who tested positive for VGKC antibodies. Symptomatic relief may be achieved with antiepileptic (antiseizure) medications, which reduce nerve excitability by blocking sodium channels.

Etiology

IS may be acquired by an autoimmune disease or cancer or inherited by a gene mutation and acquired IS can be associated with thymoma in 10%–20% of cases, and more rarely with small cell lung cancer, Hodgkin's lymphoma, and other malignancies. This condition affects the Kv1 series of fast potassium channels, while CFS may be characterized by dysfunction of the Kv7 series of slow potassium channels. [614] Evidence supports that the distal nerve close to the neuromuscular junction is where the hyperexcitability develops. Acquired IS can be associated with other autoimmune diseases, including myasthenia, rheumatoid disease, lupus, and diabetes. There has been at least one reported case of *staphylococcus aureus* bacteria or staph causing IS. [615] IS is benign except when the condition may be acquired via cancer; then survival is not necessarily guaranteed. However, if IS progresses to Morvan's syndrome (and there is no evidence that it will), then the mortality rate increases to at least 20%. [616]

More specifically, IS attacks VGKCs, the most diverse ion channels found in the human body. There are four types of ion potassium channels: [617] [618] (1) calcium-sensitive potassium channels; (2) potassium ATP channels; (3) M channel voltage-sensitive potassium channels; and (4) three types of rectifier voltage-sensitive potassium channels: Inwardly rectified, outwardly rectified, and delayed rectified.

Isaac syndrome specifically attacks the Kv1.1 ion channel, which is a delayed rectifier potassium channel. The gene KCNA1 encodes the Kv1.1 delayed rectifier potassium channel. The consequences of VGKC antibodies acting on the Kv1.1 potassium channel result in a reduction or suppression of current, causing the hyperexcitation of the peripheral nerves. More precisely, IS is caused by an IgG class 4 antibody attack against the Kv1.1 voltage-gated potassium channels (VGKC) at the neuromuscular junction. Recent theories tie IS to the VGKC antibodies reacting with two proteins called leucine-rich glioma-inactivated 1 protein (LGI1) and contactin-associated protein-2 (CASPR-2). Furthermore, "CASPR-2-IgG antibodies have been associated with chronic pain secondary to hyperexcitable nociceptive pathways, resulting in painful neuropathy." [619]

LGI1 and CASPR-2 protein function and antibody etiology are as follows. [620] LGI1 antibodies are often associated with seizures and cognitive impairment, consistent with their proximity in the central nervous system. Caspr2 proteins are found in both the central nervous system and the peripheral nervous system axons, and patients with Caspr2 antibodies may have encephalitis or acquired IS. The pathogenic mechanisms of why Caspr2 antibodies result in disease have not been proven. Caspr2 antibodies may also be associated with myasthenia gravis and thymoma, which they have recently been shown to be associated with diverse pain syndromes.

In IS, there is no change to the gating kinetics of the potassium channel (Kv1.1), nor is there any change to the sodium channel kinetics that potassium channel function may influence. That said, the dysfunction of the Kv1.1 channel happens because the density of the channel is reduced, resulting in decreased potassium current flow out of the cell. The decreased channel density theory is different from earlier theories suggesting that there may be a reduction in useful potassium channels. The decreased density of potassium channels is a phenomenon that may also occur in Guillen-Barré syndrome (GBS). [621] Since only 30 to 40% of IS patients test positive for VGKC antibodies, there must be other mechanisms causing IS that have yet to be identified.

The following is a theory I postulated from my studies. Medical articles indicate that both src tyrosine kinase and protein tyrosine phosphatase (PTP) are implicated in VGKC function and regulation. A decrease in PTP can decrease VGKC densities and, henceforth, channel currents causing muscle excitability seen in PNH disorders. In fact, when the current is reduced by 30%, the cellular membrane potential is changed by 30mV in Kv1 delayed rectifier voltage-gated potassium channels. Src tyrosine kinase also plays a role in neuromuscular activity at the neuromuscular junction, and when it is inhibited, it can develop into a rare form of myasthenia gravis (MG) called muscle-specific kinase (MuSK–MG). Interestingly, the overproduction of tyrosine kinase is also associated with cancer growth and wound healing, in particular, collagen production. As some may remember, Dupuytren's contracture is induced by an overproduction of collagen in the palms of hands. Hence, this theory provides a logical relationship between tyrosine kinase with my contracture symptoms. [622] [623] [624]

In fact, I can relate most of my symptoms to the prodigious function of Kv1.1 VGKCs. The following are specific characteristics and functions of both normal and dysfunctional Kv1.1 voltage-gated delayed rectifier potassium channels:

Normal Kv1.1 Characteristics and Function

Kv1.1 potassium channels are "a family of potassium channels that allow a sustained K^+ efflux with a delay after membrane depolarization. The outflow of potassium ions rapidly repolarizes the membrane. However, these Kv1.1 channels also play a key role in neurotransmitter release, action potential generation, and axonal impulse conduction." [625] Kv1.1 ion channels are found in every tissue within the human body. However, the quantity and distribution of the Kv1.1 ion channels can vary greatly depending on the tissue it populates. [626] It is also important to note that almost all syndromes, diseases, and disorders involving the Shaker series of potassium channels, defined as Kv1.1, Kv1.2, ... Kv1.8, all involve the Kv1.1 channel, although the other channels also appear in abundance throughout the body. [627] There are similarities in the KCNA1 and KCNQ genes. In particular, both genes form VGKC's, and there is evidence that mutations in both the

KCNA1 and KCNQ genes, which are responsible for encoding potassium channel Kv1.1 and Kv7.2, respectively, may lead to similar types of myokymia found in peripheral nerve hyperexcitation (PNH). In fact, the dysfunction of Kv7.2 and Kv1.1 may be a cause of CFS and IS, respectively. [628]

Furthermore, Kv1.1 protein channels are located in pain nociceptors; The four alpha subunits on the Kv1.1 potassium channel are primarily responsible for sensing changes in cellular membrane voltages; Kv1.1 potassium channels may be responsible for activating protein kinases such as creatine kinase (CK); and Kv1.1 channel expression may also involve cellular activities such as trafficking or the movement of the cells. [629] For instance, the Kv1.1 channel is responsible for the regulation of cell migration and proliferation in the stomach and small intestines. [630] Migration and proliferation are defined as follows. ***Migration dysfunction*** is "the production of abnormal migratory signals that may induce the migration of the wrong cell type to the wrong place, which may have catastrophic effects on tissue homeostasis and overall health." [631] [632] ***Cell proliferation*** is the addition or subtraction of cells. Millions of cells are born (cell division or replication) and die each day, and the delayed rectifier potassium channels play a huge role in this process. The body must maintain a balance between cell replication and apoptosis to maintain tissue homeostasis. Cancer is an example of cellular non-homeostasis since cancer cells replicate, but they do not die (they are immortal), and this process may be enhanced by the dysfunction of potassium channels. Other Shakur potassium channels such as Kv1.2,

Kv1.3, Kv1.4, Kv1.5, Kv1.6, Kv1.7 are also involved in cell migration and proliferation. [633] Finally, Kv1.1 potassium channels have been linked to kidney and even brain function.

Dysfunctional Kv1.1 Characteristics and Function

When Kv1.1 channels are dysfunctional many things may go wrong and are as follows. The dysfunction of a Kv1.1 potassium channel may be responsible for changes seen in the distribution, expression levels, and biophysical properties of the ion channel. [634] [635] If the sensory alpha subunits of Kv1.1 potassium channels cannot accurately sense cellular membrane voltage, it adversely affects the function of the potassium channel to both depolarize and repolarize, possibly resulting in hyper-excited muscles. A voltage sensing dysfunction may result from reduced channel expression and altered channel gating characteristics. [636] [637] Furthermore, dysfunction of the Kv1.1 channel may lead to fatigue from various mechanisms, including increased CK and "lactic acid production, pH changes, CO_2, and inorganic phosphate (Pi) accumulation." [638] Moreover dysfunction of the Kv1.1 channel may result in a change to calcium homeostasis in motor axon nerves found in the peripheral nervous system. [639] Dysfunction of the Kv1.1 potassium channel gene can act negatively on kidneys leading to hypomagnesemia or low magnesium levels. [640] Domenico Plantone outlines a plethora of possible motor, sensory, and autonomic symptoms that may happen when KV1.1 channels are dysfunctional. [641] Finally, symptoms arising from Kv1.1 dysfunction are exacerbated at cold temperatures. [642]

My Initial Diagnosis Theory

Initially, Isaac syndrome was the most logical diagnosis since it could explain most of my symptoms, including muscle hyperexcitation and the pseudo myotonia or the delayed muscle relaxation from a contracted state. Besides, from the previous sections, we learned that dysfunction of Kv.1.1 channels can plausibly explain many of my symptoms, including: [643] [644] [645] Dupuytren's contracture, worsening symptoms in cold temperatures, urinary dysfunction, gastrointestinal dysfunction, motor, sensory, and autonomic symptoms, pain, and elevated CK and lactic acid levels.

Chapter 13: Current Diagnosis Theory

I have had nine neurologists evaluate and retake my medical history. Whenever a diagnosis is elusive, having a medical history retaken by different doctors is not a bad idea. After all, a fresh set of eyes may uncover important information. Medical history is important for various reasons. For example, one important finding in my medical history indicates the neurological symptoms have both gradual onset and a gradual progression. Case in point, the gradual onset and progression may be indicative of a degenerative disease. Second, past medical history is important because neurological symptoms are often related to systemic diseases such as alcoholism and diabetes. In fact, it is important to review a patient's social history because factors such as alcoholism and other bad habits may be relevant, especially when uncovering the origination neurological symptoms. [646]

EMG Test Results

After a decade of decreased hand and feet strength, I had my third electromyography (EMG), and nerve conduction study (ENG) in September 2019. My first two EMG and ENG's were taken in November of 2008 and March of 2014, and they came back negative or inconclusive. Inconclusive indicates there may be amplitude changes or conduction velocity slowing but not enough to affect nerve function. The thought process behind another EMG and ENG was the gradual progression of the disorder may show new evidence, and that idea proved to be correct. This time both the EMG and ENG were positive and confirmed the following.

First, confirmation of *muscle atrophy* in the hands, feet, and calves was identified by the neurologist. An EMG does not identify atrophy per se, but only those abnormalities that may lead to atrophy. Part of the reason for the atrophy may be explained because I do not use these muscles as much, especially when I exercise. Cycling, especially time trialing, takes away the use of the hands, feet, and calves more so than rock climbing, hiking, or wrestling, activities I fully participated in until about seven years ago. Also, during a cycling stress test, it was determined that my water storage in my calves was deficient and that lack of oxygen could also lead to atrophy. According to a foot and lower leg study at the Huntsman games my balance results showed that I am about one standard deviation above normal. Surprisingly, the size of my muscles is about average (some are slightly above normal and others are slightly below normal). The muscle size result would seem to contradict neurologist observations of atrophy in my lower legs and feet. My feet and lower legs are very thin and lean. Since my legs and feet are much skinnier than the average athlete, that may give the false impression that there is atrophy. Conversely, persons with thicker lower legs and feet may give the false impression that their muscles are bigger than what they actually are because they have more fat. My strength results revealed that I was vastly deficient for great toe flexion and lateral toe flexion. In fact, my results were the worst of any male tested! This test may also give an impression of atrophy in the feet. That said, these strength findings are unsurprising since I have lost much flexibility and movement in my toes. Since I cannot curl my toes, I could not grasp the cord to pull the weight.

Second, the third EMG uncovered several findings, including **complex repetitive discharges** (CRDs) in one of my quad muscles (specifically, the *vastus lateralis muscle*). The CRDs were located in the same muscle where I suffer from a long-delayed muscle relaxation from a contracted state. Interestingly, the EMG report indicates that this muscle was normal. How an EMG would uncover CRDs but at the same time indicate the results are negative is a mystery. The EMG report only mentions the CRDs as a side note. CRD's is a significant finding because it may explain my increased CK, lactic acid, and fatigue in the quad muscles. CRDs are a sign of chronic denervating conditions found in disorders such as ALS or chronic myopathy diseases. Chronic myopathies with CRD's include Pompe, Becker, Duchenne, central nuclear myopathy, and various forms of idiopathic inflammatory myopathies. At the same time, since the CRDs only occur in one muscle and are not dispersed throughout the body, the finding may not be sinister but instead be brought about by some sort of compression of the nerve root at the spinal cord called radiculopathy or possibly some other unknown reason. Compressions of the spinal cord nerves can be produced by bone spurs, narrowing of the spinal column (spinal stenosis), and herniated disks.

Third, the EMG uncovered possible radiculopathy or a C8 nerve root compression causing neurological symptoms in the muscles of my hands and triceps. The findings were as follows: (1) The left and right *triceps* muscles controlled by the radial nerve originating from C6, C7, and C8 root, showed recruitment of motor units and interference pattern reduction of 25%. There were also normal to increased amplitude and duration of signals, which may indicate a reinnervation process in the triceps muscles. (2) The left and right first *dorsal interossei* (DI) hand muscle administered by the median nerve originating from the C8 and T1 root showed recruitment of motor units and interference pattern reduction of 25%. Fibrillations and positive sharp waves were identified in the left DI. There were also normal to increased amplitude and duration of signals, which may indicate a reinnervation process in the DI muscles. (3) The right *abductor pollicis brevis* (APB) hand muscle managed by the median nerve originating from the C8 and T1 root, also showed recruitment of motor units and interference pattern reduction of 25%. The left APB showed there were normal to increased amplitude and duration of signals, which may indicate a reinnervation process in the APB muscles. (4) What do the previous three points have in common? The C8 nerve root at the spinal cord, leading to the conclusion there may be compression at the C8 nerve root.

The nerve conduction study (ENG) also revealed both motor and sensory nerve concerns, in particular, in the lower arms, hands, lower legs, and feet. Specifically, the ENG identified symmetrical conduction velocity loss for motor signals traveling through the ulnar nerve from below the elbow to the hands. This type of injury can be the result of some type of demyelinating ulnar neuropathy, or it can be due to mechanical compression (or both).

Mechanical compression is produced by an external object pressing on the nerve. One possible source of symmetrical mechanical compression that originates below the elbow is riding in an aero position on a time trial bike. Please refer to Figures 5.1 and 5.2. The following are my motor conduction velocity results for the ulnar nerve, which may be a sign of early ulnar neuropathy: the right and left elbow (ulnar nerve) conduction velocity was 45 m/s, and the minimum specification is 50 m/s (a 10% slowing).

The ENG identified some mild sensory nerve abnormalities of the sural nerve (calf), and the ENG report said these results have an "uncertain clinical significance." This statement is hard to believe, considering all the other clinical findings in the same report. The sural nerve results are as follows: (1) the left calf (sural nerve) conduction velocity was 34 m/s, and the minimum specification is 35 m/s; and (2) the right calf passed but was just at the minimum specification. There was also a slight increase in the peak duration of the signal for the left calf (sural nerve).

The ENG also identified both symmetrical conduction velocity and amplitude loss for motor signals traveling through the peroneal nerve from the knee to feet. This type of injury can be the result of some type of demyelinating and or axonal neuropathy, or it can be due to mechanical compression. Symmetrical compression might result from a repetition injury. In particular, the repetitive motion of the leg muscles and joints in cycling is certainly a concern for causing a chronic injury. I complete about two million pedal revolutions or about 7,000 mi annually.

Still, a compression malfunction seems highly unlikely because the symptoms are symmetrical. Most compressions of the peroneal nerve come from pressure produced by crossed legs, resulting in an asymmetrical neuropathy, not a symmetrical neuropathy. [647] The following are my amplitude and conduction velocity results for the peroneal nerve: (1) the left ankle (peroneal nerve) has an amplitude of 1.2 mV, and the right ankle (peroneal nerve) has an amplitude of 0.3 mV. The minimum specification is 2.5 mV; (2) the left ankle (peroneal nerve) has a conduction velocity of 24 m/s, and the right ankle (peroneal nerve) shows a conduction block or 0 m/s. The minimum specification is 38 m/s. Conduction block of the right peroneal nerve may have been an issue for a long time. The one thing I remember from my second ENG was that the neurologist struggled to get a signal in my right peroneal nerve in the foot. After several attempts he never got a signal and chalked it up to me not having very much muscle mass in my feet. He said this outcome was somewhat common and he had seen similar results occur with other patients. Of course, the Huntsman study on my feet muscles would suggest my muscles are fairly normal. Hence, I am almost certain that what the neurologist found was conduction block in the peroneal nerve. The reason he did not believe the ENG result was my physical exam did not match the diagnostic finding of conduction block. If I truly had conduction block, the neurologist would expect to find more weakness in my exam, such as more limitations in my range of movement in the lower legs and feet. The reason for this discrepancy is because I am an athlete and have built up neural plasticity. If conduction block was occurring, what makes this finding interesting, the neurologist did not find any other significant nerve slowing. Thus, the disease at that time was focal, making multifocal motor neuropathy (MMN) a logical choice.

If I never found cycling, it is highly probable that instead of winning races, I would need assistance to walk (possibly a wheelchair). After all, the peroneal nerve innervates eight muscles in the lower leg and feet, including the *fibularis longus, fibularis brevis, tibialis anterior, extensor digitorum longus, extensor digitorum brevis, extensor hallucis longus, extensor hallucis brevis, and fibularis tertius* muscles. Thus, the peroneal nerve controls approximately half of the muscles in the lower legs and feet.

Finally, axonal (axonopathy) and demyelinating (myelinopathy) nerve conditions would also point to some other neuropathic disorder and not Isaac syndrome (IS). IS was the best explanation to fit my symptoms during the first five years of my diagnosis phase, but the EMG findings of CRDs as well as axonal and demyelination dysfunction ruled IS out as a logical possibility.

Now, the neurologist believes there may be several options that may explain my condition. A combination of the following conditions may provide the answer: Cramp fasciculation syndrome (CFS), radiculopathy or myelopathy, mechanical compression, multifocal motor neuropathy (MMN), and chronic inflammatory demyelinating polyneuropathy (CIDP). It is common for people with neurological disorders to contract more than one during their lifetime; people with either a compromised or aggressive immune system may be more susceptible to neurological disease. CIDP or MMN are autoimmune disorders, and therefore, there must have been an environmental trigger in the past twelve years to initiate the neuropathic symptoms (possibly heavy metal toxins, prescription drug use, or intense exercise).

Physical Exam

Below are my reflex and strength results from my last exam prior to my IVIg trial treatment:
Reflexes are graded on a 0 to 4 scale, described earlier in the text in Chapter 9 in the section on diminished reflexes. My neurologist rates my upper body deep tendon reflexes from normal to brisk (2 to 3), my patellar tendon reflex (knee) diminished (1), and my Achilles tendon reflexes from absent to reduced (0 to 1).

Strength is graded on a 0 to 5 scale, also defined earlier in the text. My neurologist rates my right- and left-hand intrinsic muscle: 4; Right and left triceps: 5-; Right and left wrist extensors: 5-; Right and left foot evertors: 4+; Fingers and toes were not measured, but I would guess my strength is, at best, a 4. Furthermore, ankle inversion and eversion muscles were not graded, and I have very little movement with these muscles. Eversion is the process to rotate the foot outward, and inversion is the process to rotate the foot inward using just the ankle joint and ankle muscles. In fact, my inversion and eversion muscle strength is probably, at best, a 3 or 4. At first glance, this does not appear to be a loss of much strength since all of the weakened muscles rates as a four or above on a scale of five. Nevertheless, remember, as discussed earlier, this is not a linear scale. Any markdown corresponds to a significant loss in strength. In other words, a rating of a four would indicate anywhere from one-third to one-half loss of strength. Generally, as reflexes diminish, so too does muscle strength, but they may or may not be diminished equally. Said differently, absent reflexes do not

necessarily indicate a loss of all strength and vice versa. My neurologist said that testing strength on athletes who have neurological disease is a difficult task because exam results may not match their diagnostic testing since they build neural plasticity by creating new pathways for muscles and the brain to communicate.

Myelopathy

Radiculopathy

Radiculopathy has the following etiology, symptoms, treatment methods, diagnosis methods, test results, and diagnosis probability: [648 649 650 651 652]

Etiology

Radiculopathy is a process in which there is a compression of the nerve root at the spinal cord. The most common place for compression of a nerve root is on the cervical spine or the lumbar spine because these sections of the spine are the most active and are, therefore, more susceptible to wear and tear. In particular, radiculopathy is common in the nerve roots between L4–L5 (L5 nerve root) or L5–S1 (S1 nerve root) on the lumbar spine and between C5–C6 (C6 nerve root) or C6–C7 (C7 nerve root) of the cervical spine. About 90% of all radiculopathies happen in the above-noted locations.

Spinal stenosis is the narrowing of the spinal canal, leading to spinal cord compression. This, too, usually happens in the cervical and lumbar regions of the spine. Causes of radiculopathy or spinal stenosis include: Age and normal wear and tear, infections such as Lyme disease, syphilis, and herpes, inflammation such as GBS, CIDP, and AIDP, malignancy (cancer) or spinal cysts, trauma or injury of the spine, and degenerative diseases of the spine.

Symptoms [653] [654]

People with radiculopathy may have symptoms such as numbness, pain, paresthesia, weakness, atrophy, and impaired reflexes. Atrophy is generally brought about from exercise intolerance to avoid pain. Since radiculopathy can affect both the sympathetic and parasympathetic nervous system, many people also have autonomic involvement. Radiculopathy may be eliminated from consideration for purely motor symptoms that may suggest spinal muscle atrophy or ALS or when there is pain in the absence of weakness, which may indicate another musculoskeletal ailment. The location of neurological symptoms depends on which nerve roots are affected:

- C3/C4–Pain and weakness in the shoulder muscles.

- C5–Pain, and weakness in the neck, shoulder, and lateral arm. Paresthesia in the shoulder with diminished reflexes on the deltoid and bicep muscles.
- C6–Pain, and weakness in the neck, shoulder, scapula, and forearm. Paresthesia in the fingers with diminished reflexes in the forearm, thumb, and bicep muscles.
- C7–Pain, and weakness in the neck, shoulder, scapula, and forearm. Paresthesia in the fingers with diminished reflexes in the triceps, forearms, and finger muscles.

- C8–Pain, and weakness in the neck, shoulder, scapula, and forearm. Paresthesia in the fingers with diminished reflexes in the triceps, forearms, hands, and little finger muscles.
- L3–Pain, weakness, and diminished reflexes in the quadriceps muscles.
- L4–Pain, and weakness in the hip and thigh. Paresthesia in the thigh with diminished reflexes in the quadriceps, calf, and feet muscles.
- L5–Pain, and weakness in the thigh, calf, and foot. Paresthesia in the calf and foot with diminished reflexes in the quadriceps, hamstring, calve, and big toe muscles.
- S1–Pain, and weakness in the thigh leg, and heel. Paresthesia in the calf and foot with diminished reflexes in the quadriceps, hamstring, calf, and little toe muscles.

Treatment Methods

Radiculopathy treatment generally starts with rest, anti-inflammatory medications, and steroids. When more conservative methods of treatment fail, then surgery is a last resort. With that said, data indicate that the long-term effects of surgery are not any better than other treatment methods. Surgery is necessary once pain disappears, but weakness persists, indicating the nerve is almost dead or when lumbar radiculopathy produces severe bladder and bowel autonomic dysfunction.

Diagnosis Methods

An MRI of the spine can determine radiculopathy or spinal stenosis. Radiculopathy is often misdiagnosed as peripheral neuropathy since they both have similar symptoms, including pain, fatigue, paresthesia, burning sensation, and other motor and sensory symptoms.

Test Results

A C-Spine MRI uncovered benign perineural cysts on the C4 to T3 vertebrae. Perineural cysts are generally non-symptomatic, but, at times, they can be problematic when they are large and compress spinal nerves. To be more precise about the MRI findings, small perineural cysts were found at C4 and C5; normal size cysts were discovered at C5 and C6 as well as C6 and C7; and large cysts were found at C7 and T1, T1 and T2, and T2 and T3 on both the right and left sides of the vertebrae. Specifically, perineural cysts are filled with spinal fluid and are only systematic in about 1% of all cases. The cysts can be drained, but that is only a temporary fix because they can refill with fluid. Thus, if the cysts are systematic, the only way to permanently alleviate the pain and discomfort is to remove the cysts surgically. It was difficult to discern if the cysts were symptomatic, but the finding was unusual for a few reasons: (1) spinal cysts are unusual in the C-spine and are more common in the L or S spine; (2) the sheer number of cysts the MRI revealed; and (3) the size of some of the cysts, especially in the C8 region. Large cysts may be problematic because there is a better chance, they will compress the nerve root.

To determine if the perineurial cysts are systematic, the neurologist ordered a lumbar spine (L-spine) MRI. If perineural cysts exist in the L-spine, then the assumption that the cysts are causing symptoms in my arms, hands, feet, and lower legs is plausible.

An L-Spine MRI came back negative, and that result was odd since perineural cysts, as mentioned above, are more common in the L-spine than the C-spine. Thus, radiculopathy is not the reason for any of the denervation occurring in my quad muscles or any of the symptoms in the lower limbs or feet. It also led the neurologist to believe that the spinal cysts in the C-spine are probably not symptomatic, especially since I do not have any radiating pain associated with radiculopathy. Another important fact that led me to believe the cysts were not systematic was because I had symptoms of paresthesia in my hands 15 years ago, and an MRI on my C-spine at that time came back negative (including no cysts). Hence, I had symptoms with and without cysts. That is not to say the cysts may be exacerbating symptoms, but the consensus is they are not.

Diagnosis Probability

The results are inconclusive that I have radiculopathy since the MRI on the C-Spine came back positive for perineural cysts, while the L-Spine results were negative. Radiculopathy would make sense for many of my symptoms if there are compressions in C5–T1 as well as the L2–S2 region. Since the perineurial cysts are only located in the C5–T1 region, they cannot be the cause of all my symptoms, but they may be a source to cause or exacerbate symptoms in the hands and arms. Conversely, it is also possible the perineurial cysts are benign since they are generally not symptomatic and do not cause any radiculopathy.

Mechanical Compression [655]

Etiology

M*echanical compression* is an external force applied to a nerve that can result in abnormal signal transmission. Symptoms from most peripheral nerve compressions are focal or asymmetrical and are brought about by mechanical pressure, while generalized or symmetrical compressions are probably the outcome of some toxin, inflammation, tumor, or infection. Therefore, most neuropathies associated with nerves, such as the ulnar, median, or peroneal nerve, are focal disorders. Mechanical compression is more likely to happen in nerves that have been demyelinated and lack insulation protection. A mechanical compression can lead to nerve demyelination as well as axonal damage. If the source of mechanical compression ceases, nerve myelin and axonal damage can be reversed. Common nerve compression locations are found on the following nerves (nerve roots): Suprascapular nerve (C4–C6), auxiliary nerve (C5–C6), thoracic nerve (C5–C7), musculocutaneous nerve (C5–C7), radial nerve (C5–C8), median nerve (C5–T1), ulnar nerve (C8–T1), genitofemoral and ilioinguinal nerves (L1–L2), lateral femoral cutaneous nerve (L2–L3), femoral nerve (L1–L4), gluteal nerves (L4–S2), sciatic nerve (L4–S3), peroneal nerve (L4–S2), and tibial nerve (L4–S3).

Diagnosis Probability

Mechanical compressions are generally asymmetrical and are very rarely symmetrical. None the less, symmetrical mechanical compression may happen when riding in a time trial position, which places a significant amount of mechanical force on both arms just below the elbows. The

ulnar nerve (C5–T1) is responsible for motor and sensory function for the muscles of the upper arm, hand, and fingers. Since demyelinated nerves increase the probability of mechanical compression, it is distinctly possible that time trialing may be causing or exacerbating the neuropathy damage of the ulnar nerve, but there no conclusive evidence to support this theory.

Neuropathy

Neuropathy, like other diseases and disorders, is characterized by sensory localization. Sensory localization is the pattern and distribution of symptoms. My symptoms mimic general distal neuropathies such as peripheral or polyneuropathy, whose sensory localization pattern for symptoms is both symmetrical and distal. Said differently, peripheral or polyneuropathy symptoms have a sensory localization pattern similar to wearing gloves and knee-high socks, which fits length-dependent axonal neuropathies. That said, the pattern and distribution for generalized distal neuropathies can be vastly different, especially if demyelination of the axons is involved. In generalized distal neuropathies, vibration sensation is often affected first, but, in many cases, all sensory systems are impaired (exteroceptive, proprioceptive, and interoceptive). Moreover, most generalized distal neuropathies impair both motor, sensory, and autonomic nerves. Furthermore, generalized distal neuropathies may affect large nerve fibers such as in Sjögren's syndrome, small nerve fibers such as in hereditary forms of neuropathy, or both. Large fiber neuropathies generally affect reflexes, while small fiber neuropathies affect pain and temperature sensation. [656]

Peripheral Neuropathy (PN)

PN encompasses many different kinds of neuropathy such as Charcot–Marie–Tooth disease (CMTD), chronic inflammatory demyelinating polyneuropathy (CIDP), and multifocal motor neuropathy (MMN) are discussed later. Below are the epidemiology facts, symptoms, etiology, diagnosis methods, treatment methods, test results, and pain analysis for PN:

Epidemiology [657]

Neuropathy means having damaged nerves. Most cases of neuropathy are called axonal neuropathy, which indicates there is damage to the nerve axon but not to the myelin sheath. Neuropathic pain is said to inflict up to 5% of the population, and up to 20% of those inflicted apply for disability insurance within two years of being diagnosed. Up to 60% of patients with neuropathic pain are depressed, and only about 25% obtain quality sleep on a consistent basis.

Symptoms [658] [659]

Early symptoms appear both symmetrically and distally, usually in the toes or lower limbs. Symptoms can affect motor, sensory, and autonomic nerve function, and may be characterized by paresthesia in the feet, loss of vibration sensation distally, and weakness. Additionally, as the condition worsens, the symptoms can spread to the upper limbs.

Numerous forms of PN, especially diabetic, attack the autonomic system. ***Diabetic neuropathy*** is characterized by (1) symmetrical, distal, and mostly sensory symptoms; (2) impaired perception of vibration in the toes and feet, loss of Achilles reflex, burning sensations, paresthesia, tingling, and numbness; and (3) weakness and atrophy usually do not present in diabetic neuropathy cases.

Alcohol-induced PN has additional symptoms that may mimic those found in thiamine or vitamin B deficiency. Intense sensory symptoms include leg pain from cramping as well as paresthesia, and the symptoms are generally symmetrical, distal, and include an absent Achilles reflex. Touch and vibration sensations diminish distally, and the calves are tender to touch.

Diagnostic Methods [660]

First, cerebrospinal fluid (CSF) can reveal elevated proteins. Second, conduction studies indicate slow signal velocities for demyelinated polyneuropathy but only mildly slow or normal velocities for axonal polyneuropathy. Axonal polyneuropathy indicates a decrease in signal amplitude as the signal propagates through the muscles. Third, an EMG reveals evidence of denervation or altered potentials. Finally, sural nerve biopsies are generally not recommended for neuropathy because the biopsy itself can make symptoms worse.

Etiology or Causation [661]

Common causes of polyneuropathy are genetics, inflammation, autoimmune disease, cirrhosis, hypothyroidism, GBS, CIDP, MMN, CMTD, malnutrition (gastritis and vitamin B-12), diabetes, gout, alcoholism, gluten sensitivities, infection (hepatitis, mumps, chickenpox, diphtheria, mononucleosis, spotted fever, botulism, and leprosy), arterial disease, toxic substances (ethanol, lead, arsenic, and thallium), prescription drugs (antiviral), and cancer. [662]

Acquired polyneuropathies have an environmental etiology. However, causation is not uncovered in over 30% of all cases. Inherited neuropathies have no underlining environmental explanations because it originates from gene mutations handed down from generation to generation. Since 30% of people with peripheral polyneuropathy have an unidentified etiology, it is very difficult to find symptom relief for those patients. Furthermore, even if the cause has been identified, such as alcohol or drug addiction, pregnancy, a vaccine, a virus, or a prescription drug, the symptoms may persist once the cause is removed. Most damaged nerves can regenerate, but the regenerated nerves are never as good as the original nerve fibers.

Demyelinating polyneuropathies are usually brought about by autoimmune disorders when either white blood cells or immunoglobulins attack the myelin and sometimes the axons of nerve cells. Evidence suggests that voltage-gated sodium channel (VGSC) dysfunction may trigger or exacerbate symptoms of peripheral polyneuropathy. [663]

Peripheral polyneuropathy may originate from an accumulation of VGSCs not only at the site of an injury but in the dorsal root of the spinal nerve. [664] Four sodium channels are of particular interest: Nav 1.3, Nav1.8, Nav1.9, and Nav1.7. Some evidence supports a relationship between neuropathic pain and abnormal distribution of Nav1.8 and Nav1.9 VGSCs after a nerve injury. The Nav1.7 (SCN9A gene) plays an important role in small fiber neuropathy (SFN) and enhanced neuropathic pain, including burning pain and swelling of the hands and feet. In fact, the opposite may be true since a mutation in the SCN9A gene may cause some people to never to feel pain. [665] The SCN3A gene (Nav1.3) may also play a role in peripheral neuropathy, but its role is not clear. Some evidence indicates that both N-type and T-type calcium channels may play a role in neuropathic symptoms associated with cancers or diseases such as HIV and AIDS. However, most of the information about sodium channels and their role in polyneuropathy symptoms has been proven on animals, but not on humans at this point. [666]

Test Results

I tested negative for a small fiber neuropathy (SFN) skin biopsy test, which specifically checks for epidermal nerve fiber density and sweat gland nerve fiber density anomalies. Briefly, ***small fiber neuropathy*** refers to dysfunction of small unmyelinated nerve fibers responsible for pain and temperature sensation, and it may or may not be associated with large nerve fibers. SFN is characterized by burning feet and distal symptoms. SFN presents with some of the same manifestations of both acquired or hereditary polyneuropathies.

Cerebrospinal fluid (CSF) is a common neurological test, and its extraction from the spinal cord is sometimes known as a lumbar puncture or spinal tap. CSF testing includes color evaluation (should be clear), CSF pressure (specification: 50 to 200 mm of H2O), white blood cell count, glucose levels (specification: 50 to 80 milligrams/deciliter, mg/dL), IgG levels (specification: less than 8.5 mg/dL), and protein levels (specification: 15 to 60 mg/dL). CSF tests can detect most demyelinating degenerative diseases such as MS, GBS, and CIDP since proteins are elevated in about 90% of all cases. Elevated proteins (more than 45 mg/dL) may also indicate other dysfunctions such as tumors, infections, stroke, connective tissue disorders, and cardiovascular disease. [667] My results came back normal for all CSF tests: CSF fluid (clear), white blood cell count, CSF pressure, total proteins (22 mg/dL), IgG proteins (1 mg/dL), and glucose levels (51mg/dL).

Pain

A common symptom of peripheral neuropathy is pain. The International Association for the Study of Pain defines neuropathic pain as "pain initiated or caused by a primary lesion or dysfunction in the nervous system." Neuropathic pain has often been described as a shooting, burning, lancinating, prickling, electrical, tingling, numbness, paresthesia, and other types of sensations. Furthermore, "The numerous features of neuropathic pain can complicate an accurate clinical diagnosis." [668]

The neuropathy and chronic pain relationship to the immune system are still a mystery. The medical community has devised pathological theories to link neuropathy and

pain are as follows: [669] ***Cytokines*** are proteins produced by inflamed tissue, and they have been shown to link the immune system with the nervous system to modulate pain. Cytokines can come in numerous varieties, and the three primary proinflammatory ones are interleukin-1 (IL-1), interleukin-6 (IL-6), and interleukin-18 (IL-18). IL-1, IL-6, and IL-18 are associated with not only inflammation but autoimmune diseases, and it is, therefore, hypothesized they are associated with neuronopathic pain. ***Chemokines*** are
also produced in inflamed tissue and are responsible for wound healing. Chemokines appear in the cells of both the central and peripheral nervous systems. Although their role in neuropathic pain is not fully understood, many have postulated links between the two. ***Nerve growth factor (NGF)*** proteins and the nonapeptide bradykinin are linked to neuropathic pain when they are released from damaged or inflamed tissue.

To counteract pain-producing agents, the body also produces anti-inflammatory cytokines such as IL-4, IL-10, and IL-13. The body also produces what is known as leukocyte derived opioid peptides to counteract pain. Many patients dealing with a compromised immune system may have a low CD4 lymphocyte (helper T-cells) cell count and are, therefore, unable to manufacture opioid peptides to fight pain.

Autoimmune conditions with links to neuropathic pain include several serious diseases and disorders such as Addison's disease, Alzheimer's disease, asthma, Celiac disease, chronic fatigue syndrome, Crohn's disease, eczema, Graves' disease, Hashimoto's thyroiditis, lupus, multiple sclerosis, Parkinson's disease, pernicious anemia, psoriasis, Raynaud's disease, rheumatoid arthritis, scleroderma, diabetes, and vitiligo. [670]

A typical pain response to neuropathy includes the release of proinflammatory cytokines such as interleukins and other substances like nerve growth factor (NGF) to the target region. When there is an accumulation of pro-inflammatory substances such as interleukins and nerve growth factors, then adjacent uninjured nerves may be affected, which leads to more activity in the central nervous system. However, those mechanisms that may initiate the neuropathy symptoms may not be the same as those mechanisms that sustain neuropathy symptoms. That said, evidence suggests, "Nerve growth factor can initiate long-lasting changes to peripheral nerves to promote and sustain an enhanced pain state." [671]

Treatment Methods for Pain and Neuropathy [672]

One proposed solution to counter the problem of a low CD4 cell count (helper T-cells) is to produce and release opioid-containing leukocytes through gene therapy. Additionally, immune suppression drugs may be helpful to alleviate symptoms, including pain, but they will make it easier for the patient to acquire a cold, flu, virus, or bacterial infection. Interestingly, IVIg and plasma exchange can treat neuropathy when it is triggered by an autoimmune disease characterized by immunoglobulin proteins acting as the antibody. Pain therapies using sodium channel blocker medications have been disappointing to this juncture. Carbamazepine is known to work as a sodium channel blocker, and it reduces my pain. [673]

Hereditary Polyneuropathy or Charcot–Marie–Tooth Disease (CMTD) [674] [675]

There are seven types or classes of *hereditary motor and sensory neuropathies (HMSN)*. The most common is Type I, which is also referred to as *Charcot–Marie–Tooth Disease (CMTD)*. Below are the epidemiology facts, etiology, symptoms, diagnosis methods, treatment methods, and diagnosis probability for HMSN:

Epidemiology

CMTD is the most common hereditary polyneuropathy and has a prevalence rate of 2 in 100,000. The age of onset varies, but, for most, HMSN-type onset occurs between 20 and 50. Most classes of HMSN are autosomal dominant, which denotes one gene pair is mutated, and one is normal. Types 6 and 7 HNSM are autosomal recessive, indicating that both genes in the pair are mutated.

Etiology or Causation

At least five genetic mutations have been uncovered, with 70 to 80% of the cases due to the peripheral myelin protein 22 gene (PMP22) on chromosome 17.

Symptoms

Sensory: Classes 1, 5, 6, and 7 have little to no symptoms for the toes and fingers; Type 2 has mild symptoms for the toes and fingers, and Types 3 and 4 have significant symptoms for the toes and fingers. Atrophy and weakness: Class 1 symptoms are located in the hands, feet (high arch), calves, peroneal muscles, and forearms; Type 2 symptoms are located in the feet (high arch) and calves, Type 3 symptoms are rapidly progressive in legs and hands, and Types 4, 5, 6, and 7 symptoms are located in the feet and hands. Reflexes: All classes present with absent reflexes in the Achilles tendon but preserved elsewhere. HNSM is characterized by thickened peripheral nerves in class 1, 3, and 4, hearing loss in class 4, and vision loss in class 6. CMTD (Type 1) patients see a very slow progression, and patients usually work until normal retirement age.

Diagnosis

Several tests are available to diagnose this condition. First, it is possible to undergo genetic testing and consider family history. Second, sural nerve biopsy reveals the effects of a cyclical process acting on the nerves, including axon degeneration, demyelination, and remyelination. An onion-skin structure appears on the sural nerve initiated by the repetitive process of demyelination and remyelination of Schwann cells. Third, an EMG can uncover chronic denervation in affected muscles. Finally, a nerve conduction study (ENG) can reveal varying conduction velocities depending on the class of HMSN: Types 5 and 6 have normal results, Types 2, 5, and 6 have mildly slow results, Type 7 shows slowed results, Types 1 and 4 show significantly slowed results, and Type 3 has severely slow results.

Treatment Methods

Treatment for hereditary disorders is usually limited to treating symptoms such as pain.

Diagnosis Probability

I have no family history of any neurological dysfunction. That said, a word of caution is warranted about easily dismissing hereditary diseases because negative family history is not always negative. Case in point, my mother died very young (so did her siblings and her mother), so she may not have had the opportunity for a late-onset hereditary disorder to develop. Furthermore, many people with CMTD may not view their symptoms as abnormal, and therefore, they may not seek medical assistance. [676] Furthermore, one of my neurologists pointed out that I have "fairly high arches" indicating that CMTD may be a remote possibility. For the above reasons, I was tested for the CMTD gene mutation, and it came back negative.

Chronic Inflammatory Demyelinating Polyneuropathy (CIDP) [677 678 679 680]

The following are some common epidemiology, symptoms, etiology, diagnosis methods, treatment methods, and diagnosis probability for CIDP.

Epidemiology

CIDP is more common in men by a 2 to 1 ratio, and the onset age is about 50. High creatine kinase presents in one-third of all cases. Up to 33% of those initially undiagnosed cases of neuropathy are CIDP.

Symptoms

CIDP affects both motor and sensory nerves, as well as myelin sheaths of nerves. Numbness is present in up to 80% of the patients, and weakness and incoordination are common; up to 50% of patients have painful paresthesia. Additionally, reduced tendon reflexes, muscle weakness, and muscle atrophy are present in the affected areas. CIDP can be progressive, or it can take the relapsing-remitting course. Symptoms can be asymmetrical or symmetrical and distal or proximal; though less common, CIDP can also have axonal involvement (axonopathy). Weakness and autonomic dysfunction are less severe but last longer than GBS. Finally, there is generally cranial nerve involvement.

Etiology or Causation

When the myelin sheath of a nerve is destroyed, the consequences of decreased path resistance and increased capacitance are signal leakage. The consequences of signal leakage are as follows: [681] (1) signal strength degrades traveling the length of the nerve, making it incapable of depolarizing cells to carry the signal to its final destination; (2) blocking uninsulated nerves is easier when they are under mechanical pressure; (3) signals jump from one nerve fiber to another (interference); and (4) damaged nerve signals may run in opposite directions of what is normal.

CIDP is autoimmune, but the pathogenesis of CIDP is unknown and not fully understood. [682] It may be brought about by immunoglobulins binding with other healthy cells such as contactin associated protein 1 (CASPR-1) or M protein. The process of nerve demyelination has varying results, including inflammation, vitamin B deficiency, genetic defects, or autoimmune disease. Additionally, CIDP may be triggered by exposure to medications such as antibiotics or antivirals as well as exposure to toxins such as alcohol and heavy metals. The demyelination of axons is accomplished by macrophage cells. CIDP is the result of the immune system attacking the myelin sheaths of the peripheral nerves. CIDP is not the same as multiple sclerosis (MS) because, in MS, the immune system attacks the myelin sheaths of the central nervous system. The condition is linked to autoimmune disorders of the digestive system, Sjögren's syndrome, and infections. [683]

There are many variants of CIDP. For instance, CIDP can be asymmetrical, symmetrical, distal, or proximal. Some forms of CIDP are purely motor, such as multifocal motor neuropathy (MMN), while other forms are purely sensory such as chronic immune, sensory polyradiculoneuropathy (CISP). Finally, some forms of CIDP are both sensory and motor, such as classic CIDP, multifocal acquired demyelinating sensory and motor neuropathy (MADSAM), or distal acquired demyelinating symmetric neuropathy (DADS).

Treatment Methods

IVIg treatment or plasma exchange work best to alleviate and remove symptoms. That said, it should be pointed out that although IVIg will quickly resolve demyelination damage, it takes longer to repair axonal damage. Axons in the peripheral nervous system can regenerate (unlike nerves in the central nervous system), but the rate of regrowth is slow. Axons regenerate at a rate of about 1 mm per day but keep in mind that regenerated nerves are never as good as the original nerve fibers. Immunosuppressants and steroid treatments such as prednisone may alleviate symptoms.

Diagnosis Methods

CIDP patients present with high levels of proinflammatory cytokines such as interleukins (IL-1) and elevated protein levels are present in the cerebral spinal fluid (CSF) in about 90% of the cases. Nerve conduction studies (ENG) uncover slowed velocities and possibly an absent or delayed F wave. The EMG may also reveal decreased amplitudes and abnormal spontaneous muscle activity.

Diagnosis Probability

When Isaac syndrome was eliminated as a potential diagnosis, then CIDP, or some form of CIDP, seemed highly probable to explain at least part of my condition. Although I tested negative for elevated CSF proteins, which present in about 90% of the cases, my EMG findings do suggest some form of neuropathy. Furthermore, CIDP may not explain the CRD's in my quad muscles and symptoms such as muscle hyperactivity. No environmental cause has been identified for triggering my CIDP, but that is fairly common for many CIDP cases. That said, my medical history does include several potential environmental triggers such as alcohol abuse, potential exposure to toxins, prescription drug use, and intense exercise that could have triggered CIDP.

Guillain-Barré Syndrome (GBS)

The following are some common symptoms, etiology, diagnosis methods, treatment methods, and diagnosis probability for GBS: [684 685 686 687]

Symptoms

GBS and its derivatives are complex and can lead to muscle weakness, hyporeflexia, sensory symptoms, distal paresthesia, sensory disturbances, autonomic nervous system dysfunction, and periodic paralysis. GBS may have symptoms affecting both the myelin or axons of nerves. There are many variants of GBS, and some may be pure sensory, pure motor, or pure autonomic.

The severity of GBS cases fluctuates greatly with some mild and others that may result in death. Severe cases affect the upper limbs, respiratory system, diaphragm, and cranial nerves innervating the head and neck. GBS may affect both the peripheral and cranial nerves and result in autonomic instability, including fluctuations in both heart rate (cardiac arrhythmia) and blood pressure. Moreover, sodium deficiency is common, while bladder involvement is rare in GBS. The condition may also be associated with autoimmune autonomic neuropathy whose symptoms include lightheadedness, gastrointestinal dysfunction, heat intolerance, dry mouth, sexual dysfunction, hyperhidrosis, bladder malfunction, numbness, tingling, paresthesia, and dysesthesia. *Dysesthesia* refers to abnormal senses, which can include pain. [688] [689]

Etiology or Causation

GBS may involve lymphocytic inflammation or antibodies that can attack myelinated nerves of the peripheral nervous system. GBS may also be brought about when the complement system disrupts sodium channel function leading to nerve failure and muscle weakness. The complement system response can also destroy the myelin sheath of axons, resulting in a demyelinating polyneuropathy. Various antibodies may be involved, including IgG or T-cells, which attack the lymph system. [690] GBS is also different from multiple sclerosis in that it attacks the peripheral nerves and not the nerves in the central nervous system.

Some theories link GBS to the flu since many people had the flu a month prior to developing GBS symptoms. In some cases, GBS was proceeded by mycoplasma pneumonia or by a virus such as the flu, chickenpox, mumps, hepatitis, HIV, or Epstein-Barr. [691] One hypothesis for GBS is an increase of inorganic phosphate in the mitochondria called hypophosphatemia. The consequences of hypophosphatemia may be muscle pain as well as adverse effects on the cardio and respiratory systems. [692] Other immune-mediated neuropathies, such as acute autonomic neuropathy, may also fall under the GBS spectrum. [693]

Both GBS and CIDP are associated with nerve compression or radiculopathy. The most common type of neuropathy associated with GBS is an ***acute inflammatory demyelinating polyradiculoneuropathy (AIDP)***. AIDP symptoms include severe weakness, numbness, paresthesia, incoordination, vibration sensation, tingling, and sensory dysfunction. However, digestive system involvement does not happen in AIDP. [694]

Diagnosis Methods

GBS presents with elevated proteins in the cerebrospinal fluid (CSF). A spinal MRI may show nerve root enhancement or radiculopathy.

Treatment Methods

Plasma exchange and immunoglobulin treatments may lead to a complete recovery, but the recovery is generally partial in most people afflicted with autoimmune autonomic neuropathy. AIDP also responds well to both plasma exchange and immunoglobulin treatments.

Diagnosis Probability

It is unlikely that I have GBS since I tested negative for elevated CSF proteins and both C and L-spine MRIs showed no definitive signs of radiculopathy. Furthermore, symptoms for GBS usually begin soon after a trigger. In other words, symptom onset for GBS is abrupt and is clearly understood. The onset of symptoms is slowly progressive for neuropathy and, therefore, the trigger is not obvious, and sometimes it is never identified. Hence, neuropathy is a more logical explanation than GBS for my illness.

Multifocal Motor Neuropathy (MMN)

The following are some epidemiology facts, symptoms, etiology, treatment methods, test results, and diagnosis probability of MMN: [695] [696]

Epidemiology

MMN affects men more than women (2:1). The prevalence of MMN is only about 1 in every 200,000 people or only about 1,500 individuals in the United States.

Symptoms

MMN symptoms include fasciculations, cramps, weakness, atrophy, fatigue, symptoms are exacerbated by cold, asymmetrical symptoms, slowly or rapidly progressive, reflexes are preserved to the level of strength, sensory nerves are normal, or vibration sensations may be diminished, it usually affects the upper limbs more than the lower limbs, and elevated CK and M protein are common. Symptoms rarely affect the cranial nerves, respiratory nerves, or cardio nerves. If denervation happens, it usually presents in the lower legs, feet, lower arms, and hands. Finger extension may be compromised as well as difficulty extending wrists backward (wrist drop). There may also be reduced mobility of the toes, as well as difficulty performing tasks that require fine motor skills, such as picking up pills or coins. Conduction block of nerve signals is common in MMN.

Etiology

One theory suggests that anti-GM1 antibodies affect peripheral nerve sodium channels at the neuromuscular junction in about 60% of all cases. [697] Other theories insist the anti-GM1 antibodies may affect the function of other proteins.

Diagnostic Methods [698] [699]

GM1 is a toxin, and accumulation of it could lead to death. GM1 antibody accumulation is not severe until it attacks motoneurons, causing MMN symptoms. There are several variants of anti-GM1 antibodies, which can include all IgG classes or IgM. IgM is the immunoglobulin class associated with MMN. The effect of the different IgG classes on anti-GM1 antibodies is still not completely understood. Anti-GM1 antibodies are sometimes but rarely associated with ALS and GBS, and are said to only attack motor nerves. However, there have been a few papers suggesting that anti-GM1 antibodies can affect a variety of sensory nerves. Finally, anti-GM1 antibodies can have both a hypo and hyperexcitation effect on muscles.

Treatment Methods

MMN is an autoimmune disorder, and it can be treated effectively with IVIg treatments. [700] Norman Latov suggests that about one-third of all autoimmune neuropathies that react positively to IVIg therapy can be resolved after several treatments. The other two-thirds symptoms may reoccur and need further maintenance treatments of IVIg. [701] MMN usually requires maintenance treatments to slow its progression. Antiseizure medications are also used to treat symptoms associated with MMN. [702] MMN does not respond to immunosuppressant treatments, steroid treatments such as prednisone, or plasma exchange. In fact, these treatments can make the disease worse.

Test Results

Anti-GM1 are ganglioside antibodies and lead to a variety of conditions and diseases, especially neuropathy such as multifocal motor neuropathy (MMN). The blood test for these antibodies came back with an intermediate or equivocal reading: [703] Asialo-GM1 antibodies, IgG-IgM: 33 IV, GM1 antibodies, IgG-IgM: 35 IV, GD1b antibodies, IgG-IgM: 36 IV, GD1a antibodies, IgG-IgM: 26 IV, and GQ1b antibodies, IgG-IgM: 5 IV

The Mayo Clinic defines these blood tests as follows: Ganglioside antibodies are associated with diverse peripheral neuropathies. Elevated antibody levels to ganglioside-monosialic acid (GM1) and the neutral glycolipid, asialo-GM1, are associated with motor or sensorimotor neuropathies, particularly multifocal motor neuropathy. Anti-GM1 may occur as IgM (polyclonal or monoclonal) or IgG antibodies. These antibodies may also be found in patients with diverse connective tissue diseases as well as normal individuals. GD1a antibodies are associated with different variants of Guillain-Barré syndrome (GBS), particularly acute motor axonal neuropathy, while GD1b antibodies are predominantly found in sensory ataxic neuropathy syndrome. Anti-GQ1b antibodies are seen in more than 80% of patients with Miller-Fisher syndrome and may be elevated in GBS patients with ophthalmoplegia.

The "1a" or "1b" designations in the test results refer to the type of nerve fibers involved in the antibody attack. Again, nerve fibers are classified by size with Type I (1) being the largest and Type IV (4) being the smallest. The "a" and "b" designations refer to the origination or location of the nerve fibers such as in the skeleton muscle fibers for Type "a" and in the Golgi tendon organs (GTO) nerve fibers for Type "b." [704]

Antibody readings above 50 IV indicate illness, and readings below 30 IV are normal. Intermediate readings between 30 IV and 50 IV may or may not indicate an illness (the readings are equivocal). Thus, these blood tests might rule out multifocal motor neuropathy (MMN), but then again, they may not, so the tests are inconclusive. Furthermore, only about 50% of people with MMN test positive for the GM1 antibody. Interestingly, GD1b was also equivocal for sensory ataxic neuropathy syndrome. Of course, most people with ataxic neuropathy syndrome have dysfunction in the cerebellum region of the brain. Ataxia symptoms include incoordination, balance dysfunction, and seizures, which do not fit my symptoms. Therefore, I am very skeptical that any of the equivocal antibody measurements in these tests are symptomatic since I do not have ataxia or any upper motor neuron symptoms. The equivocal readings may simply be the result of my very low titer concentrations for immunoglobulins: IgM: 50 milligrams / deciliter - mg/dL (Specification 35 to 263), IgG: 699 mg/dL (Specification 768 to 1632), and IgA: 83 mg/dL (Specification 68 to 408)

Diagnosis Probability

There is a very high likelihood that I have MMN since I tested equivocal for the GM1antibodies, and MMN can present without elevated CSF proteins. Furthermore, MMN is associated with hyperexcited muscles and can encompass symptoms of CFS. Although there are some conflicts between my symptoms and typical MMN symptoms, such as my symptoms are symmetrical, they are more active in the legs than arms, and they also exist in the upper leg. That said, it is possible for people with MMN to present with symmetrical symptoms and more symptom prevalence in the legs, including in the upper leg. Another symptom conflict is that MMN does not affect either sensory or autonomic nerves. It is possible that my autonomic IBS symptoms may be mutually exclusive to the neurological issue caused by, for instance, being on omeprazole for a long time. At the same time, GM1 antibodies in GBS affect the digestive system, and more recent papers are concluding that GM1 antibodies may indeed affect sensory nerves. Moreover, the link that MMN does not affect sensory nerves and, therefore, has very little pain associated with the disorder makes very little sense. After all, MMN is linked to cramps, muscle fatigue, and disability, which are painful.

Myopathy

A myopathy is a muscle disease. The differential diagnosis for CRDs encompasses various myopathies, ALS, and radiculopathy. My EMG tested 18 muscles with only one positive for CRDs and denervation. This led the neurologist to believe that it is unlikely that I have a myopathy because the CRDs are not widespread. Besides, my ENG and EMG indicate more significant signs pointing to a nerve disorder, not a muscle disorder. CRDs may also be the manifestation of spinal stenosis or radiculopathy, which can be verified with an MRI of the spine. Since the MRI came back negative, the cause of the CRDs remains unexplained. [705]

Myopathies have the following characteristics or symptoms: [706] [707] [708] Very slow progression, profound weakness is generally proximal and symmetric, reflexes diminish or disappear when weakness is severe, sensations and autonomic function are generally unaffected, contractures generally develop over the course of the disorder, creatine kinase (CK) concentrations are normal, gait is often abnormal, atrophy is not present unless the weakness is severe, myotonia's are common, coordination is usually unaffected, and finally, myopathy may be brought about by some medications, including statins for high cholesterol.

Arguably, my symptoms track all of the above points except myopathies only present with motor and not sensory symptoms, profound and severe weakness, and proximal weakness. Chronic CRDs are an indication of chronic denervating conditions such as ALS or chronic myopathies found in the following diseases, including Pompe, Becker, Duchenne, central nuclear myopathy, and various forms of idiopathic inflammatory myopathies. Since myopathies have not been completely ruled out of my diagnosis, to be thorough, all conditions that present with CRDs are evaluated for differential diagnosis in the remainder of this section.

Pompe Disease

The following is a brief explanation of symptoms, etiology, diagnosis methods, similar disorders, and diagnosis probability of Pompe disease: [709] [710] [711]

Symptoms

Pompe disease symptoms include symmetrical muscle weakness in the legs and trunk, especially in the muscles controlling breathing, which can eventually lead to respiratory failure. Inhibited breathing leads to exercise intolerance. A buildup of glycogen is common in various muscles and organs, which can result in an enlarged heart and liver.

Etiology

There are three forms of Pompe disease: *classic infant-onset*, *non-classic infant onset*, and *late-onset* in adulthood. *Pompe disease* is an inherited disorder classified by the buildup of glycogen (complex sugars) in the cells of organs and muscles. Pompe disease originates from a mutation to the GAA gene, which is responsible for producing the enzyme acid maltase whose function is to break down glycogen. The disease is inherited via an autosomal recessive mutation. Endocrine disorders, such as deficiencies with glycogen storage, enzymes, and lipid function, can mimic hereditary Pompe myopathy diseases. For example, the thyroid regulates muscle protein synthesis and, therefore, conditions such as hypothyroidism can mimic Pompe disease.

Diagnostic Methods

Pompe disease produces denervation and CRDs, which may be observed on an EMG. Alternatively, Pompe disease may be diagnosed through a genetic blood test. A muscle biopsy uncovers glycogen accumulation in the muscles and increased acid maltase activity in leukocytes. Finally, Pompe may present with elevated CK.

Similar Disorders

There are several similar glycogen deficiency disorders, such as Tarui disease. ***Tarui disease*** is a deficiency in the enzyme phosphofructokinase, which is needed to breakdown glycogen. Symptoms from Tarui disease include muscle stiffness, pain, and weakness during exercise. Pompe disease is similar to ***acid maltase deficiency***, which also presents with a glycogen accumulation in the muscles and organs. ***Forbes disease*** is similar to Tarui disease, but it affects the debrancher enzyme. Forbes disease originates from a mutation with the AGL gene, and its symptoms affect both skeletal muscles, liver, and sometimes the heart. The onset of Forbes disease is usually very early in life.

Diagnosis Probability

I do not have Pompe, Tarui, or Forbes diseases because I do not suffer from the inability to breakdown glycogen for energy, which would prevent me from competing or doing any anaerobic exercise. [712] Also, I am unaware of anyone in my family history with a genetic glycogen disorder. Moreover, since Pompe disease is inherited with an autosomal recessive pattern, this signifies that both parents must carry one copy of the mutated gene, which is extremely unlikely. Incidentally, I tested negative for the GAA gene as well as glycogen storage deficiencies associated with the GSD1a and GSD2 genes.

Duchenne and Becker Muscular Dystrophy

Duchenne and Becker muscular dystrophy have the following definitions for symptoms, etiology, diagnosis methods, similar disorders, and diagnosis probability: [713] [714] [715] [716]

Symptoms

Generally, symptoms start with hypertrophy of the calves and progressive weakness and atrophy around the pelvis and girdle region. Symptoms include adverse effects on the cardiovascular system. More specifically, cardiomyopathy may present, which prevents the heart from efficiently pumping blood. As the disorder progresses, the heart can become enlarged, and symptoms may include irregular heartbeat, shortness of breath, fatigue, and swelling in the legs and feet. Duchenne and Becker are classified as myotonias with pain, cataracts, and gastrointestinal dysfunction. Some cases of Duchenne may present with cognitive defects, such as limited learning capabilities. Weakness and atrophy may also affect the face, neck, fingers, ankles, or proximal limbs. Finally, a waddling gait may develop from both muscle weakness and scoliosis of the spine.

Etiology

Duchenne prevalence is about ten times higher than Becker, which is a much milder version of the disorder. Duchenne onset is in the first decade, and affected people generally only live to be in their 20s; however, those with Becker have a later onset and can live beyond 50. Mutations of the dystrophin (DMD) gene result in both Duchenne and Becker's muscular dystrophy. DMD plays a role in muscle cell development. More specifically, dystrophin lends mechanical support to the sarcolemma from the forces of muscle contraction. [717] Duchenne inhibits the production of dystrophin while Becker limits the production of dystrophin. Since dystrophin is associated with the brain, many inflicted with Duchenne also have mental defects.

Diagnostic Methods

First, Duchenne has markedly elevated CK. Second, an EMG usually shows short and low amplitude motor unit responses. Third, a muscle biopsy may uncover varying fiber sizes, fibrosis, and fatty tissue infiltration—finally, genetic testing for DMD gene mutation.

Similar Disorders [718][719]

There are symptom similarities between Duchenne and Becker and myotonia disorders characterized by muscle stiffness instead of muscle weakness, including myotonia chloride and sodium channel mutations.

Diagnosis Probability

I do not have Duchenne / Becker dystrophy because I tested negative for the DMD gene mutation.

Centronuclear Myopathy

The following is a brief explanation of symptoms, etiology, diagnosis methods, and diagnosis probability: [720]

Symptoms

Centronuclear myopathy (CNM) is characterized by muscle weakness and atrophy and can lead to requiring assistance to walk. The onset of CNM can happen at any age, and the severity differs in affected individuals. CNM does not affect the cardiovascular system or a person's intellectual capabilities, but it may produce some respiratory dysfunction (mild to severe). Facial muscle weakness symptoms mimic myasthenia gravis (MG). Pseudohypertrophy is common.

Etiology

The origins of the disease are from genetic mutations of the DNM2, BIN1, or TTN genes. DNM2 and BIN1 genes are important for the regulation of actin proteins and transverse muscle tubules (T tubules), which transmit electrical impulses for muscle contractions. TTN is the gene that encodes the protein titin, which is also essential for muscle contractions. Some cases of CNM have no mutations of DNM2, BIN1, or TTN, and their etiology is unknown.

Diagnosis Methods

In CNM, muscle cell nuclei are located at the center of the cell instead of on the periphery of the cell. A muscle biopsy can determine if the muscle cells are organized properly; genetic testing for BIN1, DNM2, and TTN mutations are possible.

Diagnosis Probability

It is unlikely I have CNM because I tested negative for the BIN1, DM2, and TTN gene mutations.

Idiopathic Inflammatory Myopathies [721 722 723]

Idiopathic inflammatory myopathies (IIM) have the following epidemiology facts, symptoms, etiology, treatment methods, different types of IIM, and diagnosis probability:

Epidemiology

The onset of IIM can happen at any age, but it usually has a bimodal distribution with onset starting between the ages of 5 and 15 or 40 and 60.

Symptoms

Inflammatory myopathies are characterized by muscle weakness, generally with elevated creatine kinase (CK) levels.

Etiology

The term idiopathic indicates that the origins of IIM are unknown. IIM disorders may be an association with both genetic mutations and environmental factors. For instance, it is theorized that IIM may be an autoimmune disorder brought about by a genetic dysfunction in major histocompatibility complex (MHC) proteins. Certain environmental factors may contribute to IIM, such as infections, certain medications, and even excessive sunlight.

Diagnosis Methods

An EMG can show signs of CRDs and possible fibrillations, whereas blood work can reveal elevated CK levels.

Treatment Methods

Although IIM is thought to be an autoimmune disorder, immune replacement therapies such as IVIg and plasma exchange usually fail to alleviate symptoms in most cases. Steroid therapy may help some patients but beware of steroid side effects that include gastrointestinal malfunction, insomnia, cataracts, and diabetes.

Different Types of IIM

There are three types of idiopathic inflammatory myopathies (IIM).

The first is ***Polymyositis (PM).*** Polymyositis (PM) and dermatomyositis (DM) are disorders induced by inflammation of the muscle fibers. PM and DM occur because affected muscles are attacked by T-cells and macrophages. PM involves weakness of the proximal muscles such as the hips, thighs, upper arms, and neck. Symptoms for PM are symmetric, and they can affect the lungs and cardio system and may result from a malignancy or an autoimmune disease. PM affects mostly women under 50, and it may be treated with steroids or IVIg. Muscle weakness from PM may also inhibit swallowing and make breathing difficult, and pseudohypertrophy is common.

The second type is *Dermatomyositis (DM),* which has the same symptoms as PM, but DM also has skin defects, including a red rash on the eyelids, elbows, knees, and knuckles. DM may also produce painful calcium deposits, especially on the knuckles. Males over 40 with DM have a 20–30% incidence rate of carcinoma. Furthermore, different antibodies may be present in DM than PM. In PM, ANA antibodies may be present, while in DM, anti-tRNA (transfer RNA), anti- MI2, anti-NXP2 (if there is a malignancy), and anti-TIF-1 (if there is a malignancy) may be present.

The third type is *Sporadic inclusion body myositis (SIBM)*, whose symptoms include muscle weakness of the arms, fingers, ankles, face, and thighs. Sporadic indicates that the disorder occurs in individuals with no family history of the disease. At the same time, people with SIBM probably have a family member with an autoimmune disease. SIBM patients may also have impaired swallowing. Symptoms may start asymmetrically but can become symmetrical, and pseudohypertrophy of the muscles is common. Unfortunately, there is no known treatment for SIBM.

Diagnosis Probability

IIM symptoms do not align with my symptoms, such as those affecting the cardio and respiratory systems, skin rashes, pseudohypertrophy, and symptoms affecting the bulbar muscles. Furthermore, these disorders usually affect women more so than men.

ALS

Many people are already familiar with the devastating muscle-wasting symptoms of ALS, and its etiology was outlined earlier (reactive oxide species, ROS). The following is a diagnosis probability as to why I do not have ALS. First, ALS generally begins with focal or asymmetrical motor symptoms such as beginning in one foot or hand. Second, ALS patients can present with complex repetitive discharges (CRDs) on an EMG along with signs of atrophy. In fact, these are big factors in an ALS diagnosis. However, my symptoms and progression have been going on for a long time. ALS is a brutal disease and moves quickly, with patients dying within four years. My hand, feet, and calf atrophy can be explained by both less usage and from peroneal, sural, and ulnar nerve damage from neuropathy. Moreover, my atrophy is not associated with the muscle where the CRD's are located. Third, the presence of CRD's is not enough to diagnose a person with ALS. An ALS diagnosis would require CRD's to be associated with several muscles, several nerve roots, and at least three extremities. [724] Finally, atrophy does not automatically indicate ALS since atrophy is a symptom of many less sinister disorders.

My Diagnosis

The first step in the differential diagnosis is to distinguish between disorders of the CNS and PNS. From Table 13.1, my symptoms track much closer to a PNS disorder except for autonomic dysfunction. However, it is quite possible that my autonomic circumstances have a completely different and mutually exclusive manifestation beyond any neurological disease. As we have already learned, some medications, such as proton inhibitors and excessive antibiotic use, may lead to digestive dysfunction.

Table 13.1: Clinical Features of Central Nervous System Versus Peripheral Nervous System Diseases [725]

Central Nervous System Disease (CNS, Upper Motor Neurons)	Peripheral Nervous System Disease (PNS, Lower Motor Neurons)
No Pain, Asymmetrical Weakness and Sensory Loss	Pain, Symmetric or Focal Weakness
Hyperreflexia, Spasticity, and Hypotonia	Glove, Knee-High Sock Sensory Loss
Abnormal Movements, Seizures, Headache	Hyporeflexia
Bowel, Bladder, or Sexual Dysfunction	Myotonia

Bulbar Muscle Involvement	Atrophy
Dementia	Increased CK
Altered Mental Status	Abnormal EMG
Abnormal EEG, Head, and Spine MRI	

Step two of the differential diagnosis process for a neurological disease is the evaluation and comparison of both muscle disease and peripheral neuropathy patterns outlined in Tables 13.2 and 13.3, respectively.

Table 13.2: Clinical Patterns of Muscles Disorders [726]

Muscle Disease Pattern	Weakness	Symptoms	Diagnosis
MP1– Limb-Girdle	P, S		Most myopathies acquired or hereditary, Limb-Girdle
MP2 – Distal	D, S	E	Distal myopathies and some neuropathies
MP3– Proximal Arm / Distal Leg	P (arm), D (leg), S		Emery–Dreifuss dystrophy, Acid Maltase, Scapuloperoneal dystrophy
MP4– Distal Arm, Proximal Leg	P (leg), D (arm), A		Idiopathic Inflammatory Myopathies, Myotonic Dystrophy
MP5 – Ocular	P, A (MG), S (others)		MG, Myotonic Dystrophy, Mitochondria

MP6– Symmetric Sensory Loss and Upper Motor Neuron Signs	P, S	E, T	MG, ALS
MP7– Symmetric Weakness, no Sensory loss	P, S		MG, LEMS, ALS
MP8– Episodic Weakness, Pain	P, S	E, T	Drug or Toxin
MP9– Episodic Weakness unrelated to exercise	P, S	E, With and Without T	Channelopathies, Periodic Paralysis
MP10– Stiffness and inability to relax		E, With and Without T	Channelopathies, Periodic Paralysis, Rippling Muscle Disease, Stiff

			Person Syndrome

Table 13.2 Key: MP–Muscle Pattern, P–Proximal, D–Distal, A–Asymmetrical, S–Symmetrical, E–Episodic (symptoms come and go), T–Trigger (predisposition to acquire the disorder via some environmental factor), MG–Myasthenia Gravis, LEMS–Lambert Eaton Myasthenia Syndrome, and ALS–Amyotrophic Lateral Sclerosis.

It is fairly obvious that my symptoms do not align or track with the ten recognized muscle disease patterns since my symptoms are mostly distal, they are not episodic, and no trigger has been conclusively identified.

Table 13.3: Clinical Patterns of Peripheral Neuropathy [727]

Neuropathy Pattern	Weakness	Symptoms	Diagnosis
NP1–Symmetric proximal and distal weakness with sensory loss	P, D, S	SS, Some AS	Guillen-Barré Syndrome (GBS), Chronic Inflammatory Demyelinating Polyneuropathy (CIDP)
NP2–Distal sensory loss with and without weakness	D, S	SS	Hereditary Motor and Sensory Neuropathy (HMSN), Cryptogenic Sensory,

			Polyneuropathy (CSPN), Sensory Polyneuropathy
NP3–Distal weakness with sensory loss	D, A	SS	Multifocal Acquired Demyelinating Sensory and Motor (MADSAM)
NP4– Asymmetric proximal and distal weakness with sensory loss	P, D, A	SS, Some AS	Polyradiculopat hy
NP5– Asymmetric distal weakness with or without sensory loss	D, A	SS, UMD	ALS, Multifocal Motor Neuropathy (MMN)
NP6– Symmetric sensory loss and upper neuron signs	D, S	SS, PL, UMN	Vitamin B-12 or Copper Deficiencies
NP7–	P, D, S	SS	Hereditary

Symmetric weakness with or without sensory loss			Motor and Sensory Neuropathy (HMSN)
NP8– Symmetric weakness	P (Neck, Bulbar Muscles), S	UMN	ALS
NP9– Asymmetric proprioceptiv e loss with or without weakness	A	SS, PL	Sensory Neuropathy
NP10– Autonomic Dysfunction		AS	Hereditary Sensory and Autonomic Neuropathy (HSAN), Diabetic Neuropathy, GBS, Some CIDP
NP11–My Neurological Pattern	P, D, S	SS, AS	Fits closest to Radiculopathy, GBS, CIDP, and HMSN.

Table 13.3 Key: NP–Neuropathy Pattern, P–Proximal, D–Distal, A–Asymmetrical, S–Symmetrical, SS–Sensory Symptoms, PL - Proprioceptive Loss (Balance and

Coordination), UMN–Upper Motor Neuron Loss, and AS–Autonomic Symptoms.

NP11 from Table 13.3 is my neurological pattern. NP11 closely resembles radiculopathy, but spine MRIs have eliminated that option from consideration. CIDP and GBS resemble my symptom pattern, including presenting with symptoms both proximally and distally as well as some autonomic symptoms. However, generally, both CIDP and GBS present with high CSF proteins. That said, about 10% of all cases of CIDP or GBS can have normal CSF proteins. GBS may be eliminated from consideration because the onset is usually abrupt with severe symptoms, while my symptom onset and progression have been very slow. Hence, the cause of GBS can generally be identified because symptoms will appear a few weeks after some trigger, such as an illness. Furthermore, GBS has a higher probability of causing a respiratory malfunction.

Hereditary forms of neuropathy (HMSN) also resemble my pattern of symptoms, with the exception of autonomic symptoms. That said, there is no evidence of any hereditary forms of neuropathy in my family history, and I tested negative for CMTD and, therefore, HMSN could be eliminated from consideration in the differential diagnosis process. In fact, I tested negative for 109 different gene mutations that are involved in neuromuscular function.

Of course, none of the above neuropathies explain my muscle hyperexcitation, such as fasciculations and cramping. Thus, it may be distinctly possible that I have both CFS and some unidentified neuropathy, probably CIDP or MMN. MMN is a possibility for a few reasons. First, CFS proteins are usually normal, second MMN may encompass CFS symptoms, and finally, I tested equivocal for MMN antibodies. At the same time, my symptoms do not fit the MMN neuropathy pattern in Table 13.3, but there are rare instances when MMN can present with sensory and symmetrical symptoms. The bottom line, my diagnosis is probably CFS, CIDP or MMN.

Diagnosis Discussion

My response to IVIg treatment (discussed in the next section) may certainly suggest that I have MMN and not CIDP. My response to IVIg may, at best, slow progression and that resembles how MMN responds. CIDP responds better to IVIg and many times the treatment can cure the disease. Hence, CIDP is probably not a logical diagnosis. MMN does not explain my symptoms of hyperexcited muscles (cramping, fasciculations, etc.). Although MMN symptoms may be comprised of both fasciculations and cramping, MMN does not explain fasciculations and cramping in proximal areas since MMN is a distal disorder. MMN also does not explain the chronic denervation in my quad muscles. Thus, my disorder may be comprised of both MMN and CFS. CFS would explain the proximal hyperexcited muscle issues and may even explain the chronic denervation process in my quad muscles.

The denervation process in the quadricep muscle may be the biggest mystery of my neurological disorder. The denervation process visually appears to be myotonia, but on an EMG, it appears as myopathy. However, as we learned, the denervation process is not a myotonia and may not be a myopathy. Furthermore, it is unclear whether the denervation found in the quadricep muscle results from

CIDP or MMN. The myotonia mimicking phenomenon may be explained because denervation may result from alterations in the dynamics of ion function. For instance, when potassium ion gradients are disturbed, leading to less intercellular and more extracellular potassium, it increases muscle excitability. [728]

There is also evidence that when chlorine ion conductance is decreased that it can produce muscle hyperexcitation, possibly mimicking myotonia. Thus, it is distinctly possible that environmental factors such as a lifetime of vigorous exercise altered muscle gene expression leading to changes in ion dynamics, creating not only hyperexcitable muscles but a denervating process. [729] The bottom line is that the denervating process may be part of the CFS and my hyperexcitable muscles. That said, I would not be surprised to find out that I have both a neuropathy and a myopathy at some point in the future.

I have theorized that I was born with naturally excitable muscles. Thus, I believe that I have two mutually exclusive disorders (MMN and CFS) not only because my muscle hyperexcitation occurs in my proximal muscles, but because my hyperexcited muscles are worse in my endurance trained leg muscles. In other words, since my leg muscles respond favorably to endurance training, this has made them more hyperexcitable and therefore, my legs get the brunt of my CFS symptoms. Remember, endurance training can change the dynamics of ion channels by increasing the threshold voltage of ion channels. Increased threshold voltages mean muscles are more efficient because they contract faster, but at the same time, they become susceptible to fasciculations since there is a smaller margin of error for muscle cells to depolarize. Furthermore, since cycling reduced the use of my lower leg and foot muscles, it consequently correlated to a reduction in CFS symptoms in those areas. That said, it is certainly possible MMN may be exacerbating the effects of muscle hyperexcitation in distal locations.

The above paragraph would lead many to think that if I quit endurance training, it would relieve my hyperexcited muscles. These persons may be correct in that assessment, especially considering how cycling reduced the hyperexcitability in my lower legs and feet. However, the irony of my situation is that I also theorized that exercise, especially endurance training, increases neural plasticity to overcome MMN demyelination symptoms of muscle weakness. In fact, since my muscles react slightly favorably to endurance training, I am willing to bet that strenuous exercise can open more efficient and additional pathways for the muscles to communicate with the brain than moderate exercise. Just as a highly trained brain can increase the opportunities for neural pathways, it makes sense that the same is true is for highly trained muscles. Thus, quitting endurance training would improve my hyperexcitable muscles but the cost would be dramatic because it would increase the effects of much more debilitating MMN symptoms.

Furthermore, there is evidence that strenuous exercise can minimize the effects of MMN antibodies. More precisely, anti GM1 antibodies bind with the nodes of Ranvier of motor nerves causing both axonal and demyelinating damage. EPO production may reverse the inhibitory effects of GM1 antibodies because they bind with EPO receptors. [730] This information would lead one to conclude that strenuous exercise (increases EPO production) may block some of the inhibitory effects of GM1 antibodies. Remember, EPO is secreted by the kidneys in response to cellular hypoxia that may be caused by disease or exercise. Thus, EPO production is increased proportionally to the level of the intensity of the exercise. The bottom line, strenuous exercise may inhibit GM1 antibodies much more effectively than moderate exercise or sedentary lifestyles. Moreover, this may explain why my GM1 antibodies are equivocal and not over specification.

It is remotely possible that symptoms in the hands and arms may be exacerbated by perineural spinal cysts and an ulnar mechanical compression from riding a time trial bike. I probably have naturally hyperexcitable muscles whose condition was exacerbated from a lifetime of vigorous exercise and other environmental factors. Autonomic symptoms may or may not be the result of my neurological disorder. It is possible that some autonomic symptoms may be mutually exclusive and the result of other environmental factors, such as the impact of food sensitivities, vigorous exercise, or prescription drugs on digestive function.

My current diagnosis from my neurologist is some unidentified sensory and motor neuropathy, possibly MMN, as well as CFS. But it is quite conceivable what I have is unknown. If I do not have CIDP or MMN, then I have some unidentified chronic, axonal, demyelinating, symmetrical, denervating, sensory, motor, and autonomic polyneuropathy. This definition means: (1) Unidentified, cryptogenic, or idiopathic means the etiology is unknown; (2) chronic expresses that the symptoms are always present, and they are progressive; (3) axonal (axonopathy) and demyelinating (myelinopathy) denotes the symptoms affect both unmyelinated and myelinated nerve fibers; (4) symmetrical connotates that the symptoms occur on both sides of the body; (5) sensory, motor, and autonomic signifies that the symptoms affect sensory, motor, and autonomic function, which may also indicate cranial nerve involvement; and (6) denervating means the process of denervating motor units is ongoing.

After 13 years, nine neurologists, and dozens of tests costing hundreds of thousands of dollars, I still do not have a concrete diagnosis, possibly because science has not caught up to what I have. If that is true, I have earned the right to name my disorder if it is not CIDP or MMN. I dubbed my disorder chronic idiopathic prodigious and ubiquitous polyneuropathy (CIPUP). Idiopathic indicates that the etiology of the disorder is not known. Prodigious and ubiquitous suggests that symptoms are vast and appear throughout the body. More specifically, prodigious denotes the symptoms not only encompasses those that fall under the neuropathy umbrella but even some that do not, such as symptoms found in myopathies (denervation), myotonias (contractures, symptoms improving with repetition, or worsening in the cold), and neuromuscular disorders (fasciculations and cramping). Ubiquitous signifies that the symptoms are present everywhere, such as: (1) Muscle involvement in symmetrical, proximal, and distal locations; (2) involvement of both cranial and peripheral nerves, (3) involvement of both skeleton and smooth muscles; (4) involvement of both large and small nerve fibers; (5) involvement of nerves, muscles, and the neuromuscular junction; (6) involvement of sensory, motor, and autonomic nerves; and (7) involvement of both unmyelinated and myelinated nerve fibers.

One trait that I admire about my current neurologist is that she does not have an ego. She understands that my case is unusual and is willing to seek help from other doctors who specialize in neuromuscular disorders. Knowing that my symptoms do not fit any one diagnosis, she sent me to seek a second opinion. The second opinion neurologist is not so sure my current neurologists' diagnosis is correct, but he did not rule it out. The second opinion neurologist would like to collaborate with my current neurologist and check a few more potential avenues, such as a more detailed neuromuscular genetic analysis, before deciding on a diagnosis. The bottom line, I am living proof that knowledge of autoimmune and neurological diseases are still in their infancy and there is a long way to go before timely and accurate diagnosis are routine. Stay tuned as the story of my neurological disorder continues to change.

Treatment Options

IVIg

IVIg is an intravenous treatment of immunoglobulins obtained from the blood plasma of thousands of healthy people. IVIg comprises primarily IgG (95%-98%) and only trace amounts of IgM and IgA. The IgG subclass concentrations of IVIg are similar to those IgG subclass percentages found in the human body. IVIg treatment is similar to a blood transfusion. Although IVIg may be the only thing that can help slow the progression of my disorder, coverage was initially denied by my insurance company. Sure, there was a good chance the IVIg would not help me at all, but something that has a remote chance of working should not be denied. Of course, this outcome was protested by my doctor, and after several months of wheeling and dealing, it was reluctantly approved. The plan was to put me through four consecutive days of IVIg treatments (loading dose of 2 grams/kilogram) followed by one treatment every two weeks for three months (maintenance dose of 0.5 grams/kilogram). For example, since I weigh 75 kilograms, my initial treatment dose was 150 grams over four days, and my follow-up treatment dose was 37.5 grams in one day. Since IVIg comes in 20-gram bottles, my dosage was rounded to 40 grams per day. Hence, my initial treatment load was 160 grams total, and my follow-up treatment load was 40 grams. As a side note, one 20-gram bottle of IVIg is expensed at about 7,500 dollars.

There are three manufacturers of IVIg, and the brand I was initially given was called *Gammagard Liquid*. The side-effects were fairly severe, resulting in minor flu-like symptoms, skin rash (eczema), very high blood pressure (hypertension), and extreme headaches where it hurt to open or move my eyes. The interesting side-effect that I had was chest discomfort. Chest discomfort is not a common side-effect of IVIg, but lo and behold, in one Gammagard Liquid clinical trial of 44 patients with multifocal motor neuropathy (MMN), it showed that chest discomfort was the second most common symptom. What made this finding interesting is that in two other Gammagard Liquid clinical trials of random patients (no particular diagnosis), it does not list chest discomfort as a side-effect. In fact, there are 21 possible side-effects that occurred in at least 5% of the patients in the clinical trials, and chest discomfort is not one of them. Does this suggest chest discomfort is a unique symptom for people with MMN? I do not know, but that is food for thought and may indicate that I have MMN. Yes, this is a very loose relationship, but when you are trying to find answers, it is easy to grasp at straws. Gammagard Liquid clinical trials on MMN patients showed strength and neurological acuity decreased during treatment periods, but the decrease was not nearly to the extent seen in the control group who were given a placebo. In other words, IVIg slowed the progression of MMN, but it did not improve the patient's overall condition.

After six treatments, I was transferred to another brand of IVIg called *Privigen* to see if I respond better with fewer side-effects. Privigen shares similar side effects as Gammagard, such as headache, influenza, and skin rash. Privigen conducted clinical trials 'on chronic inflammatory demyelinating polyneuropathy (CIDP) patients studying the impact of Privigen treatment on the inflammatory neuropathy cause and treatment (INCAT) test. The INCAT test is used in many neuropathy clinical trials to measure both arm and leg disability. INCAT scores range from 0 or no disability to 12 or severe disability. CIDP patients in the clinical trial showed, on average, a 1.4-point improvement in their INCAT score after an extensive Privigen treatment over a year. Likewise, patients also showed a considerable 14-point improvement in grip strength in both the dominant and non-dominant hands. Unlike Gammagard studies on MMN, Privigen studies on CIDP show an overall improvement and not just a decline in the progression of the disorder. In fact, most clinical trials show CIDP patients respond much better to IVIg than MMN patients. Unfortunately, the eczema skin rash from the Privigen was very significant. The allergic reactions were bad enough to have my neurologist cancel any further IVIg treatments. In a post-IVIg examination (7 months after my pre-IVIg examination), it was determined that my strength was "a little better" in the feet but the same in the hands. Additionally, my reflexes remained the same.

Subcutaneous immunoglobulin (SCIg) treatments are infusions of immunoglobulin under the skin instead of through the veins. SCIg treatments are required more often than IVIg, but for many it helps to mitigate adverse side-effects. And when adverse side effects occur, many times they are localized to the infusion site area. For properly trained persons, SCIg has the added benefit that infusions may be self-administered in the confines of their home. [731] SCIg may be in my future if IVIg adjustments to the product type, infusion rate, saline quantity, and prednisone treatment fail to mitigate my adverse side effects.

Other Options

Other treatment options for CIDP encompass both steroid (prednisone) and or immune suppressants. However, prednisone is known to make cases of MMN worse, and immune suppressants are generally ineffective at fighting MMN. Complicating matters is that prednisone is also a banned substance for competitive cycling. Nevertheless, prednisone is a legal substance in the offseason, and people can race so long as the drug clears the system (prednisone has a fairly short half-life of only a few hours). Since my neurologist believes what I have is

MMN, the only effective treatment option I have is IVIg. In the future, if my strength starts to decline, the plan is to obtain a lower dosage of IVIg maintenance treatments with prednisone to lessen the severity of the eczema outbreaks. Moreover, my only option is to receive these IVIg treatments in the cycling offseason because of both the legality of prednisone and the major IVIg
side-effects complicating training. The choice of bad side effects or wasting away does not sound good, but I am grateful to have at least one option.

Summary

My fitness level is better than over 99% of the people above 50 years of age. So, the question that has to be asked is, why do healthy people become sick? It all comes down to genes and what is called the prevention paradox. The prevention paradox states, "A healthy lifestyle measure that reduces the risk for the entire population may offer little or no benefit to any given individual." In fact, some healthy lifestyle measures can make some people sick and trigger autoimmune disease. Vaccines, exercise, supplements, widely-used prescription drugs, and even healthy diets can have a negligible or negative effect on some people. In the near future, it may be commonplace to have the complete genetic makeup to identify potential mutations that may be lurking behind a seemingly healthy person. For instance, vaccinations are beneficial to 99.9% of the public, but to the remaining 0.1% of the public (including healthy people), some vaccines may trigger autoimmune disease. [732]

There are some important points to summarize about my disorder, diagnosis, and journey. At first, I was bitter and angry about my misdiagnosis, mismanagement, and lack of a true diagnosis. Obviously, the sooner a condition is diagnosed, the sooner it can be treated. The longer the diagnosis takes, the more permanent the neurological damage may become, and the situation is more difficult to correct. My situation is analogous to someone falsely imprisoned. Let me explain. When someone is in prison, they lose most of their freedoms. They lose the freedom to travel, play activities they enjoy, to work a job of their choosing, and to enjoy family. Now, consider a situation when a person is wrongly accused of a crime and placed in prison. Having a neurological condition is similar, but it is not quite as severe. That said, people with any medical ailment become prisoners of their own bodies and also lose freedoms. For example, I lost the freedom to rock climb, mountaineer, wrestle, do woodwork, run, and work. These freedoms are not by any stretch of the imagination as bad as losing family, work, and travel; nevertheless, we take much for granted. [733] The misdiagnosis and mismanagement of my disorder have, in effect, left me as a prisoner to my own body. Maybe it is not fair, just as it not fair to be wrongly convicted. However, after considerable consideration, I would not change these events; they happened for a reason. The adversity of my neurological condition taught me: (1) to evolve, learn new information, and write books about it; (2) to help educate others in need; (3) to be humble, grateful, patient, and willing to make the most of each day; (4) be a better person for the greater good of society; and (5) to achieve childhood dreams and become a state and national champion cyclist.

Some may argue that cycling competition does not support the philosophy or narrative of being a better person for the greater good of society. Some would even argue that cycling competition is narcissistic. I would strongly disagree for numerous reasons. First, all people have a fundamental right to play, which promotes other fundamental rights such as building family and friendships, the social glue that holds society together. Conversely, in our current high-tech society, people are becoming less social and more politically charged. Second, cycling and competition support the natural law fundamental right to obtain knowledge. Cycling, especially time trialing, is an activity supported by scientific technology for training and aerodynamics, which exerts brain function, unlike other useless technology activities. Third, competition teaches individuals not only how to accept defeat and cope with adversity, but to build a life plan by setting and achieving goals. Fourth, cycling and competition keeps people healthy, which is important to maintain lower healthcare costs for everyone. America is a sick country both mentally and physically, especially with high tech fostering inactivity and bolstering obesity. Cycling and competition are more inspiring and motivational than high technology behaviors of playing games, useless texts, and selfies. Finally, environmentalists would also support cycling over driving cars for the greater good of the planet to control carbon emissions.

The following are the benefits I garnered from my neurological disorder: *Gratitude, Eliminating Fear, and Acceptance*: I remind myself every day I am a lucky person. I do not have amyotrophic lateral sclerosis (ALS) or multiple sclerosis (MS), and there are literally millions of people around the globe suffering from ailments far worse than mine. We take so much for granted, but I now realize that I won the lottery when I was born in this great nation. I did not have a storybook childhood, but this country afforded me opportunities that billions will never have. For example, I received an engineering degree, own a great home, have a wonderful wife, and have great family and friends; I have also traveled around the country and globe, seen views in my climbing adventures that most people can only dream about, and have always had a job that pays well. My life has been great, and I plan to live each day to its fullest.

Evolving Personally: I am a better person wanting to help others who suffer from PNH and others who are less fortunate than myself. In particular, I correspond with several individuals each week who suffer from fear and anxiety brought about by PNH or neuropathy. For instance, one person I corresponded with wrote this thoughtful note to me: "I just wanted to say thank you for your encouragement during probably the darkest time of my life when there seemed to be only a spark of light here and there, and you were one of those sparks." There is no better feeling then being able to help another person in need.

Evolving Athletically: I would have never competed in cycling if I did not have PNH or some other neurological disorder. I fulfilled my childhood dreams by winning both state and national senior games championships in cycling and authoring several books. Furthermore, I cherish cycling much more than my previous activities because I know freedoms can be taken away at any moment. I do not feel I missed out, nor do I remain bitter about losing the opportunity to finish other goals such as climbing the highest point in every state (only Alaska remains) and all the fourteen thousand-foot peaks in Colorado (about 20 remain).

Goal-setting: With the progression of my disorder, I evolved my cycling regimen to encompass fewer hours of training and fewer intense rides, but I have still been able to compete and enjoy cycling.

Living Life to its Fullest, Education, Advocacy, and Eliminating Fear: In my many hours resting from fatigue, I learned United States history, constitutional law, and medicine to understand my disorder to advocate for my healthcare and eliminate the fear factor.

The positive effects of my disorder on cycling are purely mental such as increased grit, perseverance, resilience, and mental toughness. For example, the disorder enhances or increases pain tolerance for training and racing. Positive effects from cycling on the neurological condition include maintaining balance and strength through the development of new or alternate pathways for the brain to communicate with muscles and tendons.

However, the negative effects of the disorder on cycling encompass numerous physical limitations, including balance and strength. In fact, neurological disease is counteracting what training is attempting to accomplish. The negative effects of my disorder on cycling and vice versa are physical and include enhanced symptoms such as stiffness, fasciculations, fatigue, and pain. That said, fatigue seems to be the biggest factor.

The bottom line, it is possible to improve athletically over the age of 50 with a debilitating neurological condition. Furthermore, improvement may come in the absence of athletic genes (or slightly favorable). I achieved athletic success with a debilitating neurological condition for four reasons. First, training techniques can alter muscle protein composition overcoming physical limitations. Second, training can teach the body to bypass diseased cells by creating alternate neural pathways for the brain and muscles to communicate. Third, cycling is the great equalizer in sports. What I mean by this is that cycling is a sport that enables older individuals and people with disabilities to remain fast and competitive. Finally, disease influences personality traits such as resiliency, grit, and mental toughness to overcome physical limitations such as pain.

A Summary of Life Lessons, Facts, and Observations:

- The good news is that people are living longer, the bad news is people are suffering from higher rates of morbidity.
- About 1 in 13 Americans or 25 million people in the United States suffer from neurological disorders.
- To date, about 600 rare diseases have been identified. A rare disease inflicts fewer than 200,000 persons in the United States, which account for nearly 25 million illnesses.
- The medical arena did not believe autoimmune disorders were possible just 60 to 70 years ago. Thus, science has been trying to catch up to identify and understand these diseases.
- It is estimated that 50 to 100 million Americans deal with some sort of chronic pain.
- America is a sick country and it is causing healthcare costs to skyrocket.
- Neurological disease does not have be the end, but instead it can be a new beginning.
- There is no magic formula to end adversity and pain. Only hard work and sacrifice is the best solution to the problem.
- Most neurological disorders cannot be cured. That said, many symptoms can be treated with modest results.
- Natural treatment methods for symptoms, such as exercise and diet, are more advisable then taking

drugs that can have long term negative epigenetic effects.

- Since the medical community treats the symptoms and not the illness, this allows people to live longer but the quality of life is reduced.
- Competition is good because it motivates people to set goals and build structure in their lives.
- For a given competition, winning and success means something different to each person.
- A coach or trainer who devises a unique plan tailored to your needs may help you attain your goals.
- Evolving and adaption to adversity does not mean to quit, but instead means doing less or changing to another activity.
- Stress and adversity are not necessarily all bad. Stress can improve one's health and strengthen the immune system. Strengthening the immune system from stressful experiences stems from resiliency that educates the body to fight future stress and pain.
- Acute stress is more healthy than chronic stress.
- Chronic stress can initiate both the aging process and disease as well as exacerbate existing symptoms.
- Do something every day that takes you out of your comfort zone.
- Learn something new every day. A stronger and more diverse brain can increase the chances

muscles can find new pathways to communicate with the brain.

- Always advocate strongly for your medical care. Do not hesitate to make changes.
- Acceptance does not mean giving up trying to find relief and answers, it simply suggests moving forward and not dwelling on the negative aspects of the adversity we face.
- Sometimes in order to go faster and get stronger you have to go slower. Rest is important.
- Keep a journal, it is therapeutic.
- A good attitude is pushing the envelope by focusing on the positives instead of harping on the negatives.
- Proactive behavior is being practical which means focusing on the present and future and forgetting the past.
- Always strive to do more and don't settle for the expectations of authors, doctors, friends, family, teachers, and bosses. Be an overachiever.
- Fatigue gets a bad rap, but it is necessary for muscle and cardiovascular gains.
- Beware of analysis paralysis by overanalyzing data from workouts and races.
- Exercise can make epigenetic changes to genes which enables the brain and muscles to bypass diseased tissue by creating new and alternate pathways.
- Practice and train alone for the best gains.
- Training and practicing always beat talent until talent begins to practice and train.

- Good athletic genes do not guarantee success without having the right attitude.
- Cycling is the great equalizer of endurance sports.
- Endurance athletes cannot become elite if they are unable to suffer during workouts and races.
- Train at low altitude and sleep high altitude for the best endurance gains.
- Body type is an important factor when determining the most ideal sport for an athlete.
- Luck plays a huge role in who becomes an elite endurance athlete.
- Contrary to public opinion, pedal technique in endurance cycling is not overly important.
- Race to how you feel and not to technology.
- Always use more effort on the high resistance portions of a race (into the wind or uphill).
- A proper bike fit may help you avoid pain during exercise.
- Human diversity or phenotype is characterized more by differences in our bacteria composition as well as epigenetic alterations than our genetic composition.
- Change warmup methodology to match the weather conditions.
- A slow cadence riding uphill increases the number of slow twitch type I muscle fibers that are essential for endurance racing.
- Every person has flawed genes. Thus, it is true, no one is perfect.
- Be humble with your success and pay it forward.

- Our mission on this planet is to become a better person for the greater good of society.
- Training and racing schedule flexibility are okay since many paths lead to the same goals.
- Avoid boredom because there is truth to the statement of "being bored to death".
- Never be satisfied with past achievements, always strive to meet new goals and expectations.
- Focus on things you can control with yourself and not on things we cannot control.
- Be grateful for what we have and never obsess over what we do not have.
- Confidence may be the single most important variable to success because without confidence, motivation, a positive attitude, and perseverance are impossible.
- Mental toughness is synonymous with resiliency. Forgoing mental training is an unfortunate oversight by many athletes and persons suffering from pain or neurological disease.
- Stay busy because distractions are the best way to deal with stress, pain, and fear.
- Keep moving to avoid atrophy, weakness, and becoming overweight. Remember, endurance exercise has more positive effects on the body, including the brain, than weight training since a higher body mass index (BMI) equates to a decrease in brain volume. [734]
- Enhance the senses of touch, smell, hearing, sight, and taste to dull the sensation of pain.

- Neurological patients live in fear that their disorder may be something more sinister.
- Muscle fatigue and muscle weakness are not the same thing. Fatigue are tired muscles; whereas, weakness is a loss of strength.
- Atrophy is muscle wasting and weakness and can be caused by inactivity from exercise intolerance and not from a sinister neurological disorder.
- Bravery is defined as perseverance in the presence of fear. Bravery can be learned through epigenetic changes.
- The correct response to fear, stress, adversity, and pain should be motivation and not long-term depression.
- Pain is necessary for life to exist. Without pain, humans could not survive.
- When fear and depression take over, rational thought is lost and mental illness is not far behind.
- Knowledge, a healthy diet, and exercise can conquer fear, stress, and pain.
- Cognitive expectations may intensify pain. For instance, if a person has an expectation that their pain will be relieved, it may not feel as bad as when they may know there is no relief for their pain.
- Negativity transforms pain into suffering and suffering comes from uncertainty. Thus, many of us may unnecessarily exaggerate our pain instead of trying to put it into perspective.
- Negative emotions can turn pain into suffering. Try to stay even-keeled by not berating oneself for

failing to meet some goals and not by congratulating oneself too much for doing well.

- As bad as you think you may be suffering, remember there are millions more going through more difficult times and experiences. This is a dramatic coping strategy to deal with pain.

- One mistake made by most people with chronic pain is that they tend to be overcautious and rest too much. Very few sufferers of chronic pain try to do too much.

- Pain tolerance is the duration of time and intensity of pain an individual endures before the initiation of a pain response and this varies significantly among persons. That said, pain tolerance can be improved.

- It is never too early to start the bucket list.

- It is never too early to plan for retirement and illness.

- The goal should be to understand your medical ailment better than the doctors.

- Misdiagnosis of neurological disorders is common and a correct diagnosis can take years.

- The most common reason for misdiagnosis is a premature closure of a case before all the facts are uncovered.

- The most common misdiagnosis of neurological disorders is something called functional neurological disorders (FND).

- Misdiagnosis can also occur because the neurologist gives little credence to any sensory symptoms they cannot see or measure.

- Athletes are difficult to diagnose with neurological disease because their physical exam and diagnostic EMG results do not align.
- Live life to the fullest.
- Take one day at a time.
- Americans need to realize they are very fortunate and won the lottery when they were born in the United States. The same is true for persons born in other free and industrialized societies.
- We can change or reverse bad outcomes for our destiny by changing habits to make epigenetic alterations in our genes.
- Our environment plays a bigger role in our destiny than our genes.
- Environmental factors such as exercise and a proper diet can slow the aging process and ward off disease.
- People can improve at a sport, such as cycling, after the age of 50.
- Focus and goals should be concentrated on improvement instead of trying to maintain a status quo.
- Nothing worth achieving is never easy.
- If you live with pain regardless of your activity level, then you may as well exercise.
- We never realize how much we miss something until that freedom is taken away.
- Experts claim it takes the average person 10,000 hours of training and practice (10 years) to master a sport or activity.

- According to Devin Starlanyl: "We cannot know other people's experiences simply by observing them, just as our internal strife remains largely invisible to onlookers."
- Genome testing allows patients to understand and identify which foods and prescription drugs they metabolize efficiently and those they do not.
- Genome testing can also identify how the body may respond to different types of exercise such as endurance or strength training.
- 23 genes have been identified that may impact endurance athletics. At best, a person may have a dozen favorable gene expressions for endurance training.
- Success in athletics and overcoming health issues largely depends on a person's support system (family, friends, community, etc.).
- Surround yourself with inspirational people.
- Ignore but forgive naysayers.
- The positive effects vigorous exercise has on the muscles includes improved muscle force and power through adaptations to neural, muscle, balance, force transmission, and muscle contraction kinetic physiology which can be attributed to increased muscle fiber size and recruitment.
- Muscle fiber protein adaptations are vast and complex from exercise and training. What's more, adaptions occur in both healthy innervated muscles as well as diseased denervated muscles.

- Nearly all people respond positively to a healthy diet and moderate exercise. There are rare cases of persons responding negatively to some healthy foods and strenuous exercise.
- The prevention paradox states "a healthy lifestyle measure that reduces the risk for the entire population may offer little or no benefit to any given individual."
- It has been theorized that strenuous exercise can increase the chances of having hyperexcited muscles that more readily twitch and cramp.
- Type A personalities may be more at risk to have hyperexcited muscles.
- Our genetic makeup or expression is a culmination of all our life experiences and the experiences of our parents, and we often pass this on to our children.
- When our genetic expression is incompatible or mismatches with environmental conditions, then disease may be the outcome.
- There is a good chance you will die from a disease caused by genetic mismatches with the environment.
- When muscles are affected in all four limbs then there are generally four potential reasons: Myelopathy, myopathy, a neuromuscular junction disorder, and peripheral neuropathy.
- Myelopathy or radiculopathy is a compression of the spinal nerve roots or spinal cord and usually results in no fasciculations, increased reflexes,

normal muscle tone, pain, some sensory involvement, and often digestive and bladder dysfunction.

- Myopathy generally presents with proximal weakness and atrophy, normal reflexes, normal sensory function, no pain, and generally the bulbar muscles are spared. Myopathies are also characterized by a significant loss of muscle power despite minimal weakness and atrophy. Myopathies generally affect proximal muscles; whereas, distal myopathies affecting the hands and feet are very rare.

- Neuromuscular junction disorders generally present with proximal weakness, fatigue, normal muscle tone, sometimes fasciculations are present, spared sensory nerves, normal reflexes, no pain, and bulbar muscle involvement.

- Peripheral neuropathy generally presents in distal muscles with weakness and atrophy, fasciculations may be present, reflexes are diminished or absent, pain, sensory loss, and the bladder and digestive system are usually not affected.

- 2 in 5 medical papers lack a sufficient sample size. What's more, many medical papers are biased or skewed to defend whomever may sponsor the study.

- Statistical significance and correlation do not necessarily mean practical significance.

- Do not blame or take your unfortunate circumstances out on others.

- Cyclists and motorists need to learn to respect each other and share the road.

Patrick Bohan

Appendix I: Epidemiology Study of PNH

I conclude this book with a 2014 paper that I wrote, with the help of Mitra Wagner, about peripheral nerve hyperexcitation (PNH) disorders. The paper was specifically a statistical analysis or an epidemiology study about PNH.

The reason there is little information on PNH is simple: The medical profession believes these disorders are no big deal since they are "benign," and this paper is trying to change that perception. After all, we must look out for ourselves when the medical industry is failing us. Besides, I found it was best to put all that anxiety and energy I was wasting complaining to find those answers that no one else is seeking.

Abstract

The purpose of this paper is to present an epidemiology study about peripheral nerve hyperexcitation disorders (PNH), which encompasses benign fasciculation syndrome (BFS), cramp fasciculation syndrome (CFS), Isaacs syndrome (IS), and Morvan's syndrome (MoS). In particular, the goal of the paper is twofold. First, the paper presents a statistical analysis of various PNH parameters classified into seven groups. PNH parameter classification and definitions are outlined in the "Results" section (Table A.1 through A.7). Second, to find if a correlation exists between any two PNH parameters (Table A.8 to A.14).

The method to collect data was via an internet survey that was developed on Google Drive. Data were obtained from 527 people over three years. Of the 527 responses, 438 were evaluated within this paper. Hence, 89 survey entries were omitted as outliers for a variety of reasons, which will be defined later. The data were analyzed for: (1) Statistical averages, means, and standard deviations. (2) Linear regression analysis determined parameter t-statistics and ρ to identify statistical or practical significance between the various PNH parameters. (3) Data points with high statistical significance were evaluated further using a Spearman correlation method to determine if there is any correlation.

To conclude, the paper tackles the following questions, conclusions, and discussions: (1) The fallacies about survey usefulness and accuracy; (2) the inadequacies of control studies, clinical trials, and patient observation; (3) the paper investigates PNH disorder's misconceptions; (4) the paper attempts to identify a true definition of BFS, CFS, IS, and MoS.; and (5) the paper discusses why PNH symptoms and remedy effectiveness are uniquely individualized.

Introduction

Defining and understanding neurological disorders can be medically challenging. In fact, it can be an outright mystery. Peripheral nerve hyperexcitation (PNH) is a disorder characterized by fasciculations or muscle twitching for unexplained reasons. Other PNH symptoms may include muscle fatigue, cramps, pins and needles, paresthesia, muscle vibrations, headaches, itching, sensitivity to temperatures, numbness, muscle stiffness, muscle soreness, myotonia, fear, depression, and pain. [1] PNH etiology is not entirely understood, demonstrating a clear need for this study. One etiology theory suggests that

BFS or PNH may involve the voltage-gated potassium channel (VGKC) at the neuromuscular junction and its inability to properly close its gates when a motor nerve impulse reaches the nerve terminal, resulting in hyperexcitable muscle fibers. [2] The dysfunction of the VGKC is what results in involuntary impulses that consequently stimulate the nerve endings, causing them to fire and twitch. Another etiology theory postulates PNH may arise from a decreased density of the VGKC, which inhibits potassium current flow. [1, 3, 4]

PNH disorders are understudied and misunderstood, especially amongst those chronically afflicted by the syndrome. Unfortunately, this lack of knowledge leads to several common misconceptions about PNH. The first misconception is that chronic BFS is not physically or mentally debilitating. One study claims that up to 1% of the population may suffer from PNH. [6] PNH, for most people, is benign and insignificant, but those individuals with chronic symptoms 24/7, PNH can wreak havoc on their lives. Like other neurological disorders, there is no known cure for PNH. While this disorder is considered "benign," it contains very real symptoms, and, in some cases, these symptoms are both psychologically and physically debilitating. [5] The debilitation factor is primarily due to the chronic and progressive nature of the disorder in some individuals. Neurologists and doctors often tell PNH patients that their symptoms are "not debilitating." This assumption is a common misconception about the disorder. The statistical analysis of PNH from the survey proves that symptoms in many people are chronic (high frequency and intensity), progressive, and physically debilitating.

Moreover, chronic PNH is also mentally debilitating. Based on a Microsoft research study conducted by White and Horvitz, there is a 50% probability that a quick internet search on "muscle twitching" leads them to sites related to amyotrophic lateral sclerosis (ALS). This results in a great deal of distress and fear for the individual knowing the relationship between twitching and ALS. Furthermore, chronic PNH patients are prone to coping with anxiety and fear since their early-onset symptoms are similar to other crippling disorders such as Parkinson's disease, multiple sclerosis (MS), and brain tumors. Moreover, because of their symptoms, many PNH patients have often undergone advanced medical testing, including magnetic resonance imaging (MRI) on the brain as well as electromyography (EMG) to rule out other, more serious, neurological disorders. [1]

Thus, the biggest misconception of PNH is that it is benign. In fact, chronic PNH patients have similar symptoms to other progressive neurological disorders, including peripheral neuropathy, fibromyalgia, reflex sympathetic dystrophy (RSD), stiff person syndrome, continuous muscle fiber activity, and continuous motor nerve discharges. [1] Therefore, remedies to relieve PNH symptoms are exactly the same as those remedies used for other neurological disorders. [1] Furthermore, if PNH is always benign in the eyes of most neurologists, then why do people with PNH experience advanced medical testing and take powerful medications such as anti-seizure, anti-depressant, sleeping pills, benzodiazepines, muscle relaxants, and other strong medications to relieve symptoms? The answer is because there are people with extreme chronic cases of PNH.

The next misconception is that PNH can grow into ALS or some more sinister disorder. This misconception is driven by a fairly recent study indicating individuals who started with twitching and cramping symptoms but developed ALS years later. [7] While these cases are extremely rare, the knowledge of them can produce continual anxiety, fear, and depression in the chronic PNH patient. At the same time, this paper shows why the case studies about PNH developing into more sinister diseases are flawed. In fact, at this time, there is no evidence that PNH patients are any more likely to acquire other more serious neurological disorders, such as ALS or MS, than any person without PNH. [4] What people need to understand is if these case studies on PNH developing into ALS had any credence, then neurologists would be studying instead of ignoring PNH patients.

There are a vast number of definitions of the different types of PNH, which creates a great deal of confusion and leads to further misconceptions. The following are PNH definitions used by this text: First, BFS encompasses one symptom: Fasciculations or muscle twitching. Second, when symptoms become more chronic and painful, marked by cramping or muscle stiffness, then the patient has CFS. BFS and CFS are acquired disorders attacking the motor and sometimes the sensory nerves. Third, *Isaac syndrome (IS)* may be acquired or hereditary. Acquired IS may be brought about by an autoimmune dysfunction and, therefore, symptoms expand to include the autonomic nervous system that controls cardiovascular, gastrointestinal, and respiratory functions. IS can also produce myotonia or a delayed relaxation from a contracted state. Acquired IS can be contracted via carcinoma of the thymus or lung. Hereditary IS may be characterized by a mutation of the KCNA1 gene that encodes the VGKC. [20]. Fourth, *Morvan's syndrome (MoS)* is when the disorder affects not only the peripheral nerves but the nerves in the central nervous system leading to more advanced symptoms, including psychosis. IS and MoS are very rare and probably affect fewer than one thousand people in the United States.

Since IS and MoS are very rare, and the data reveal that over 99% of the survey participants have more than one symptom, it reasonable to conclude that most of the survey participants have CFS. In fact, most papers on PNH do not even mention BFS. Hence, if patients are misdiagnosed with BFS instead of CFS, this will lead to a disconnect or misconception between patient and medical professionals and possibly explaining why doctors tell their patients what they have is no big deal. [15, 16, 17] I also believe that PNH disorders have evolved in the age of booming autoimmune disorders and, therefore, have more complex symptoms and become more chronic. I have no solid evidence to support this hypothesis, but it would go a long way to explain why doctors are may be quick to classify people with BFS than CFS and why they label it as no big deal. The only evidence I had to formulate the growing chronic nature of BFS is that older individuals who have had BFS for a long time show a strong correlation to twitching symptoms, but younger individuals who have not had PNH symptoms very long show no strong correlation to any particular symptom. These data would seem to indicate that young people have a large array of symptoms. Furthermore, there is a strong correlation to suggest that stress-induced PNH or stress that exacerbates PNH symptoms happens in younger people, possibly causing epigenetic changes never seen in older PNH patients. After all, if the environmental factors triggering PNH are different than they were a few decades ago, then one would suspect the manifestation of the syndrome symptoms would also be different.

Methods

The following sections cover the methods used to collect and analyze the survey data. Methods discussed in this section are as follows: Study Criteria, PNH Support Groups, Survey Data Information and Definitions, Sample Size Requirements, and Data Analysis information, respectively.

Study Criteria

The online survey meets human research criteria as outlined by the "Committee on Human Experimentation" and the "Helsinki Declaration of 1975" for the following reasons: (1) The survey was anonymous; (2) participation in the survey was voluntary; (3) the privacy and confidentiality of the participants is maintained and protected; and (4) survey participants were notified in advance that results would be shared publicly

Furthermore, other important facts guarantee the results are unbiased and accurate, and they are as follows: First, all tabulated data in this paper are original. Second, the survey and subsequent data were not a clinical trial. Third, since there was more than adequate survey participation data (527 participants) to guarantee both a high confidence level and interval, the data were carefully cleaned for potential outliers that may incorrectly skew the results. Finally, the authors of this paper have no conflicts of interest and, thus, no information to disclose. The authors are independent and have no affiliation to any university, group, organization, or company; there was no funding for this project.

PNH Support Groups

People were contacted through the following PNH social network forums to participate in the survey:

- Facebook: https://www.facebook.com/#!/groups/88467288815/
- Internet: http://www.nextination.com/aboutbfs/

Survey Data Information and Definitions

Information regarding survey data gathering and methods are listed below:

- A survey was developed in Google Docs and is accessible at the following link:
  - https://spreadsheets.google.com/spreadsheet/viewform?hl=en_US&authkey=CJvBgaQM&formkey=dElCQkFBRWlvY1ZSTThKTmNsbEg4d0E6MQ#gid=0
- The Survey can also be reached from the author's BFS webpage:
  - http://patrickbohan.elementfx.com/BFS.htm. Click on the link "BFS Survey."
- The raw data for the survey results appear on the author's web page:

- o http://patrickbohan.elementfx.com/BFS.htm.
  Click on the "Survey Data Summary" link.
- The above link will open an Excel file. For specific information about the data included within any of the Excel file worksheets, please contact the author.
- Since the survey data are mostly comprised of a rank-order system (using a 1–10 scale), the Spearman method of correlation is used. [8, 9]

Sample Size Requirements

What is the correct sample size for a survey study? To understand this, it is imperative to determine (estimate) how many people suffer from severe and chronic PNH symptoms (population size). According to the Center for Disease Control (CDC), about 1 in 10,000 people in the United States have ALS, and about 1 in 600 people have Parkinson's disease. At these rates, as many as 700,000 people around the globe can have ALS and 12 million people can have Parkinson's disease. If the rate of chronic PNH is comparable to the rate of ALS and even Parkinson's disease, the sample size of the survey would need to be at least 384 people to tolerate a 5% error (confidence interval) and a 95% confidence level. There are dozens of online calculators available to compute and verify these calculations (see footnote 18). Hence, our current sample size of 438 meets this criterion. [18] However, for parameters found within the remedy effectiveness classification, the confidence interval may surge to 5.5% to 9%, depending on the reduced sample size (see Table A.12) for each remedy effectiveness parameter. The increase in the confidence interval for remedy effectiveness parameters is explained in detail in the next section on "Data Analysis."

Data Analysis

The data were initially analyzed to determine outliers. This analysis was twofold. First, survey participants who had three responses outside +/- 3 standard deviations of the normalized response were marked as outliers. For example, it is easy to understand that remedy effectiveness and symptom severity are inversely proportional. One would think if a medication is somewhat effective, then symptom intensity and frequency should be lower. The outlier analysis eliminated those responses where a survey participant may claim to be getting optimum alleviation from certain medications but at the same time show no relief from symptom intensity or frequency. Since this person's answers may not be completely logical, rational, or reasonable, they were eliminated from the survey data analysis.

Second, the survey encompassed control questions to eliminate survey participant responses from the data analysis who have not met at least two of the following conditions: (1) diagnosed with PNH by a physician; (2) symptoms serious enough to warrant an EMG; and (3) symptoms serious enough to warrant an MRI.

When modeling variables using a linear regression model, there are two sets of variables: x and y. Only one variable is allowed for y in a linear regression analysis, but multiple variables can be used for x so long as there are more equations than unknowns. A linear regression model for each parameter (y) was computed with the other 55 parameters (x) to calculate t-statistics and p and determine statistical significance. Thus, 55 linear regression models were computed from the data results (one for each parameter or y variable). These 55 models have very low adjusted R^2 values (the results are not linear) and are, therefore, not very good models to predict future outcomes. [8] However, t-statistic and ρ values obtained from linear regression models are a good measure of statistical significance between any two parameters. For example, on data with large sample sizes, t-statistic results that have outcomes greater than the absolute value of two usually designates strong statistical significance between variables (over a 95% probability, or a ρ result of less than 0.05).

A Spearman correlation study was used to calculate the correlation between any two parameters with a high statistical significance. Spearman correlation results are as follows: [9] (1) the absolute value of 0.5 to 1 represents a strong correlation; (2) the absolute value of 0.3 to 0.5 represents a moderate correlation; (3) the absolute value of 0.1 to 0.3 represents a weak correlation; and (4) the absolute value of 0 to 0.1 represents no correlation.

When remedy effectiveness parameters were the y variable, the raw data used to calculate the results was modified. Since most of the survey participants have not tried all the remedies listed in the survey, these nonresponses were removed from remedy effectiveness linear regression model computations. Hence, data for these results need an asterisk because their sample size is much smaller–anywhere from 119 to 321 (Please see Table A.12). Thus, the confidence interval (or error) for these parameters may increase to as much as 9% because of the smaller sample sizes. In other words, for Table A.12, ρ is greater than 0.05, even when t-statistic values are greater than the absolute value of 2. Moreover, the data for these parameters have less statistical significance than the data from those parameters found in the other six tables.

Finally, potassium channel blocker medications and acupuncture remedy effectiveness parameters were removed entirely from the survey data results because they had fewer than 30 responses.

Results

The following section, Parameter Classifications and Parameter Definitions, list the parameter classifications and definitions in Table A.1 through Table A.7. For example, from Table A.1, one may surmise that "General Information" is a parameter classification and "Age" is one parameter represented under "General Information." The result for the "Age" parameter depends on how survey participants answered the question: "What is the age of the survey participant?":

Parameter Classifications and Parameter Definitions

Table A.1: General Information Parameter Classification

Parameter	Survey Question
Age	What is the age of the survey participant?
Gender	What is the gender of the survey participant (male or female)?
Region	What continent does the survey participant reside in?
MRI	Did the survey participant have an MRI (Yes or No)?
EMG	Did the survey participant have an

	EMG (Yes or No)?
Years Diagnosed	How many years ago was the survey participant diagnosed with PNH?
Years with PNH Symptoms	How many years has the survey participant had PNH symptoms?

Table A.2: Symptom Stressors Parameter Classification (Answers provided on a scale of 1 to 10)

Parameter	Survey Question
Sickness 1	What intensity and frequency are PNH symptoms exacerbated by an illness?
Exercise 1	What intensity and frequency are PNH symptoms exacerbated by exercise?
Stress / Anxiety 1	What intensity and frequency are PNH symptoms exacerbated by stress or anxiety?

Table A.3: Symptom Parameter Classification (Answers provided on a scale of 1 to 10)

Parameter	Survey Question
Twitching	What frequency and intensity do survey participants have twitching?
Pins and Needles	What frequency and intensity do survey participants have pins and needles?
Cramps	What frequency and intensity do survey participants have cramps?
Muscle Fatigue and Weakness	What frequency and intensity do survey participants have muscle

	fatigue and weakness?
Headaches	What frequency and intensity do survey participants have headaches?
Itching	What frequency and intensity do survey participants have itching?
Numbness	What frequency and intensity do survey participants have numbness?
Vibration Sensations	What frequency and intensity do survey participants have vibration sensations?
Pain and Soreness	What frequency and intensity do survey participants have pain and soreness?
Sensitivity to Temperatures	What frequency and intensity do survey participants have a sensitivity to temperatures?

Table A.4: Body Region Affected by Symptom Parameter Classification (Answers provided on a scale of 1 to 10)

Parameter	Survey Question
Feet	What frequency and intensity do survey participants have symptoms in the feet?
Lower Leg	What frequency and intensity do survey participants have symptoms in the lower leg?
Upper Leg	What frequency and intensity do survey participants have symptoms in the upper leg?

Buttock / Hips	What frequency and intensity do survey participants have symptoms in the buttock/hips?
Back	What frequency and intensity do survey participants have symptoms in the back?
Abdomen	What frequency and intensity do survey participants have symptoms in the abdomen?
Chest	What frequency and intensity do survey participants have symptoms in the chest?
Neck and Head	What frequency and intensity do survey participants have symptoms in the neck and head?
Arms and Shoulders	What frequency and intensity do survey participants have symptoms in the arms and shoulders?
Hands	What frequency and intensity do survey participants have symptoms in the hands?

Table A.5: Remedy Effectiveness Parameter Classification (Answers provided on a scale of 1 to 10)

Parameter	Survey Question
Anti-Seizure Medication	Do anti-seizure prescription drugs improve symptoms?
Anti-Depressant Medication	Do anti-depressant prescription drugs improve symptoms?
Sleeping Pill Medication	Do sleeping pill prescription drugs improve symptoms?
Muscle Relaxant	Do muscle relaxant prescription

Medication	drugs improve symptoms?
Benzodiazepine Medication	Do benzodiazepine prescription drugs improve symptoms?
Homeopathic Treatments	Do homeopathic treatments (i.e., acupuncture) improve symptoms?
Supplements	Do supplements (i.e., vitamins) improve symptoms?
Diet	Did a change to a healthier diet improve symptoms?
Massage	Does massage improve symptoms?
Yoga	Does yoga improve symptoms?

Table A.6: Miscellaneous Information Parameter Classification

Parameter	Survey Question
Remedies	Did any remedies tried by the survey participant make symptoms worse? (Yes or No)
Missing	Are any potential remedies missing from the survey list? (Yes or No)
Time	Are symptoms getting worse or better over time? (1 to 10 Scale)
Day	What time of day are symptoms worse? (Morning, Day, Evening)
Altitude	Do symptoms get worse at altitude? (Yes or No)

Table A.7: Causation Parameter Classification (Answers are provided as a Yes or No)

Parameter	Survey Questions
Chemicals	Does the survey participant feel any

	exposure to toxins may have produced their PNH symptoms?
Other	Does the survey participant feel something not listed in the survey may have induced their PNH symptoms?
History	Does the survey participant feel a family history of neurological disease may have produced their PNH symptoms?
Vaccine	Does the survey participant feel a vaccine may have caused their PNH symptoms?
Illness	Does the survey participant feel an illness may have induced their PNH symptoms?
Stress and Anxiety	Does the survey participant feel that stress and anxiety may have produced their PNH symptoms?
Prescription Drugs	Does the survey participant feel a prescription drug may have caused their PNH symptoms?
Spine and Neck Injury	Does the survey participant feel a spine or neck injury may have induced their PNH symptoms?
Exercise	Does the survey participant feel intense exercise may have produced their PNH symptoms?

General Statistics

The mean age of survey participants was 39.7 years old, with a standard deviation of 10.1 years, and 63% of the survey participants were male (37% female). Ninety-one percent of the survey participants were diagnosed with at least BFS. About 66% of the survey participants were from North America, 24% from Europe, 4% from South America, 4% from Asia, and about 1% from Africa. On average, patients had lived with symptoms for about 4.5 years, and it was about 2.6 years, on average, since they were diagnosed with some type of PNH disorder. Nearly 80% of the survey participants had an EMG, and 64% had an MRI.

As far as etiology is concerned (participants could choose more than one), stress was the leading reason at 71%, illness (30%), exercise (25%), prescription drugs (20%), hereditary (20%), some other cause (19%), spine/neck injury (10%), vaccine (9%), and exposure to toxins (4%). Concerning symptoms, 99% of the participants have twitching, vibration sensation (84%), muscle pain and soreness (82%), pins and needles (79%), muscle fatigue and weakness (78%), muscle stiffness (76%), cramps (70%), numbness (67%), sensitivity to temperatures (57%), headaches (51%), and itching (44%). Finally, with regard to body regions affected by symptoms, nearly 100% of participants have symptoms in their feet, lower leg (97%), upper leg (93%), arms and shoulders (90%), hands (85%), hip and buttock (83%), back (77%), neck and head (77%), chest (75%), and abdomen (60%).

Of course, the above data or information does not indicate the frequency or intensity of the symptoms, nor does it indicate the frequency or intensity at which specific body areas are affected. Intensity and frequency data were determined to be as follows.

The participants rated twitching with an average frequency and intensity of 7.6 out of 10, vibration sensation (4.8), muscle pain and soreness (4.8), pins and needles (4), muscle fatigue and weakness (4.4), muscle stiffness (4.3), cramps (3.6), numbness (3.1), sensitivity to temperatures (3.4), headaches (2.6), and itching (2.4). For example, a survey participant, on average, will have twitching symptoms about 76% of the time. The standard deviation for symptom frequency and intensity ranges from 2-3 for each symptom. The high variance illustrates the results varied considerably for each participant.

As far as body region frequency and intensity is concerned, the average survey participant rated symptoms in their feet (5.7 out of 10), lower leg (7.4), upper leg (5.3), arms and shoulders (5.1), hands (4.7), hip and buttock (4), back (3.5), neck and head (3.8), chest (2.8), and abdomen (3.1). For example, a survey participant, on average, will have symptoms in their lower leg 74% of the time. The standard deviation for body region frequency and intensity was 2-3 for each parameter. This, too, also illustrates the results varied considerably for each participant.

PNH symptoms for survey participants is very serious because it is not generalized to one region. Of the ten regions of the body, the average survey participant has symptoms in over eight of them with an average frequency and intensity of 4.1 out of 10. This finding illustrates that people will have symptoms body-wide all day long (24 / 7) with an intensity of 4.1. Even worse, the amount of relief from prescription drugs and other treatment options (of those who tried the survey treatment options) only ranged from 1.8 (homeopathic treatments like acupuncture) to 3.8

(benzodiazepines) on a scale of 10. Sleeping pills were the second most effective remedy with a mere impact of 2.8. Hence, the top two most effective remedies work to inebriate the patient making their quality of life worse, not better.

About 12% of the participants said a potential remedy made them feel significantly worse (increasing symptoms or creating new side effects), and another 10% claim to have found a helpful remedy that was not on the survey list. On a 10-point scale, with 5 indicating no change in symptoms, 1-4 indicating symptoms are improving over time, and 6-10 indicating symptoms are getting worse, the average was 5.6, indicating that overall symptoms for survey participants are progressively getting worse, but very slowly. About 40% of survey participants indicate symptoms are worse at night, 33% indicate symptoms are worse in the morning, and about 26% indicate symptoms are worse during the day. I suspect the reason for this result is because people are more active during the day and are too busy to feel their symptoms. Staying busy is important for reducing symptoms. The ***symptom stressors,*** or factors that exacerbate symptoms reveal, on average, that an illness may elevate symptom intensity and frequency about 3.5 out of 10, exercise (5.5–this is exercise intolerance), and stress (6.8).

Correlation Results
Spearman Correlation Study

The tabulated results in Tables A.8 through A.14 are reported as follows: First, results in bold fonts indicate a strong Spearman correlation (values greater than the absolute value of 0.5). Second, results in italic fonts indicate a moderate Spearman correlation (values greater than the absolute value of 0.3 and less than the absolute value of 0.5). Third, normal font indicates only a weak correlation (values greater than the absolute value of 0.1 and less than the absolute value of 0.3). Fourth, results not tabulated have no correlation. Only results with some correlation are tabulated. Finally, a minus sign (-) before the result indicates a negative correlation, while no sign indicates a positive correlation. A positive correlation indicates the two parameters track proportionally, and a negative correlation (minus sign) denotes the two parameters are inversely proportional.

Table A.8: General Information Classification

Parameter (y Variable)	Parameters with Weak, Moderate, and Strong Correlation (x Variables)
Age	Years with PNH Symptoms, -Stress / Anxiety, History, -Stress Anxiety 1, Muscle Stiffness, Lower Leg
Gender *	Region, -Feet, Lower Leg, -Hip Buttock
Region *	Gender, Stress Anxiety, -History, -Muscle Relaxant, -Diet, -Remedies
Years Diagnosed	**Years with PNH Symptoms**, EMG, -Stress / Anxiety, Exercise1, Lower Leg, Anti-Seizure
Years with PNH Symptoms	Age, **Years Diagnosed**, -Stress Anxiety, Exercise1, -Stress Anxiety1, Twitching, Sensitivity to Temperatures, Lower Leg, Time

EMG	Years Diagnosed, MRI, Sickness, -Stress / Anxiety, -Stress Anxiety1, Back, Anti-Seizure, Benzodiazepine
MRI	EMG, Prescription Drugs, Spine and Neck Injury, Pins and Needles, Cramps, Diet, Remedies

*: Note–For the gender and region parameters in Table A.8, negative correlation represents women (gender) and people residing in North America (region), while positive correlation represents men (gender) and people residing outside North America (region).

Overall, women are more affected by symptoms in their hips, buttock, and feet, while men are more likely to feel symptoms in their lower legs. Men with PNH symptoms are more prevalent outside the United States. Stress and anxiety-induced PNH is more common outside the United States, but hereditary forms of PNH are more common in the United States. Muscle relaxants and dietary changes are more effective in resolving symptoms for PNH patients in the United States. Dietary changes make sense since Americans consume more sugar and processed foods than any country around the globe. United States survey participants are more likely to try remedies missing from this survey. It is also important to keep in mind that the correlation for the gender and region parameters are of the weak variety. For example, we can conclude it is a weak trend that women have more symptoms in the hips, buttocks, and feet than men, but it is certainly not guaranteed to be the situation all the time.

From Table A.8, the "Years with PNH Symptoms" parameter is evaluated for correlation. Generally, older respondents in the survey have had PNH symptoms longer (Age). People who have had PNH symptoms a long time are less likely to have stress or anxiety induced PNH (Stress Anxiety). Stress is less likely to exacerbate symptoms in people who have had PNH for a long period of time (Stress Anxiety 1). Twitching and sensitivity to temperature symptoms are more common for people who have had PNH for a long time (Twitching and Sensitivity to Temperatures). Symptoms for people who have had PNH for a long time will predominately exist in the lower legs (Lower leg), and their symptoms progressively worsen over time (Time). All of the correlation for the Years with PNH Symptoms parameter is of the weak variety. The only strong correlation found in Table A.8 is that people who have had PNH symptoms a long time have also been diagnosed with PNH for a longer period of time (Years Diagnosed).

Table A.9: Symptom Stressor Classification

Parameter or Variable	Parameters with Weak, Moderate, and Strong Correlation
Sickness1	*Sickness*, Exercise1, Stress / Anxiety1, Missing
Exercise1	Years Diagnosed, Years with PNH Symptoms, Exercise, Other, Sickness1, Stress / Anxiety1, -Anti-Depressant, -Muscle Relaxant
Stress / Anxiety1	-Age, -Years with PNH Symptoms, -EMG, *Stress / Anxiety*, -Other, Sickness1, Diet,

	Benzodiazepine

From Table A.9, correlation for the "Stress / Anxiety 1" parameter is examined. Stress or anxiety is more likely to exacerbate symptoms in younger people (-Age) and people who have not had PNH symptoms for very long (-Years with PNH Symptoms). People whose symptoms may be exacerbated by stress are less likely to get an EMG (-EMG). People whose symptoms may be exacerbated by stress are more likely to have PNH symptoms triggered by stress (stress / anxiety). This parameter has a moderate correlation. People whose symptoms are exacerbated by stress may also have symptoms exacerbated by an illness (sickness 1). People whose symptoms may be exacerbated by stress are less likely to have another trigger (-other) that is not listed in the survey. Diet and benzodiazepine medications may work best to control symptoms exacerbated by stress. Apart from stress or an illness exacerbating PNH symptoms in people who have PNH symptoms triggered by stress and illness respectively (moderate correlation), all the other correlation found in Table A.9 is of the weak variety.

Table A.10: Symptom Classification

Parameter or Variable	Parameters with Weak, Moderate, and Strong Correlation
Twitching	Years with PNH Symptoms, Stress / Anxiety, Pins and Needles, **Lower Leg**, -Anti-Depressant, -Diet, -Benzodiazepine, *Time*
Pins and Needles	MRI, Twitching, *Numbness*, *Vibration / Buzzing Sensation*, Feet

Cramps	MRI, *Numbness, Muscle Pain and Soreness*, Lower Leg
Muscle Fatigue and Weakness	**Muscle Stiffness, Muscle Pain and Soreness**, Feet, Lower Leg, Anti-Seizure, Massage
Headaches	Itching, Neck / Head
Itching	-Exercise, Headaches, Muscle Stiffness, Sensitivity to Temperatures, Neck / Head
Numbness	*Pins and Needles, Cramps, Muscle Stiffness,* Sensitivity to Temperatures, Anti-Depressant
Muscle Stiffness	Age, **Muscle Fatigue and Weakness**, Itching, *Numbness*, **Muscle Pain and Soreness**, Diet
Vibration/Buzzing Sensation	-Vaccine, *Pins and Needles, Feet,* - Muscle Relaxant, Benzodiazepines
Muscle Pain / Soreness	*Cramps*, **Muscle Fatigue and Weakness, Muscle Stiffness**, *Sensitivity to Temperatures, Hands*, Anti-Depressants
Sensitivity to Temperatures	Years with PNH Symptoms, Itching, Numbness, *Muscle Pain and Soreness*, Homeopathic Treatments

From Table A.10, the "Twitching" symptom is examined for correlation trends. Twitching (fasciculation) symptoms will worsen for most PNH patients over time (moderate correlation). Twitching symptoms are commonly triggered by stress or anxiety. People who have twitching as a symptom may also experience pins and needles as a secondary symptom. There is a strong correlation to support that twitching will generally occur in the lower leg. Remedies such as anti-depressant medications, dietary changes, and benzodiazepine medications do not alleviate twitching symptoms. Conversely, no remedy was found to help twitching symptoms, which is unsurprising since twitching was not only the most common symptom but the symptom with the most frequency and intensity.

There are several parameters with a moderate to strong correlation in Table A.10. Not surprisingly, symptoms such as muscle fatigue, weakness, stiffness, pain, and soreness are all closely related. I purposely grouped fatigue and weakness into the same category, although they are two vastly different symptoms. Most people incorrectly relate fatigue to weakness; fatigue is being tired, and weakness refers to a loss of strength. To avoid any confusion from the survey participants, I grouped the two symptoms together. Also, not surprisingly, symptoms such as cramps, numbness, and sensitivity to temperatures have some moderate correlation with parameters such as muscle pain and soreness. Other strong trends make sense as well, such as vibration and buzzing sensations occurring in the feet and also being associated with pins and needles. Cramps are associated with numbness, muscle pain, and muscle soreness (moderate correlation). Muscle pain and soreness are more commonly related to the hands (moderate correlation).

Table A.11: Body Region Classification

Parameter or Variable	Parameters with Weak, Moderate, and Strong Correlation
Feet	-Gender, Spine or Neck Injury, Pins

	and Needles, Muscle Fatigue and Weakness, *Vibration / Buzzing Sensation, Lower Leg, Hands*
Lower Leg	Age, Gender, Years Diagnosed, Years with BFS Symptoms, **Twitching**, Cramps, Muscle Fatigue and Weakness, *Feet*, -Arms / Shoulders
Upper Leg	*Hip / Buttock, Abdomen*, Arms / Shoulders
Hip / Buttock Region	-Gender, *Upper Leg*, **Back**
Back	EMG, **Hip / Buttock, Abdomen**, *Chest, Arms / Shoulder*, Anti-Seizure
Abdomen	*Upper Leg*, **Back, Chest**, -Yoga
Chest	*Back*, **Abdomen**, Neck Head, Arms / Shoulder, Anti-Seizure
Neck / Head	Headaches, Itching, *Chest, Hands, Arms / Shoulder*, Massage, Remedies
Hands	Sickness, *Muscle Pain and Soreness, Feet, Neck / Head, Arms / Shoulders*
Arms / Shoulder	-Lower Leg, Upper / Leg, *Back, Chest, Neck / Head, Hands*

From Table A.11, the "Lower Leg" and "Feet" parameters are examined for correlation. Symptoms in the lower leg are most likely to affect older male PNH patients.

Twitching is the primary symptom in the lower leg (strong correlation) along with secondary symptoms of cramping and muscle fatigue, and weakness. People with lower leg symptoms are less likely to have PNH symptoms in the arms and shoulders but are highly likely to also have symptoms in the feet (moderate correlation). The feet parameter is interesting because it affects mostly women, and it is associated with muscle fatigue, weakness, pins and needles, and a vibration sensation (moderate correlation). A spine or neck injury is a common trigger for feet symptoms, and there is a moderate correlation that PNH symptoms will also affect the hands if a person's feet also have symptoms.

Strong correlation trends from Table A.11 are as follows: It is no surprise that symptoms in the chest, back, hip, buttock, and abdomen are closely related since they are all proximal regions of the body. There is a moderate correlation between symptoms in the arms and shoulders with the hands, the upper leg with the hip and buttock, the arms and shoulders with the back, and feet and lower legs. As far as symptoms in the hands and feet being closely related is unsurprising, although they are not close in proximity. This phenomenon is explained because axonal peripheral neuropathy symptoms generally start in the longest nerves (length dependent). Obviously, both the hands and feet have long nerves since nerves originate from the spine.

*Table A.12: Remedy Effectiveness Classification *

Parameter or Variable	Parameters with Weak, Moderate, and Strong Correlation

Anti-Seizure	Years Diagnosed, EMG, -Spine or Neck Injury, Sickness, Exercise, Muscle Fatigue and Weakness, Back, -Chest
Anti-Depressants	-Exercise1, -Twitching, Numbness, Muscle Pain and Soreness
Sleeping Pills	Exercise
Muscle Relaxants	-Region, History, Exercise1, -Vibration / Buzzing Sensation
Homeopathic Treatments	Sensitivity to Temperatures, Missing
Supplements	Stress / Anxiety1, -Twitching, Muscle Stiffness, Neck / Head
Diet	-Region, MRI
Massage	Sickness, Exercise, Stress / Anxiety1, Muscle Fatigue and Weakness, Neck / Head
Yoga	-Abdomen, -Remedies
Benzodiazepine Drugs	EMG, Stress Anxiety, -Twitching, Vibration / Buzzing Sensation

Note* The sample size is smaller for remedy effectiveness parameters since most survey participants have not tried all the remedy solutions. Sample sizes are as follows: Anti-Seizure 137, Anti-Depressants 177, Sleeping pills 121, Muscle Relaxants 119, Homeopathic Treatments 131, Supplements 322, Diet 221, Massage 209, Yoga 124, and Benzodiazepine Medications 199.

From Table A.12, the "Anti-Seizure" parameter is evaluated for correlation: People are more likely to find relief from anti-seizure medications after having been diagnosed with PNH for a long period of time. People who are more likely to find relief from anti-seizure medication have had an EMG. Anti-seizure medications may be more effective for people whose PNH symptoms were triggered by an illness or exercise, and they experience muscle fatigue and weakness as a symptom. Anti-seizure medications may help people find relief from symptoms that occur in the back, but people on anti-seizure medications are less likely to find relief for symptoms in the chest. It is not surprising that people who have had a spine and neck injury induce symptoms that are less likely to find relief from anti-seizure medication. Since most PNH remedies do not work very well, it is not surprising there is not any moderate or strong correlation within this group of parameters.

Table *A.13: Various of Miscellaneous Classification*

Parameter or Variable	Parameters with Weak, Moderate, and Strong Correlation
Remedies	-Region, MRI, Chemicals, Prescription Drugs, Neck / Head, -Yoga, Missing, Altitude
Time	Years with PNH Symptoms, *Twitching*
Day	No Correlation
Missing	Vaccine, Sickness, Sickness1, Homeopathic Treatments, Remedies

| Altitude | Sickness, Supplements, Remedies |

From Table A.13, the "Remedies" parameter is investigated for correlation. People from North America are more likely to have tried a remedy that has made their PNH symptoms worse, and that may be one reason why they are more likely to have had an MRI. People with chemical or prescription drug-induced PNH are more likely to have tried a remedy that has made their symptoms worse. PNH patients trying remedies that make their symptoms worse are more likely to have symptoms in the neck and head region of the body. This result may indicate that people are getting a headache as a side-effect. Yoga is not helpful for people who tried survey remedies that make them feel worse. People who feel worse from a survey remedy are more likely to try unlisted survey treatments to find relief. People who have tried remedies that make their PNH symptoms worse also claim altitude or low pressure can make their symptoms worse. The only moderate correlation found in Table A.13 is that twitching symptoms will tend to worsen over time.

Table A.14: Cause or Trigger Classification

Parameter or Variable	Parameters with Weak, Moderate, and Strong Correlation
Flu Shot / Vaccine	Chemicals, -Vibration / Buzzing Sensation, Missing
Chemicals	Vaccine, Prescription Drugs, Spine or Neck Injury, Remedies
Prescription Drugs	MRI, Chemicals, Sickness, Remedies

Spine and Neck Injury	MRI, Chemicals, Feet, -Anti-Seizure
Sickness	EMG, Prescription Drugs, *Sickness1*, Hands, Anti-Seizure, Massage, Missing, Altitude
Exercise	Stress Anxiety, Exercise1, -Itching, Anti-Seizure, Sleeping Pills, Massage
Stress / Anxiety	-Age, Region, -Years Diagnosed, -Years with PNH Symptoms, -EMG, Exercise, *Stress / Anxiety 1*, -Twitching, Massage
History	Age, -Region, Muscle Relaxant
Other	Exercise1, -Stress / Anxiety1

From Table A.14, the "Stress and Anxiety" parameter is examined for correlation. Stress-induced PNH is more likely to happen in younger patients who have not had symptoms for a very long time. People with stress-induced PNH tend to reside in Europe and are less likely to have had an EMG. Stress will exacerbate symptoms (moderate correlation) for people with stress-induced PNH. Twitching symptoms are less severe in stress-induced PNH. Massage works best to alleviate symptoms for stress-induced PNH. People with stress-induced PNH also feel that exercise may have triggered their symptoms. This result may indicate that these persons may get stressed out from competition and trying to excel at a sport. The only other parameter in

Table A.14 with any moderate correlation is that PNH symptoms triggered by illness may also have symptoms exacerbated by illness.

The above examples should help the reader interpret all correlation data in the above tables.

Conclusions and Discussions

Is a Survey Reliable?

Medical professionals believe the only acceptable publications are studies encompassing a control group, clinical trial, or observation of patients. However, there are several important reasons why surveys should not be ignored.

First, most medical research papers or clinical trials are mathematically flawed. One reference estimates that two in five medical research papers have an inadequate sample size. [9] On the other hand, this survey study meets the guidelines for a 95% confidence level and a 5% confidence interval because it has surpassed a sample size of 384. To dismiss this survey as insignificant is the same as dismissing the voice of 25 million people. Furthermore, most medical studies using "acceptable methods" are statistically flawed, and most doctors that read these medical research papers do not know they are flawed. According to one reference, "The increasing volume of research by the medical community often leads to increasing numbers of contradictory findings and conclusions. Although the differences observed may represent true differences, the results also may differ because of sampling variability as all studies are performed on a limited number of specimens or patients. When planning a study reporting differences among groups of patients or describing some variable in a single group, the sample size should be considered because it allows the researcher to control for the risk of reporting a false-negative finding (Type II error) or to estimate the precision his or her experiment will yield. Equally important, readers of medical journals should understand sample size because such understanding is essential to interpret the relevance of a finding with regard to their own patients." Furthermore, the paper concludes, "We believe correct planning of experiments is an ethical issue of concern to the entire community." [9]

Second, doctors question whether survey participants are truthful and accurate with their responses. To avoid that dilemma, this study eliminates outliers (i.e., questionable responses that are beyond 3 standard deviations of the mean). Since we know very little about PNH, it can be argued that all the information in this writing is statistically and practically significant regardless of no, weak, moderate, or strong correlation findings. Said differently, regardless of correlation findings, this study contributes to the body of evidence for PNH. Third, some people argue that my lack of a medical degree disqualifies me from publishing a medical paper. However, there is nothing medical about this paper. This paper is merely a thorough statistical or epidemiological analysis of a medical problem that we know very little about PNH. Any discussions about associating PNH to medical conditions are a hypothesis; the paper is not reporting these medical findings as fact. Surveys are cost-effective, while controlled studies and clinical trials can be cost-prohibitive. Fourth, doesn't it make sense to find statistical significance, practical significance, and correlation from a survey before moving on to an expensive clinical trial? One would hope so. Fifth, surveys can also collect data globally, while controlled studies and clinical trials can limit data collection to localized regions. For instance, this study uncovered that stress-related PNH is statistically significant outside North America, while people with PNH who have a family history of neurological disease are more likely to reside within North America. In fact, one-third of the survey participants in this paper are located outside of North America. The bottom line, proximity restrictions can hide relevant results.

Sixth, observation of PNH patients has a limited benefit since most patients look normal and exhibit few symptoms that can be viewed. For example, sensory symptoms cannot be observed. In other words, doctors can only rate a PNH patient's sensory symptoms based on their response to questions–similar to a survey or questionnaire. In fact, since neurologists cannot visually confirm certain symptoms, they may misdiagnose PNH as BFS instead of CFS. Furthermore, patient observation can also be influenced by stress. Case in point, patients commonly present with elevated blood pressure when they visit the doctor due to anxiety.

Seventh, in an anonymous survey, the person analyzing the data is not influenced by human bias. However, in clinical research trials, bias and opinion are routinely injected in these studies by medical personnel. One study of 21 clinical trials found, "On average, non-blinded assessors of subjective binary outcomes generated substantially biased effect estimates in randomized clinical trials, exaggerating odds ratios by 36%." [10] A biased outcome can be eliminated in a double-blinded and controlled clinical trial.

Eighth, there is also evidence that money used to fund clinical trials by industry and the government can bias outcomes: "Thus, although there is little direct evidence that industry sponsorship has led to a deliberate skewing of the results or reporting, there are multiple cases in which industry and government sponsors have withheld important study results and in which the conclusions presented in the reports appear to overstate the study findings. The risk of undue influence in research exists." [11]

Misconceptions about PNH

The data refute two myths about PNH. The first myth is that PNH is the same for everyone–easy to live with and "no big deal." For most individuals, it is true, PNH is no big deal and easy to live with, but many chronic sufferers from this disorder feel ignored. The data in this survey uncover a chronic version of PNH. The data suggest people in the survey are affected by, on average, 7.7 of 11 symptoms over approximately 80% of their bodies with an average frequency and intensity for each symptom of 4.1 out of 10.   From these data, we can conclude that the people in this survey suffer from chronic PNH because many probably live with symptoms 24/7 throughout their entire body. Even worse, the best remedies for relieving symptoms inebriate sufferers (i.e., sleeping pills for 2.8 out of 10 and benzodiazepine medications for 3.8 out of 10. The other remedies in the survey help about 2 to 2.5 out of 10). Nearly 50% of the participants in the survey have had both an MRI and EMG, and over 85% have had either an

EMG or MRI. This is significant because only people with chronic PNH symptoms would be subject to such expensive testing to rule out other more serious neurological conditions.

None of these findings should be surprising since the people taking this survey belong to a PNH social networking site. People will only go to these forums if they have a chronic condition for which they cannot find appropriate relief or answers. This explains why only two survey participants out of 438 report twitching (fasciculations) as their only symptom. Thus, there is a chronic aspect to PNH that is being understated, underrepresented and ignored. After all, if the symptoms were inconsequential or insignificant, then it is unlikely a person would reach out for assistance. Thus, the findings for this paper overwhelmingly represent individuals chronically inflicted with PNH (CFS) and not those who are only mildly inflicted with PNH symptoms (BFS). This is important for several reasons. It proves there is a disconnect between doctors and patients when mild and chronic patients are categorically considered one and the same. Additionally, since the data in this survey are skewed toward those with chronic PNH, more studies would be needed to understand the statistical significance behind those with milder forms of PNH, such as BFS.

The second myth is that PNH is always "benign," which the data refute. In medicine, benign means that there is "no danger to health; not recurrent or progressive; not malignant." While BFS is considered "benign" because it will not kill those afflicted, it contains very real symptoms that, in many cases, are both psychologically and physically debilitating (Kincaid JC, Muscle Pain, Fatigue, and Fasciculations, Neurology Clinic 1997). Fasciculations alone are harmless, but when coupled with chronic symptoms, BFS can wreak havoc on a person's life. Coupled with increased stress, less sleep, and exacerbated symptoms, in my humble opinion, this disorder is debilitating and, without doubt, can decrease the life expectancy of sufferers. The decrease in life expectancy is due to the fact that most people with PNH disorders fail to exercise because they have exercise intolerance and depression. Said differently, PNH disorders can progress, and the data support this finding. The survey results show that only stress-induced PNH patients can adequately control their symptoms over time. Patients with PNH etiology induced by anything other than stress will see their symptoms progressively worsen over time.

Since these patients' symptoms are progressive; therefore, by definition, PNH is not "benign" in all circumstances. A better name would be progressive fasciculation disorder (PFD) for chronic sufferers of PNH that is not stress-induced. Alternatively, better yet, patients can be diagnosed properly with CFS instead of being misdiagnosed with BFS. There are better avenues for doctors to take with BFS patients. One reference on neurological bedside manner and etiquette explained a doctor's function: "Never reject the patient's own interpretation of his or her symptoms, even if it seems implausible or absurd." Furthermore, "The patient has a right to be told what your findings are and what they imply about his or her illness. Explain these matters truthfully, in language, the patient can understand, and with due respect for his or her feelings." Moreover, "Every patient has the right to be treated courteously and tactfully and to have the physician's full attention for an adequate period of time." Unfortunately, many doctors diagnosing patients with BFS and PNH disorders do not follow this advice. [21] Another source indicates that not only is patient history and their description of symptoms the most important facet of the diagnosis process, but doctors interrupt patients during their explanation of symptoms nearly 50% of the time, usually within 18 s. [19]

Multiple Triggers or Causes?

There are nine suggested etiology or causation paths for participants to choose from in this survey. Causation possibilities are environmental factors that may trigger or exacerbate the PNH symptoms. Oftentimes, patients believe they have had more than one causation over the course of their lives. For instance, with the author's own experience with PNH, I believe there may have been a multitude of triggers for my symptoms, including exercise (high altitude climbing and mountaineering), sickness (had a gamma globulin deficiency that resulted in staph infections as a youth), prescription drugs (regular use of antibiotics for folliculitis, statins, and allergy medications), exposure to toxins, and like others surveyed, had experienced a great deal of stress. I even had potential environmental triggers not mentioned in the survey, such as alcohol abuse and child abuse, to name a few. On average, a survey participant selected 2.1 of the potential triggers.

It is possible that once afflicted with PNH that the introduction of new environmental triggers exacerbates current symptoms and possibly introduce new symptoms. This should be explored further. The vast number of options for individual trigger possibilities is what may make PNH distinctive in each patient (different symptoms and remedy effectiveness). Considering this uniqueness in this umbrella diagnosis, it is no surprise that it is difficult to cure or find solutions to alleviate symptoms. While PNH is benign (in the sense that it is not deadly), it is still an illness for which its patients would benefit from an effective treatment.

It should be pointed out that potential triggers were purposely omitted from this survey, such as substance and domestic abuse. [2] Social triggers are important to understand, but I did not want to frighten potential participants away because they felt the survey was becoming too personal or checking into illegal activity. Conversely, many people have found the use of medical marijuana as an effective remedy, and it was purposely omitted as a potential remedy because marijuana is a controlled substance that is illegal in the United States [2] The omission of illegal activities and social environmental factors from the list of causes and remedies may partly explain why nearly 20% of survey participants had potential causation not listed in the survey and another 12% of survey participants finding a useful remedy not listed in the survey.

Statistical Significance, Practical Significance, and Correlation

No survey discussion is complete without a discussion on statistics. Statistics can be vastly confusing and open to multiple interpretations. Statistical significance between parameters does not imply practical significance.

Sometimes commonsense is needed to determine practical significance from statistical significance. However, a survey on a complicated subject, which we know little about, such as PNH, makes it more difficult to decipher practical significance. Given that we know little about PNH, one could conclude any statistical significance is also practical significance. That said, mathematically speaking, it is true that large sample sizes (like this study) may reveal statistical significance but very little practical significance. [12] However, the goal of this paper is to report the data and statistical significance. It is the job of medical professionals who not only pose theories from these data but to test the theories for robustness to determine if the data have practical significance. In other words, since I am not trying to prove any theories, I am not determining any practical significance, just statistical significance.

A strong correlation does not imply statistical significance, especially if the sample size is small. Conversely, statistical significance may not imply a strong correlation; it may only occur because the sample size is large. Hence, it important to report statistical significance, sample size, and correlation, together as one item, to determine practical significance. [12] In this survey, since the sample size is large, the data fail to indicate numerous occurrences of strong correlation, but mostly weak correlation–yet these data can be of practical significance to some medical researchers. Weak correlation, strong statistical significance, and the large sample size is usually better than weak statistical significance, small sample size, and strong correlation. [12] All parameters outlined in Tables A.8 through Table A.14 not only have some level of correlation but also have strong statistical significance (p-value of less than 0.05), indicating the results are reliable. The only exception is Table A.12, whose variables have much smaller sample sizes, which is important to note for others using those data to find practical significance. The bottom line, I am not attempting to find practical significance. The job of finding practical significance resides with those medical professionals who generate and prove theories with the enclosed information and data. [12]

Are People Commonly Misdiagnosed with PNH?

There are four types of peripheral nerve hyperexcitation (PNH) syndromes. The simplest form is BFS, and people with this should only experience one symptom: muscle twitching. That said, the data suggest that many PNH patients diagnosed with BFS experience other symptoms. Thus, these patients have been misdiagnosed and more likely to have cramp fasciculation syndrome (CFS) since Isaac syndrome and Morvan syndrome are very rare. This would go a long way to explain the disconnect between PNH patient symptoms and what advice they were hearing from neurologists. The tendency to misdiagnose BFS may explain why doctors were telling patients what they have is "no big deal" and why they failed to provide them any advice to alleviate symptoms. According to the survey data, the following findings can be reported: (1) The 438 people experience, on average, 7.7 of the 11 listed symptoms with an average frequency and intensity of a 4.1 out of 10 for each symptom; (2) only 2 of 438 people experience twitching as their only symptom; (3) only 13 of the 438 people experience two or fewer symptoms; and (4) only 12 of the 438 people experience symptoms in fewer than 8 of the 10 body regions surveyed. The average person experiences symptoms in 8.4 of the 10 body regions.

Thus, the following conclusions can be made: First, two individuals in the survey have BFS and 436 people in the survey probably have CFS. My diagnosis changed from BFS to CFS after seeing a fourth neurologist, although my symptoms remained constant. Second, the confusion over PNH classifications explains why so many people may be misdiagnosed with BFS when they have some other form of PNH. Finally, these results are unsurprising since people who reach out to social media forums about PNH are more likely to have more bothersome symptoms.

Why do neurologists misdiagnose so many patients with BFS? This is a difficult question to answer but here are a few of my thoughts on the subject: Confusion over the symptoms that may encompass the different PNH disorders. Furthermore, BFS is a convenient diagnosis when neurologists are uncertain about the etiology. Moreover, it is possible that the exposure to more environmental triggers (stress, drugs, toxins, etc.) has formulated epigenetic changes altering the etiology of PNH patients as they were understood just a few decades ago.

Fasciculations or muscle twitching is a symptom that can be viewed both visually and confirmed by an EMG. Other symptoms such as pins and needles, cramps, muscle fatigue and weakness, headaches, itching, numbness, muscle stiffness, muscle pain and soreness, muscle buzzing or vibration sensation, and sensitivity to temperatures are more difficult symptoms to verify and are primarily subject to patient input. Hence, it may be possible that neurologists only diagnose what can be verified through technology and observation.

Neurological diagnosis is very difficult, so misdiagnoses are common. As rule of thumb, if a diagnosis does not fit at least three of the top five symptoms or characteristics of a disease, it is probably incorrect. Only about two-thirds of initial neurological diagnoses are correct and MG and GBS are two of the most common to be misdiagnosed. Interestingly, the diagnosis success rate was not much different for junior residents, senior residents, and staff neurologist. MG patients generally see five to seven physicians before a correct diagnosis is made. People with GBS who suffer from severe respiratory dysfunction are sent home from emergency care multiple times before a correct diagnosis is made. MS diagnosis takes, on average, 3.5 years because a patient may be referred to two to three non-neurological physicians before finally being referred to neurologist to be properly diagnosed. [19]

Neurologists fail to maintain a professional relationship with patients. Neurologist should "maintain a lively interest in patients as people" for several reasons. It allows doctors to confirm if their diagnosis passes the test of time. It provides doctors the opportunity to determine a diagnosis if they have not been able to find a conclusive diagnosis during the initial diagnostic tests. For those reasons, it is proper etiquette to maintain contact with patients. [19]

The most common misdiagnosis of neurological symptoms is something called functional neurological disorders (FND). FND misdiagnosis may find a person suffering from "hysteria," stress, anxiety, or depression instead of neurological disease. FND misdiagnosis is more common in young women. An FND misdiagnosis is a common reason for medical malpractice lawsuits when patients have real neurological problems. Approximately 1 in 20 patients is diagnosed with FND. [19] FND may be a common misdiagnosis of PNH since stress and anxiety are common triggers. That said, patients with BFS or PNH have very real symptoms regardless if they were brought about by stress, anxiety, or depression. These patients deserve a physician's full attention until symptoms are fully understood and they have been corrected or reduced.

Paper Acknowledgements

The authors would like to thank our fellow PNH patients for taking part in this survey and study. Due to their participation a significant sample size was obtained for this study and subsequently brought forth pertinent statistical information about the PNH ailment.

Book Acknowledgements

I would like to thank my wife, Molly, and my best friends Andrew and Dave for providing me with love and inspiration in the pursuit of my goals I. I would also like to thank my brother, Bruce, who always inspires me with his vast wealth of knowledge. I also need to mention my other siblings, Greg, who inspires me because he lives with constant chronic pain; Matthew, who inspires through his fearless uniqueness; And Ashley, who inspires through her toughness and strong work ethic. I cannot express in words how instrumental my stepmom, Denise, has been in my life. She has unquestionably had the most positive influence on my life. I also wrote this text in loving memory of both my father, William, and my mother,

Beverly. I want to thank my cycling coaches, Earl and Al, and cycling friends, Dick, Mark, Donna, Ericka, and Curtis for having more faith and confidence in my abilities than I do. Finally, I would like to thank my great medical providers (doctors and nurses) that fought for me and helped me through some difficult times, including Thomas, Teerin, Suzanne, Catherine, and Rhoda.

A special thank you to all those that helped me complete this project and to bring more attention to neurological and autoimmune disease: Ross Teggatz, Rex Teggatz, Maureen Durkin, Molly Bohan, Andy Lowther, Leon Damonze, Shawn Gillis (Absolute Bikes), Matt Wells and Lindsey Lighthizer (Black Burro Bikes), Joe Parkin and Simon Stewart (Boneshaker Cycles), Michelle Wolins (Big Ring Cycles), Michelle Main, Carl Newberg, Mark Wolfe, Stephen Seccombe, Deborah and Ken Miller, Al Senft (https://www.sustainableendurancecoaching.com/), Ashley Bohan, Ashley McCain, Bruce Bohan, Carl Newberg, Carlos Alers, Chris Pearson, D'Arcy Straub, Dave Snyder, David Briggs, David Hart, Denise Bohan, Don Ladwig, Earl Walker, Eduardo Bartolome, Elizabeth Galloway, Erica Carvin, Geert Geysen, Harry Aronis, Jeanne Cotter, John Ledford, Kaye Vansinckle, Ken Agee, Linda Benson, Lisa Yancey, Margaret Gill, Mark Culver, Michael Lively, Mike Skorcz, Mitra Wagner, Peter Wimberg, Chris Aronis, Richard Stewart, Richard Antley, Romy Maxwell, Sean Pieper, Shawn Askinosie, Theresa Grillo, and Vernon Jones. I would also like to thank the following organizations for their support: (1) Racer X cycling club https://racerxcycling.com/road/; (2) The Foundation for Peripheral Neuropathy https://www.foundationforpn.org/;

and (3) GBS and CIDP International Foundation
https://www.gbs-cidp.org/

Paper Endnotes, Book References, and Book Endnotes can be found at: https//www.patrickbohan.com/book-research

---

Made in the USA
Middletown, DE
05 April 2021